DRUGS IN NURSING PRACTICE
A HANDBOOK
OF DRUGS

THIS BOOK IS DEDICATED TO
James Crooks CBE
1919–1983

DRUGS IN NURSING PRACTICE
A HANDBOOK OF DRUGS

C. R. Henney RGN SCM
Research Officer (Nursing), Tayside Health Board and Research Fellow, Department of Pharmacology and Therapeutics, University of Dundee

R. J. Dow BSc MB MRCP(UK)
Formerly Senior Registrar, Department of Pharmacology and Therapeutics, University of Dundee

A. M. MacConnachie BSc(Hons) MPS
Principal Pharmacist, Drug Information and Education Services, Tayside Area Health Board, and Honorary Lecturer, Department of Pharmacology and Therapeutics, University of Dundee

The late J. Crooks MD FRCP(Ed) FRCP(G) FRCP(L) MFCM
Formerly Professor of Therapeutics, Department of Pharmacology and Therapeutics, University of Dundee

Second edition

Churchill Livingstone
EDINBURGH LONDON MELBOURNE AND NEW YORK 1986

CHURCHILL LIVINGSTONE
Medical Division of Longman Group Limited

Distributed in the United States of America by
Churchill Livingstone Inc., 1560 Broadway, New York,
N.Y. 10036, and by associated companies, branches
and representatives throughout the world.

© Longman Group Limited 1982, 1986

All rights reserved. No part of this publication
may be reproduced, stored in a retrieval system,
or transmitted in any form or by any means,
electronic, mechanical, photocopying, recording
or otherwise, without the prior permission of the
publishers (Churchill Livingstone, Robert Stevenson
House, 1–3 Baxter's Place, Leith Walk,
Edinburgh EH1 3AF).

First edition 1982
Second edition 1986

ISBN 0 443 03379 X

British Library Cataloguing in Publication Data
A Handbook of drugs.—2nd ed.
1. Drugs 2. Nursing
I. Henney, C. R. II. Drugs in nursing practice
615'.1'024613   RM12S

Library of Congress Cataloging in Publication Data
Main entry under title:
A Handbook of drugs.
  (Drugs in nursing practice)
  Rev. ed. of: Drugs in nursing practice. 1982.
  Includes index.
  1. Drugs—Handbooks, manuals, etc. 2. Pharmacology—
Handbooks, manuals, etc. 3. Nursing—Handbooks,
manuals, etc. I. Henney, C. R. II. Drugs in nursing
practice. III. Series. [DNLM: 1. Drugs—administration
& dosage—nurses' instruction. 2. Pharmacology—
nurses' instruction. QV 55 H236]
RM300.H36 1986   615'.1   85-21287

Produced by Longman Singapore Publishers (Pte) Ltd.
Printed in Singapore

Preface

The first edition of this book was prompted by our awareness of the important role which nurses have to play in the ever-expanding field of therapeutics. Modern therapeutics involves the use of a large range of powerful pharmacological substances which, as well as producing beneficial effects, have the potential to produce, on occasion, unwanted effects. Nurses working in both hospital and community are the health care professionals who have more continuous contact with patients than any others. Thus they are ideally placed to monitor drug therapy and so determine that therapeutic objectives are met as well as noting the occurrence of unwanted side-effects. Because of the special relationship of nurses with their patients, they are also likely to be considered by them as a source of information about the drugs which have been prescribed. The explosion in the number of drugs available and information about efficacy and toxicity presents nurses with the problem of ready access to a large amount of information about drugs. Such information is required if nurses are to monitor drug treatment effectively as well as provide information to patients about their drug therapy.

The aim of this book is to provide a ready reference or *aide-mémoire* for nurses, both student and qualified, in hospital and community, on drugs currently of relevance to modern nursing practice. The publication of a second edition is timely since the rate of introduction of new drugs and newer applications for existing drugs continues to increase. Changes of particular importance which have taken place include the standardisation of insulin strengths on 100 units per ml and the rapid development of more antimicrobial agents, in particular the appearance of many 'newer generation' cephalosporins. The former has major implications for the role of nurses in educating diabetic patients and the latter has given rise to newer approaches in the prevention and treatment of bacterial infections.

The layout of this book is the same as before. A section on how to use it has been included in the text and potential users are strongly recommended to consult this so that information may be obtained swiftly and effectively.

Throughout the preparation of the book, the over-riding aim was to emphasise what nurses need to know and understand about drugs in order to give the best care to their patients. In addition to information on drug presentation, action and uses and dosage, the special points of interest to nurses have been highlighted in separate 'nurse monitoring' sections. There is a section entitled 'Special Notes' and two appendices at the end of the book which deal with aspects of drug treatment of particular concern to nurses. There is also a section on weights and measures which will, we hope, be of practical value.

Finally, we wish to pay tribute to our late colleague, James Crooks, without whose vision and guidance this book would never have been produced. James Crooks was a leading authority in the field of therapeutics and he contributed much toward promoting the role of nurses in therapeutic monitoring. His untimely death was not only a great loss to the medical profession but also to the nursing and pharmaceutical professions.

Dundee, 1986   C.R.H., R.J.D., A.M.MacC.

Contents

How to use this book 1

DRUG NOTES
(arranged alphabetically by approved name) 5

SPECIAL NOTES

Note 1: Nursing aspects of intravenous infusion fluid therapy and drug additives to intravenous infusion 298

Note 2: Intravenous (parenteral) feeding 306

Note 3: Antibiotics and sulphonamides 310

Note 4: Drugs in breast milk 314

Note 5: Ophthalmic preparations 320

Note 6: Anti-cancer drugs—their safe handling 323

APPENDICES

Appendix 1: The security and administration of medicines in hospital 328

Appendix 2: Metric weights and other measures 330

INDEX OF DRUGS BY PROPRIETARY AND OTHER COMMON NAMES 335

How to use this book

This book is composed of four main sections:
1. Drug notes (arranged alphabetically by approved name)
2. Special notes
3. Appendices
4. Index of drugs by proprietary and other common names.

DRUG NOTES

This is the major part of the text and consists of a description of drugs in common usage listed in alphabetical order by approved name. When the nurse has found the individual drug about which she requires information, she will find a number of headings as follows:

a. Presentation. This describes the various preparations which are available for each drug, e.g. tablets, injections, nasal spray, suppository, pessary, ointment etc.

b. Actions and uses. Knowledge of the actions and uses of the drug enables the nurse to monitor therapy more effectively in the patient, and therefore a brief description of pharmacological action for each drug is given. In this section the different methods of administration covering the various uses of the drug or drug groups are dealt with.

c. Dosage. The doses given in this book are those commonly ordered for the different types of presentation and mode of administration. The nurse should appreciate that the doctor is not bound to give the official dose but may order more or less of any drug at his discretion. However if the nurse finds that the dose of a drug given in this book deviates from that prescribed by the doctor, it is advisable that she considers checking with the doctor that he really did intend to order that particular dose. It should be remembered that the doses for children are usually smaller than doses for adults and this also applies to the elderly in the case of many drug groups.

d. Nurse monitoring. This section highlights the important contribution which nurses can make in achieving the most effective and safe use of drugs for their patients. It deals with possible unwanted side-effects of drugs and should be consulted to ascertain the symptoms and signs of adverse drug effects which may become manifest in the patient. The detection of the more serious of these may demand immediate action by the nurse, such as advising the patient to stop taking the drug and notifying the doctor. On other occasions the occurrence would only warrant the notification of the event to the doctor and in some instances will only require explanation to the patient that the effect is not unexpected and has no serious significance. Lack of efficacy of a drug can constitute an adverse effect and may be related to an inappropriate dose, an inappropriate drug or a failure to comply with prescribing instructions. In all these circumstances the doctor should be notified.

e. General notes. Many modern drugs deteriorate with potentially serious consequences for the patient if the storage conditions are adverse. Both in the hospital and in the community the nurse has the best opportunity to monitor the storage conditions. This section provides the information which allows her to do this most effectively.

Where a large number of preparations belonging to a particular drug group exist i.e. as with the beta-adrenergic receptor blockers, the major points on the drug group concerning (b) and (d) above are included under a group heading i.e. 'beta-adrenergic receptor blockers', and thereafter when individual members of this group appear in the text readers are advised to refer back to the group heading.

SPECIAL NOTES

The second section of this book comprises the special notes. These deal with therapeutic topics of great importance to the nurse in everyday practice, and their contents are briefly as follows:

Note 1: Nursing aspects of intravenous infusion therapy and drug additives to intravenous infusions. This provides basic information on the types of intravenous infusion fluids available, and also gives practical guidance on common known interactions either between drugs and intravenous infusion fluids or between combinations of drugs in intravenous infusion fluids.

Note 2: Intravenous (parenteral) feeding. This section gives an outline of the therapeutic objectives of intravenous feeding and also gives practical guidelines as to how such a regime should be administered.

Note 3: Antibiotics and sulphonamides. This section gives a fuller outline of the action and use of antibiotics and sulphonamides. Included in this section is a list entitled 'Common infections and the organisms which may cause them'. The purpose of this list is two-fold: if a nurse finds an infection described in the main text she will be able to obtain fuller information in the list as to the types of organisms which may cause that infection. Also if an organism is referred to in the main text the nurse may gain an idea of what types of infection that organism may cause by consulting this list.

Note 4: Drugs in breast milk. In recent times there has been a trend in favour of breast feeding. As many women who may wish to breast feed may be on coincident drug therapy, and also as many women already breast feeding may require to start drug therapy, it is essential that the nurse has some idea of which drugs are either safe or unsafe or whether indeed anything is known about the particular drug's excretion in breast milk, and its likely effect on the infant.

Note 5: Ophthalmic preparations. As there is a wide variety of ophthalmic preparations an attempt has been made to summarise the various preparations available for problems which are suitably treated by topical application.

APPENDICES

The third section of the book comprises the appendices:

Appendix 1: The security and administration of medicines in hospitals. This deals with legal aspects of drug prescribing and the use of drug Kardexes.

Appendix 2: Metric weights and other measures. This section is included to allow the nurse to refer to units of weights and measures with which she may not be normally familiar, and where possible methods of conversion to more commonly recognised units are given.

INDEX OF DRUGS BY PROPRIETARY AND OTHER COMMON NAMES

The index of proprietary drug names is the fourth and last section of the book. When a nurse comes across a drug with which she is not familiar, the only fact she may know about that drug is its name. In order for the nurse to be able to use this book correctly, it is important that she understands that a single drug may have more than one name. As mentioned above, drugs are arranged in Section 1 under their approved names (the approved name being the official British name for the drug). Therefore as an initial step the nurse is advised to consult the main text at the appropriate point in the alphabetical order to see whether the drug appears in that place. If the drug is not found then it is likely that the nurse has the drug's proprietary name. The proprietary name is the name given to a drug by the company which produces it. The nurse should then refer to Section 4, the index of proprietary preparations. This is a list of proprietary names in alphabetical order and the nurse should, by using this, be able to locate the approved name and thus the drug in the main text. As the approved name in the main text is followed by current proprietary names for each drug she should immediately be able to check that she has found the correct drug. For example, if a nurse comes across a drug by the name of propranolol and searches alphabetically through the main text, she will find propranolol. However if she starts with the name Inderal she will not find it in the main text, and should then consult the index of proprietary names where she would find 'Inderal (Beta-adrenergic receptor blocking drug)—see Propranolol'. Reference in the main text to propranolol will give her all the necessary information on that drug. In addition, if she wished to read about beta-adrenergic receptor drugs as a whole, this again could be found alphabetically in the main text. As a final note, it should be remembered that a number of combinations of drugs exist and as it is impossible for them to be listed under approved names they have been included in the main text under their proprietary names. They will still however appear in the index of proprietary names and therefore should be easily found.

DRUG NOTES
(arranged alphabetically by approved name)

A

ACEBUTOLOL (Sectral)
Presentation
Capsules—100 mg, 200 mg, 400 mg
Injection—25 mg in 5 ml
Actions and uses
Acebutolol itself is a cardioselective beta-adrenoreceptor blocking drug and therefore has the advantages described in the section on beta-blockers. It is metabolised in the body to another chemical which is in fact a non-selective beta-adrenoreceptor blocking drug and this may explain why some patients are prone to develop side effects equivalent to those seen in the non-selective beta-adrenoreceptor blocking group.
Dosage
Oral Adult Dose Range is:
1. *Hypertension.* 400 mg to 800 mg daily in two divided doses. Occasionally up to 1200 mg may be required.
2. *Angina pectoris.* 200 mg twice daily. Occasionally 300 mg three times daily, with a maximum dose of up to 1200 mg per day.
3. *Cardiac dysrhythmias.* 100–200 mg two-three times daily. Occasionally up to 1200 mg in divided doses may be necessary.
4. Intravenous for emergency treatment of cardiac dysrhythmias 25 mg given over 3–5 minutes. A further three intravenous injections of the same dosage may be given over a period of up to one hour if necessary. During intravenous administration monitoring as described under the same section on Propranolol (q.v.) is necessary.

Nurse monitoring
See beta-adrenoreceptor blocking drugs.
General notes
Acebutolol capsules and injection solution may be stored at room temperature.

ACETAZOLAMIDE (Diamox)
Presentation
Tablets—250 mg
Capsules—500 mg sustained release
Injection—500 mg vials
Actions and uses
Acetazolamide affects an enzyme called carbonic anhydrase and in doing so produces three major effects:
1. It increases the urine output.
2. It decreases the flow of acqueous humour within the chamber of the eye thus reducing intra-ocular pressure.
3. By an unknown action in the brain it may reduce the frequency of seizures in epileptic patients.

In clinical practice this drug is now only used for the treatment of glaucoma.
Dosage
For the treatment of glaucoma:
Adults: 250 mg–1 g daily in divided doses or 500 mg twice daily as the slow release capsules.
Nurse monitoring
1. Side effects which occur most often in the initial stages of treatment include flushing, thirst, headache, drowsiness, dizziness, fatigue, paraesthesia, ataxia,

hyperventilation and gastrointestinal upset (anorexia, nausea and vomiting).
2. Much more rarely hypersensitivity reactions may occur leading to skin, kidney and bone marrow damage. Acetazolamide is in fact a derivative of the sulphonamide group and affects the skin, kidney and bone marrow in the same way as described for sulphonamides (q.v.).
3. Prolonged use may lead to stone formation in the kidneys with resultant ureteric colic.
4. The drug may produce an abnormality in blood biochemistry known as acidosis which can be potentially dangerous. Symptoms of this include altered consciousness—initially drowsiness and later coma and deep irregular breathing.

General notes
1. The preparation may be stored at room temperature.
2. Acetazolamide for intravenous injection is reconstituted with 5 ml of Water for Injections immediately before use.

ACETOHEXAMIDE (Dimelor)

Presentation
Tablets—500 mg
Actions and uses
See hypoglycaemic drugs, oral (1).
Dosage
250 mg–1.5 g daily as a single dose.
Nurse monitoring
See hypoglycaemic drugs, oral (1).
General notes
Tablets may be stored at room temperature.

ACETYLCYSTEINE (Airbron, Parvolex)

Presentation
Inhalation—Sterile aqueous solution of 20% in 2 ml and 10 ml vials
Injection—2 g in 10 ml
Actions and uses
1. This substance is claimed to reduce the viscosity and tenacity of sputum and, therefore, may be used to good effect to aid the resolution of acute exacerbations of chronic bronchitis and chest infections associated with cystic fibrosis.
2. Acetylcysteine is a specific antidote to paracetamol which damages the liver in overdosage, and it is administered intravenously in the treatment of paracetamol poisoning.

Dosage
1. Inhalation (to reduce viscosity and tenacity of sputum):
   a. By nebuliser: 2–5 ml of a 20% solution or 4–10 ml of a 10% solution every 4–6 hours.
   b. By direct instillation: 1–2 ml of the 10 or 20% solution may be administered every 1–4 hours.
2. Injection (to specifically treat paracetamol poisoning): Initially, 150 mg/kg body weight by intravenous infusion over 15 minutes followed by an infusion of 50 mg/kg over 4 hours. Thereafter a dose of 100 mg/kg is administered in 1 litre over the next 16 hours. This provides a total dose of 300 mg/kg in 20 hours.

Nurse monitoring
1. The following relate to the use of acetylcysteine by inhalation:
   a. As large volumes of mucus may be loosened in the airways, patients who have impaired coughing may require mechanical suction to maintain an open airway.
   b. Great care should be taken in administering this compound to asthmatics as cases of bronchospasm have occurred. If bronchospasm does occur Salbutamol or an alternative sympathomimetic aerosol should be administered.
   c. Side-effects are uncommon but include stomatitis, nausea, vomiting and coughing.
   d. During nebulisation the patient may notice a slight

disagreeable odour but this usually quickly disappears.
  e. When using a face mask stickiness may be noticed on the face. This can easily be removed by washing with warm water.
2. When administered by injection:
  a. Acetylcysteine is an effective antidote to paracetamol if administered up to 8–10 hours after poisoning. Its effectiveness rapidly diminishes thereafter. It is therefore important, if possible, to deterine the time of poisoning in relation to hospital admission.
  b. Note that the drug is incompatible with rubber and metals and for this reason plastic cannulae are used when doses are administered.
  c. The drug is generally well tolerated but a few patients are hypersensitive and skin rashes may develop. Rarely, acute anaphylaxis has occurred.

General notes
1. The drug should be stored in a cool place.
2. If only a portion of a vial is used the remainder should be stored in a refrigerator and discarded if not used within 96 hours.

ACTINOMYCIN D (Cosmegen Lyovac)

(Also described as Dactinomycin)
(See also Note 3, p. 310)

Presentation
Injection—Vials containing 0.5 mg

Actions and uses
Actinomycin is a derivative of a group of antibiotics. A simplified version of its action is as follows: Every cell has in its nucleus two strands made up of proteins known as DNA. The DNA contains all the information necessary for cell duplication. When Actinomycin combines with DNA it blocks the process of cell duplication. This drug is used with some success in three rare conditions:

1. Wilms' tumour of the kidney
2. Choriocarcinoma
3. Testicular teratomas

There is evidence to suggest that the drug is more effective if patients receive concurrent radiotherapy.

Dosage
The dose depends on the type of tumour under treatment:
1. *Adults*:
  a. The usual adult dose is 0.5 mg by intravenous injection daily for courses up to 5 days in duration. These courses are repeated at intervals of several weeks.
  b. An alternative dose of 0.01 mg/kg body weight has been used.
2. *Children*:
  a. The usual dose by intravenous injection is 0.015 mg/kg daily for courses of up to 5 days in duration.
  b. An alternative regime is to give a total dose of 2.4 mg per m^2 of body surface area over a period of one week.

Nurse monitoring
1. The drug is always given by intravenous injection and is highly irritant if it escapes from the vein.
2. During the treatment course abdominal pain, anorexia, nausea and vomiting may occur
3. Side effects which may be delayed for days or even weeks after finishing a course include bone marrow depression with anaemia, leucopenia and thrombocytopenia and resultant increased risk of severe infection and haemorrhage. Ulcerative stomatitis and dysphagia, alopecia, erythema, fever, hypocalcaemia, myalgia, malaise and gastrointestinal symptoms can also occur.
4. Skin reactions may occur with this drug and these are more common at sites where simultaneous or prior irradiation has been given.
5. The drug should never be given to patients with chickenpox as

severe or fatal generalised reaction may result.
6. The drug should never be given during pregnancy.
7. Side effects are particularly severe when given to children under the age of one.
8. The nurse should be constantly aware that most cytotoxic drugs are irritant to the skin and mucous surfaces, and are in general very toxic. Great care should therefore be exercised when handling these drugs, and in particular spillage or contamination of personnel or the environment must be avoided. If cytotoxic drugs are handled regularly it is theoretically possible that repeated skin contact or inhalation may produce systemic toxic effects and in nurses who have developed hypersensitivity, severe local and general hypersensitivity reactions.

General notes
1. Solutions for injection are prepared by adding 1.1 ml Water for Injections to each vial to give a final solution containing 0.5 mg in 1 ml. This may be injected directly or via the drip tube of a 5% dextrose or 0.9% sodium chloride infusion. Any unused solution must be discarded.
2. Actinomycin D is very corrosive to skin and soft tissue and accidental leakage following intravenous injection may cause irritation, phlebitis and cellulitis.
3. Vials containing sterile powder for injection may be stored at room temperature under dry conditions.

ACYCLOVIR (Zovirax)

Presentation
Tablets—200 mg
Injection—250 mg vials
Eye ointment—3%
Cream—5%

Actions and used
Acyclovir is an anti-viral agent which has potent activity against herpes simplex virus (H.S.V.) and is to a lesser extent active against herpes zoster virus (varicella) and possibly other viruses. In clinical practice it is used for the following:
1. Intravenously for the treatment of systemic infections due to Herpes virus.
2. Intravenously for the prevention of systemic infections due to Herpes virus following the appearance of oral and perioral herpetic lesions in immuno-suppressed patients.
3. Orally for the treatment of H.S.V. infections of the skin and mucous membranes, including genital herpes.
4. As ophthalmic ointment applied in the treatment of herpes simplex keratitis.
5. As topical cream, for the treatment of H.S.V. infections of the skin, including genital herpes.

Dosage
1. Intravenous:
Adults and children: By intravenous infusion, 5–10 mg/kg body weight is administered every 8 hours. Each infusion is administered slowly over a period of one hour.
2. Oral:
Adults: 200 mg five times daily, usually for a period of 5 days.
3. Ophthalmic:
Adults and children: Ophthalmic ointment is applied 5 times daily at intervals of 4 hours with treatment continued for at least 3 days after healing takes place.
4. Cream:
Adults and children: Apply to herpetic lesions 5 times a day and continue for at least 5 days after healing takes place.

Nurse monitoring
1. A reversible increase in blood urea and serum creatinine may occur after intravenous infusion. This effect is less marked if patients are well hydrated before treatment is administered.
2. Patients with severe renal impairment should receive a reduced dosage.
3. Acyclovir for infusion is irritant

and inflammation and ulceration may occur at injection sites if leakage from the vein into the surrounding tissues occurs. Bolus injection or rapid infusions should therefore be avoided and patients should not take solutions prepared from injection vials by mouth.
4. Topical application may be associated with skin irritancy which is usually described as a burning sensation.
5. The drug is only contraindicated in patients who have displayed previous hypersensitivity.

General notes
1. Preparations containing Acyclovir may be stored at room temperature.
2. Eye ointment should be discarded one month after opening.
3. Intravenous infusions are prepared in sodium chloride 0.9%, dextrose 5%, dextrose/saline mixtures or Hartmann's solution.

ALFACALCIDOL (One-Alpha)

This drug is also known as One-Alpha Hydroxycholecalciferol

Presentation
Capsules—0.25 μg and 1 μg

Actions and uses
The actions and uses of Alfacalcidol are in theory identical to all those described in the section on Vitamin D. In practice, however, Alfacalcidol is used mainly for the treatment of renal osteodystrophy.

Dosage
For the treatment of renal osteodystrophy:
1. In adults and children over 20 kg body weight: 1 μg initially with subsequent adjustments according to clinical and biochemical response.
2. Children under 20 kg body weight: 0.05 μg/kg per day initially with subsequent adjustments according to clinical and biochemical response.

Nurse monitoring
The nurse monitoring aspects of this drug are identical to those described for Vitamin D (q.v.). It is important to note that Alfacalcidol is the most effective preparation of Vitamin D and therefore requires careful monitoring as side effects are more likely.

General notes
The drug may be stored at room temperature.

ALGINIC ACID (Gastrocote, Gaviscon)

Presentation
Combined with various antacids in tablet, liquid and granular (sachet) form.

Actions and uses
Alginic acid forms a protective coating on the surface of gastric juice and therefore prevents reflux of gastric acid and bile into the oesophagus, and reduces the symptoms caused by such reflux. It should be used for the treatment of heartburn and dyspeptic pain when these are caused by hiatus hernia and reflux oesophagitis.

Dosage
1. *Adults*: 1–3 tablets or 10–20 ml (Gavison) after meals and at bedtime.
2. *Children*: one tablet or 5–10 ml liquid after meals and at bedtime.
3. *Infants*: a special formulation of infant Gaviscon is available for the very young. The dose is ½–1 sachet mixed with water or with made up feeds.

Nurse monitoring
This drug is not associated with troublesome side effects. It does however contain sugar and therefore if given to diabetics the amount of sugar in the preparation should be taken into account when formulating diabetic diets.

General notes
Tablets, granules and liquid preparations containing alginic acid may be stored at room temperature. Tablets and granules should be thoroughly chewed before

swallowing. The liquid may be diluted with up to an equal amount of water for ease of administration.

ALLOPURINOL (Zyloric)

Presentation
　　Tablets—100 mg, 300 mg

Actions and uses
　　If uric acid accumulates in excess in the blood, gout may be produced with subsequent arthritis, skin lesions and impairment of renal function. Increased blood urate occurs most commonly in patients suffering from classical gout and in patients with malignant disease who are treated with cytotoxic drugs or radiotherapy. In the latter case the increased urate is due to an increased destruction and turnover of cells. A less common cause of raised blood uric acid is diuretic therapy. Allopurinol may be used for the treatment of a raised blood uric acid. It acts by inhibiting one of the enzymes which take part in the production of uric acid from its constituent chemicals and it therefore reduces the total amount of uric acid produced.

Dosage
1. *Adults*:
   a. For the treatment of gout: Initially 100 mg once a day increasing to a maintenance dose of 300–400 mg per day in divided or single dosage.
   b. For treatment of hyperuricaemia in leukaemic patients: 200 mg three times a day for three days prior to treatment, then adjusted as required to a maintenance dose of 300 mg per day.
2. *Children*: Treatment of hyperuricaemia in leukaemia. Maintenance 20 mg/kg per day.

Nurse monitoring
1. When Allopurinol treatment is commenced the blood urate is likely to fall. It has been found that any change in blood urate may lead to an acute attack of gout and therefore when Allopurinol is commenced an anti-inflammatory analgesic drug is usually given concurrently for at least a month.
2. Side effects which occasionally occur with this drug are nausea, vomiting and skin rashes. Rarely severe skin reactions, fever, joint pain and eosinophilia may occur.
3. Side effects are more common in patients with kidney or liver disease and the dose should be reduced by an appropriate amount in patients with renal failure.
4. Allopurinol inhibits the liver metabolism of 6-Mercaptopurine and Azothioprine and the dosage of these drugs therefore has to be considerably reduced in such circumstances.

General notes
　　Allopurinol tablets may be stored at room temperature.

ALLYLOESTRENOL (Gestanin)

Presentation
　　Tablets—5 mg

Actions and uses
1. The actions and uses of progestational hormones are described in the section on progestational hormones.
2. In clinical practice this drug has three indications:
   a. For the treatment of habitual abortion.
   b. For the treatment of threatened abortion
   c. For the treatment of failure of nidation.

Dosage
1. For the treatment of habitual abortion—5–10 mg per day. Treatment may be continued for up to 16 weeks.
2. For the treatment of threatened abortion—5 mg three times per day for at least 5–7 days. If necessary daily dosage may be increased and the treatment period extended without risk.
3. For the treatment of failure of nidation—10–20 mg daily from

the 16th to the 26th day of each cycle until conception is achieved. Thereafter 10 mg a day for at least 16 weeks.

Nurse monitoring
1. At the recommended doses no side effects or other problems have been reported.
2. In contrast to other pregnancy-maintaining progestational agents virilisation of the fetus has not been reported with prolonged treatment.

General notes
The drug may be stored at room temperature.

ALOXIPRIN (Palaprin Forte)

Presentation
Tablets—600 mg

Actions and uses
1. Aloxiprin is converted to Aspirin and therefore its actions and uses are similar to those described for that drug (q.v.).
2. Aloxiprin is converted to Aspirin and it is therefore used in an attempt to avoid the gastric irritation which Aspirin frequently produces.

Dosage
1. *Adults*: The usual adult dose is calculated on a basis of 600 mg per 6.5 kg of body weight daily in divided doses. The precise dose may be regulated by measuring Aspirin levels.

Nurse monitoring
1. As this drug is converted to Aspirin the nurse monitoring notes on that drug are applicable.
2. As noted above this form of Aspirin may produce less frequent gastrointestinal side effects.

General notes
Aloxiprin tablets may be stored at room temperature.

ALPRAZOLAM (Xanax)

Presentation
Tablets—0.25 mg and 0.5 mg

Actions and uses
Alprazolam is a member of the benzodiazepine group (q.v.). Its principal use is in the treatment of anxiety.

Dosage
0.25–0.5 mg taken 2 or 3 times daily.

Nurse monitoring
See the section on benzodiazepines.

General notes
Tablets containing alprazolam may be stored at room temperature.

ALUMINIUM HYDROXIDE (Alu-Cap, Aludrox)

Presentation
Tablets—375 mg
Suspension/Gel—3.5–4.4% as aluminium oxide
Capsules—475 mg

Actions and uses
Aluminium hydroxide is an antacid used for the relief of dyspeptic pain and heartburn. Very high doses may in addition cure peptic ulcers, but few patients can tolerate the high doses required.
A further use of aluminium hydroxide is in chronic renal failure where there is reduced phosphate excretion by the kidney leading to high blood concentrations of phosphate. Aluminium hydroxide binds to phosphate in the gut, reducing its absorption, and thus counterbalances the effect of the reduction in its excretion.

Dosage
1. For symptomatic relief of dyspeptic symptoms: 2 tablets or 10 ml suspension, two-hourly if necessary. Alternatively 1 capsule may be taken regularly four times a day and at night on retiring.
2. For the treatment of hypophosphataemia in chronic renal failure: dosage should be individually determined.

Nurse monitoring
1. Constipation may occur. If used in combination with mangesium salts which tend to cause diarrhoea, this effect may be offset.

2. Neurological abnormalities may arise due to aluminium toxicity. This occurs only in patients with chronic renal failure who are taking very high doses.
   3. Absorption and therefore clinical effectiveness of drugs such as salicylates, digoxin and antibiotics may be impaired.

General notes
   Aluminium hydroxide preparations may be stored at room temperature. Tablets should be chewed before swallowing and the suspension/gel thoroughly shaken before each dose is taken. Capsules are swallowed whole.

AMANTADINE (Symmetrel)

Presentation
   Capsules—100 mg
   Syrup—50 mg in 5 ml

Actions and uses
   This drug was originally developed as an anti-viral agent and was initially used for prophylaxis against and treatment of influenza. It still has a role in the treatment of herpes zoster. An additional benefit which was noticed in patients treated for infection was that it improves the symptoms of Parkinson's disease. The mechanism of action of this is unknown.

Dosage
   Adults only:
   1. For Parkinson's disease: 100 mg once or twice daily.
   2. For the treatment of herpes zoster: 100 mg twice daily.
   3. For the treatment of influenza: 100 mg twice daily.

Nurse monitoring
   1. This drug should be used with great caution in patients who have a past history of convulsion.
   2. Side effects involving the central nervous system may be severe and include: nervousness, insomnia, dizziness, convulsion, behavioural disturbance and hallucinations.

General notes
   The drug may be stored at temperature.

AMIKACIN (Amikin)

(See also Note 3, p. 310)

Presentation
   Injection—500 mg in 2 ml
   100 mg in 2 ml

Actions and uses
   Amikacin is an aminoglycoside antibiotic and its actions and uses are described in the section on these antibiotics. It may be effective in the treatment of infections due to Gentamicin-resistant micro-organisms.

Dosage
   The dosage for adults and children is calculated on a basis of 15 mg/kg per day total, usually given in two divided doses by intramuscular or intravenous injections. Occasionally in adults as much as 500 mg eight hourly may be given.

Nurse monitoring
   1. The nurse monitoring notes for aminoglycoside antibiotics apply to Amikacin.
   2. Unlike Gentamicin this drug may be given effectively by intravenous infusion in either normal saline, 5% dextrose or dextrose/saline mixtures.

General notes
   1. The drug may be stored at room temperature.
   2. The drug should never be mixed prior to administration with other antibiotics.

AMILORIDE (Midamor)

Presentation
   Tablets—5 mg
   Also combined with hydrochlorothiazide in Moduretic.

Actions and uses
   Amiloride has a mild diuretic action. Its site of action is on the distal tubule. It is of little use as a diuretic alone but it may be usefully combined with thiazide diuretics as it is one of the drugs which has a potassium-conserving action, and it may therefore prevent the hypokalaemia commonly encountered when patients are given thiazide diuretics alone.

Dosage
The daily adult dose range is 5–20 mg taken as a single dose in the morning.

Nurse monitoring
1. Hyperkalaemia may occur, particularly in patients with impaired renal function. It is clinically undetectable, and extremely dangerous as it may lead to sudden death due to cardiac arrest.
2. Side effects are as follows:
   a. Anorexia, nausea, vomiting, abdominal pain, constipation or diarrhoea
   b. Dry mouth, thirst, paraesthesia, dizziness, weakness, lethargy and muscle cramps
   c. Skin rashes, itching
   d. Mental confusion and visual disturbances.
3. In common with other diuretics, Amiloride may alter blood glucose levels and therefore treatment requirements in diabetic patients may be altered.

General notes
Amiloride tablets may be stored at room temperature.

AMINOCAPROIC ACID (Epsikapron)

Presentation
Sachets—3 g
Syrup—300 mg in 1 ml

Actions and uses
One of the processes involved in the prevention of bleeding by clot formation is the production of a substance known as fibrin. Fibrin is broken down by fibrinolysin under normal circumstances as a process of healing, and also under certain pathological conditions.
Aminocaproic acid prevents the destruction of fibrin and therefore inhibits bleeding. It has been used in the treatment of haemorrhage associated with menorrhagia and IUCD insertion and in the treatment of severe haemorrhage associated with severe trauma or major surgical procedures. It is also used in the treatment of haemorrhage associated with neoplastic diseases such as metastatic carcinoma of the prostate and leukaemia.

Dosage
1. Orally:
   a. *Adults*: 3–6 g four to six times per day
   b. *Children*: 100 mg/kg four to six times per day.

Nurse monitoring
1. As this drug inhibits the degradation of fibrin there is an increased risk of thrombosis.
2. Common side effects include diarrhoea, postural hypotension, gastric pain, nasal stuffiness and increased urinary output.
3. The risk of thromboembolic disease is increased if the patient has reduced renal function or is concurrently receiving oral contraceptive therapy.

General notes
The drug may be stored at room temperature.

AMINOGLYCOSIDE ANTIBIOTICS

Amikacin
Gentamicin
Kanamycin
Streptomycin
Tobramycin
Netilmicin
(*See Note 3, p. 310 and Note 4*)

Presentation
See individual drugs.

Actions and uses
1. The aminoglycoside group of antibiotics have a predominantly bactericidal action i.e. they kill bacteria present in body tissues. They are effective against the following organisms:
   a. Gram-negative pathogens including *E. coli*, proteus species and *Pseudomonas aeruginosa*
   b. *Haemophilus influenza*
   c. *Neisseria meningitidis*.
It is important to note that in recent years many organisms have developed resistance to

drugs of this group.
These drugs are not sufficiently well absorbed to make oral administration effective. They can, therefore, only be given by the intravenous or intramuscular routes and because of this are reserved for the treatment of severe infections.

2. Superficial infections of the eye, ear and skin may be effectively treated by topical applications.

Dosage
See individual drugs.

Nurse monitoring
1. If excessive doses are administered the 8th cranial nerve may be irreversibly damaged leading to deafness and difficulty with balance. High doses may also cause renal damage. These problems may nowadays be avoided by monitoring blood concentrations of the drug and adjusting doses appropriately. However, despite this the development of hearing or balance difficulties in a patient receiving aminoglycoside antibiotics should still be taken as an indication to stop the treatment.
2. Aminoglycoside antibiotics possess moderate muscle relaxant properties which may increase the effects of muscle relaxant drugs given during surgery.
3. The aminoglycoside, gentamicin, should always be given by bolus injection and not by infusion as adequate blood levels cannot be maintained by the latter method of administration.
4. Aminoglycoside antibiotics are often given in combination with other antibiotics for the treatment of severe infections. It is important to note that they are chemically unstable and therefore may be rendered ineffective by mixing them before administration with other antibiotics, especially Penicillin and Cephalosporins.

General notes
See individual drugs.

AMINOPHYLLINE (Phyllocontin)

Presentation
Tablets—100 mg
Tablets, slow release—100 mg and 225 mg
Injection—250 mg in 10 ml
Suppositories—5 mg, 50 mg 150 mg and 360 mg

Actions and uses
Aminophylline produces three major effects which make it useful in clinical practice.
1. It produces relaxation of smooth muscle in the bronchi thus increasing airflow to the areas of oxygen exchange.
2. It stimulates the heart muscle and reduces congestion in the venous return to the heart.
3. It has a mild to moderate diuretic action.

It is used in the management of obstructive airways disease e.g. asthma and chronic bronchitis, including status asthmaticus and in particular where respiratory disease is associated with heart failure e.g. in cor pulmonale. It is also used in the management of apnoea in prematurity.

Dosage
1. *Adults*:
   a. Oral: 100–300 mg (conventional tablets) taken 3 or 4 times daily. Slow release tablets are used in a twice daily dosage of 225 mg to 450 mg.
   b. Intravenous: 250 mg to 500 mg is administered very slowly (over 10–15 minutes) by bolus injection. Alternatively, an intravenous infusion can be administered in sodium chloride 0.9% or dextrose 5% at a dosage of 500 microgram to 1 mg per kg per hour.
   c. Rectal: One or two suppositories are inserted daily, usually at night for nocturnal wheezing.
2. *Children*:
   a. Oral: Slow release tablets are used for older children 3–5 years or more, in a dose of 100–200 mg twice daily or as

a single dose at bedtime for nocturnal wheeze.
b. Intravenous: A dose of 3 mg/kg body weight by bolus injection (over 15 minutes) is used. This may be followed if necessary by maintenance infusion at a rate of 800 μg per kg per hour. Intravenous infusion has been administered in the management of apnoea in prematurity. Intramuscular injections have been given but this route is associated with extreme pain at the injection site.
c. Rectal: Up to 1 year:
12.5–25 mg
1–5 years:
50–100 mg
6–12 years:
100–200 mg

Premature infants have received 5 mg suppositories on a 6-hourly basis for prevention of attacks of apnoea. Note that suppositories may be cut with a warmed knife to obtain non-standard dosages. Cuts should be made lengthwise to obtain quarter and half suppository quantities.

Nurse monitoring
1. The above dosages are for guidance only. In practice patients should have their blood theophylline (aminophylline is converted to theophylline) levels monitored. The precise dose is that which will maintain the blood theophylline level within the therapeutic range of 55–110 micromol/litre. Levels in excess of this range are associated with C.N.S. toxicity.
2. It should be noted that certain factors may alter the theophylline blood level and might explain an apparant lack of effect or the sudden development of toxicity. Cimetidine, allopurinol and erythromycin may increase blood levels while bartiburates and cigarette smoking will reduce levels.
3. It is important to note that there is a major risk of very high (toxic) blood levels occurring rapidly after intravenous injection in patients already receiving aminophylline, theophylline or other drugs of this type by the oral or rectal routes. Intravenous injections should be avoided or given with extreme caution in these cases and it is important to determine in advance the patient's current drug therapy.
4. Gastrointestinal irritation is a major problem with oral therapy, particularly when conventional tablets are taken. It is much less likely if slow release tablets are used and patients who complain of dyspepsia may benefit from a change of theophylline preparation.
5. Suppositories are also irritant and frequently produce proctitis.
6. The other major side effect which frequently occurs with blood levels in excess of the therapeutic range is C.N.S. stimulation. This produces anxiety, confusion and restlessness and patients may complain of vertigo and show marked hyperventilation.

General notes
1. Preparations containing aminophylline may be stored at room temperature.
2. Suppositories must be kept in a cool place and not close to a radiator or other direct heat source since they are designed to melt at temperatures approaching body heat.

AMIODARONE (Cordarone X)
Presentation
Tablets—200 mg.
Injection—150 mg in 3 ml.
Actions and uses
Amiodarone is used for the treatment of cardiac dysrhythmias including paroxysmal supraventricular, nodal and ventricular tachycardias, atrial flutter and atrial fibrillation. It may be effective in dysrhythmias resistant

to more commonly used drugs. It is thought to be of particular value in the treatment of paroxysmal arrhythmias associated with the Wolff-Parkinson-White syndrome.

Dosage
Adults:
a. The initial loading regime is 200 mg 3 times a day for 1 week. This regime may be extended if a response is not achieved.
b. To decide the maintenance dose the initial regime is gradually reduced until the lowest dose that will maintain control is obtained.

Nurse monitoring
1. During prolonged therapy patients have developed micro-crystalline deposits of the drug in the cornea. These occasionally produce impairment of vision. Regular opthalmic examinations are advised during prolonged treatment and should this side effect arise, the drug should be stopped.
2. Peripheral neuropathy and tremor have occurred. These problems may be diminished or resolved by reduction in the dose but if they persist the drug should be withdrawn.
3. Photosensitivity and pigmentation of the skin may occur. Common side effects include headaches, dizziness, nausea, vomiting and a metallic taste in the mouth. Sleep disturbance and nightmares also occur although these more frequently occur during the period of initial therapy and tend to diminish as maintenance doses are achieved.
4. The drug should be avoided or used with great caution in the following situations:
a. presence of sinus bradycardia or AV block
b. where a patient has cardiac failure not controlled by digoxin and diuretic therapy
c. patients currently receiving beta-blockers or verapamil
d. those with a history of thyroid disease.

5. It is important to recognise that the drug may increase the serum level of digoxin in patients already receiving digoxin and the patient should therefore be carefully monitored for the side effects which may arise.

General notes
1. The tablets may be stored at room temperature.
2. They should be protected from the light.

AMITRIPTYLINE (Tryptizol, Lentizol)

Presentation
Tablets—10 mg, 25 mg, 50 mg
Syrup—10 mg in 5 ml
Capsules—25 mg, 50 mg, 75 mg (all as sustained release)
Injection—10 mg in 1 ml

Actions and uses
Amitriptyine is a tricyclic antidepressant drug. Its actions and uses are described in the section on tricyclic antidepressant drugs.

Dosage
1. Orally for the treatment of depression: the usual dose range is 75-150 mg. The drug may be taken in three divided doses or as a single evening dose on retiring.
2. If given by the intramuscular or intravenous route: 20-30 mg four times daily is the usual required dose.
3. For the treatment of enuresis in children the following doses are administered:
Under 6 years: 10 mg in a single bed-time dose
6-10 years: up to 20 mg in a single bed-time dose
10-16 years: up to 50 mg in a single bed-time dose.

Nurse monitoring
As described in the section on tricyclic antidepressant drugs.

General notes
1. Preparations containing Amitriptyline may be stored at room temperature.
2. The injection solution and syrup should be protected from light.

3. For ease of administration Amitriptyline syrup may be diluted with Syrup B.P. before use but such dilutions must be used within 14 days.

AMOXYCILLIN (Amoxil)

(See Note 3, p. 310)
Presentation
Capsules—250 mg, 500 mg
Syrup—125 mg in 5 ml, 250 mg in 5 ml
Injection—vials containing 250 mg, 500 mg and 1 g

Actions and uses
Amoxycillin is an antibiotic of the Penicillin group which has actions and uses identical to Ampicillin (q.v.). It has an advantage over Ampicillin when given by the oral route in that it is better absorbed from the gastrointestinal tract and may be given less frequently. By the parenteral route, however, it has little if any advantage over Ampicillin.

Dosage
1. Oral:
   a. Adults and older children: 250–500 mg three times a day
   b. Children:
      1–7 years—125–250 mg three times a day
      Less than 1 year—62.5 mg three times per day
2. Parenteral—The parenteral dosage is identical to the oral dosage.

Nurse monitoring
The nurse monitoring notes on Ampicillin (q.v.) apply to this drug.

General notes
1. Preparations containing Amoxycillin may be stored in dry powder form at room temperature.
2. When reconstituted with Water for Injection such solutions should be used immediately and any unused portion should be discarded.
3. Intravenous infusions should be given in 500 ml of sodium chloride 0.9%, dextrose 5% or dextrose/saline mixtures in the appropriate dose over 4–6 hours.
4. Syrup and suspension once prepared should be used within seven days.

AMPHETAMINES AND RELATED DRUGS

Introduction
Because of the major problems of drug dependence and addiction associated with these drugs, discussion in this text will be restricted to an example of the group, namely Dexamphetamine sulphate (Dexedrine).

Actions and uses
The amphetamines have two major clinical effects:
1. They produce a marked depression of appetite
2. They produce a marked stimulation of neurological function.

In clinical practice they have only two indications:
1. For the treatment of narcolepsy
2. For the treatment of hyperkinetic states in children.

Dosage
1. For the treatment of narcolepsy: the recommended adult dose is 10 mg either in divided doses or as a single spansule in the morning. The dosage should be increased by 10 mg a day at weekly intervals to a maximum of 60 mg a day to obtain clinical response.
2. For the treatment of hyperkinetic states in children
   Aged 3–5: 2.5 mg a day increasing at weekly intervals by 2.5 mg.
   Aged 6 and over: 5–10 mg a day is recommended as a starting dose increasing by 5 mg at weekly intervals.
   The usual upper limit of dosage for administration to children is 20 mg per day.

Nurse monitoring
1. The administration of amphetamines is associated with a serious risk of physical and psychological dependence. The administration of this drug is therefore entirely contraindicated other than for treatment of the conditions described above.
2. Side effects include insomnia, restlessness, irritability, euphoria, tremor, dizziness, headache, dry mouth, anorexia, sweating, tachycardia, palpitation and moderate increase in blood pressure.
3. With higher doses symptoms of psychosis, indistinguishable from schizophrenia, may occur.
4. This drug should never be given to patients who are already receiving treatment with a monoamine oxidase inhibitor (q.v.) or in patients who have cardiovascular disease or hypertension or thyrotoxicosis.

General notes
The drug should be stored in a cool dry place and dispensed in moisture-proof containers.

AMPHOTERICIN B (Fungilin, Fungizone)

Presentation
Tablets—100 mg
Suspension—100 mg in 1 ml
Lozenges—10 mg
Cream, ointment, lotion and oral (dental) paste—30 mg in 1 g
Pessaries—50 mg
Injection—50 mg vials
Vaginal cream—100 mg per 4 g application

Actions and uses
1. This drug is an effective antifungal agent useful against a wide variety of yeasts and yeast-like fungi including *Candida albicans*. It is important to note that absorption from the gut is negligible even with very large doses.
2. An intravenous preparation is available which is effective against cryptococcosis (Torulopsis), North American blastomycosis, the disseminated forms of candidosis coccidiomycosis and histoplasmosis and also aspergillosis and other extremely rare fungal infections.

Dosage
1. Ointment and cream preparations should be applied two to four times daily
2. Lozenges are sucked four times daily
3. Oral suspension should be applied four times daily
4. Vaginal cream is inserted at night
5. Pessaries should be inserted at night
6. Tablets may be administered in a dose of one or two four times daily
7. Parenteral therapy: For adults and children the total daily dose should be administered by slow intravenous infusion over a period of six hours. The dosage is calculated on the basis of initially 0.25 mg/kg body weight, gradually increasing to a level of 1 mg/kg body weight depending on on individual response and tolerance.

Nurse monitoring
1. In treatment of the serious infections for which parenteral therapy is used, the duration of therapy may be extended to months and patients may require a great deal of psychological support.
2. Intravenous infusion may cause fever, rigor, headache, anorexia, weight loss, nausea, vomiting, malaise, painful muscles and joints, dyspepsia and cramping stomach pains, diarrhoea, anaemia and hypokalaemia.
3. The intravenous infusion may also cause irritation and thrombophlebitis at the injection site.
4. The intravenous infusion may cause renal failure, disturbance of cardiac rhythm, visual defects and convulsions.

5. The drug should be used with great caution in patients who are known to have kidney disease.
6. The drug should be used with great caution if other drugs known to damage the kidney are also being given, such as Gentamicin or Caphaloridine, and concurrent administration of corticosteroids is absolutely contraindicated.
7. Some gastrointestinal upset has followed the use of oral tablets which are otherwise without side effects.
8. For intravenous infusions the final concentration of solutions for infusion must not exceed 0.1 mg in 1 ml.

General notes
1. Topical preparations, tablets and suspension may be stored at room temperature.
2. Powder for infusion should be refrigerated.

AMPICILLIN (Penbritin)

(See Note 3, p. 310)

Presentation
Capsules—250 mg, 500 mg
Tablets—125 mg
Syrup and suspension—125 mg in 5 ml, 125 mg in 1.25 ml, dropper, 250 mg in 5 ml
Injection—Vials containing 250 mg and 500 mg

Actions and uses
Ampicillin is an antibiotic of the Penicillin group. It is bacteriocidal, i.e. it kills cells present in the body. It does this by interfering with the synthesis of substances necessary to maintain the bacterial cell wall and therefore causes the cells to burst. It has a wider spectrum of antibacterial activity than Benzylpenicillin (q.v.) and is effective against Gram-positive and Gram-negative cocci and some Gram-positive and Gram-negative bacilli. It is therefore used for the treatment of ear, nose and throat infections, bronchitis, pneumonia, urinary tract infection, gonorrhoea, gynaecological infections, septicaemia, peritonitis, endocarditis, meningitis, enteric fever and gastrointestinal infections when they are caused by the above organisms.

Dosage
1. Oral:
   a. Adults and older children: 250–500 mg four times a day.
   b. Children:
      1–7 years—125–250 mg four times a day.
      Children less than one year — 62.5 mg four times per day.
2. Parenteral: Parenteral doses are the same as for oral dose, although in severe illness higher doses may be used.
3. Ampicillin injection is occasionally used by local instillation either intrapleurally, intraperitoneally or intra-articularly. 500 mg in 5–10 ml of Water for Injection is given.

Nurse monitoring
1. It is important to note that Ampicillin is an effective drug when taken orally.
2. Ampicillin is associated with a low incidence of the production of skin rashes.
3. The drug may produce serious effects in the few patients who are hypersensitive to it. These range from urticaria to anaphylactic shock.
4. Diarrhoea is a common problem with Ampicillin.

General notes
1. Preparations containing Ampicillin may be stored in dry powder form at room temperature.
2. When reconstituted with Water for Injections such solutions should be used immediately and any unused portion should be discarded.
3. Intravenous infusions should be given in 500 ml of sodium chloride 0.9%, dextrose 5% or dextrose/saline mixtures in the appropriate dose over 4–6 hours.
4. Syrup and suspension once prepared should be used within seven days.

AMYLOBARBITONE (Amytal, Sodium Amytal)

Presentation
Tablets—15 mg, 30 mg, 50 mg, 100 mg and 200 mg
Tablets and capsules (as the sodium salt)—60 mg, 200 mg
Injection—250 mg, 500 mg (as the sodium salt)

Actions and uses
As described in the section on barbiturate drugs.
1. Amylobarbitone base is used for day-time sedation.
2. The sodium salt of Amylobarbitone which has a slightly more rapid onset of action than the base is taken at night as a hypnotic.

Dosage
1. For day-time sedation:
   a. 15–50 mg may be taken orally three or four times daily
   b. Up to 500 mg may be given by the intramuscular route in adults
   c. It is also possible to administer this drug by slow intravenous injection and up to 1 g may be given slowly.
2. For night sedation: Up to 200 mg may be administered as a single dose prior to retiring.

Nurse monitoring
As described in the section on barbiturates.

General notes
Capsules and tablets containing Amylobarbitone and Amylobarbitone sodium may be stored at room temperature.

ANTAZOLINE (Antistin-Privine, Otrivine-Antistin)

Presentation
Antistin-Privine—nasal drops and spray
Otrivine-Antistin—eye drops

Actions and uses
Antazoline is an antihistamine. The actions and uses of antihistamines in general are described in the section on antihistamines.
Antazoline is specifically used:
1. In eye drops for allergic ocular inflammatory conditions e.g. due to hay fever and allergic rhinitis.
2. As a nasal decongestant e.g. in the treatment of allergic rhinitis and hay fever.

Dosage
1. Nasal drops and spray used 3–4 hourly.
2. Eye drops used 2–3 times daily.

Nurse monitoring
Topical applications of antihistamine may produce skin sensitisation and subsequent eczematous and other eruptions.

General notes
The drug may be stored at room temperature.

ANTICONVULSANTS

The drugs used in the treatment of epilepsy include:
Beclamide
Carbamazepine
Clonazepam
Ethosuximide
Ethotoin
Methylphenobarbitone
Phenobarbitone
Phenytoin
Primidone
Sodium Valproate
Sulthiame
Troxidone

Presentation
See individual drugs.

Actions and uses
The epilepsies are a group of chronic disorders which may be classified as follows:
1. *Grand mal epilepsy*: In this the patient characteristically suffers repeated episodes of sudden loss of consciousness known commonly as a convulsion, accompanied by cessation of breathing, cyanosis, tongue-biting and rapid and irregular movements of the limbs. Patients frequently micturate during a convulsion and after the convulsion may remain unconscious for a number of

hours and suffer headache on recovery.
2. *Petit mal epilepsy*: This is characterised by short periods wherein although the patient does not lose consciousness or develop abnormal muscular movement they actually lose awareness of their surroundings, noticed because their teachers or parents observe that they have periods of inattention.
3. *Temporal lobe epilepsy*: This form of epilepsy does not have a characteristic clinical presentation, but takes the form of paroxysmal episodes of alteration in behaviour or personality.

All forms of epilepsy are thought to be due to abnormal bouts of electrical activity in the brain. The anticonvulsants act by suppressing the abnormal activity and thus reducing the frequency.

Dosage

See individual drugs.

Nurse monitoring

1. Anticonvulsant therapy frequently has to be taken throughout life. The nurse may play an important role in emphasising, particularly to patients who are on successful therapy and who have therefore not had a fit for some time, that tablets should be regularly taken and dosage should only be altered after consultation with medical staff.
2. The second most important point to know about any anticonvulsant treatment is that it must not under any circumstances be suddenly stopped as this may precipitate the serious and life-threatening state of status epilepticus and the patient may suffer prolonged severe and repeated episodes of convulsions.
3. The nurse may also play an important role in detecting the adverse effects of anticonvulsant treatment which are due either to excessive dosage or to side effects. These are discussed more fully under the specific drug headings.
4. It is important to note that a number of drugs may affect anticonvulsant control and frequency of convulsions and they should therefore be used with great caution in epileptic patients. These include phenothiazines (q.v.), tricyclic antidepressants (q.v.), Isoniazid and Lignocaine.
5. Epilepsy still carries, both with patients and the general public, an impression of abnormality which may lead to great social stress. The nurse may play an important role in encouraging a more enlightened approach to this illness in both patients and their relatives and the public in general.
6. Anticonvulsants can affect liver enzyme systems which are involved in the metabolism of many types of drugs. This may lead to an alteration in the effect of other drugs given to patients already receiving anticonvulsants. Examples of this are with oral contraceptives which may be ineffective if anticonvulsants are being coincidentally administered. The dosage of anticoagulants may also have to be altered.

ANTIHISTAMINES

Introduction

This group of drugs comprises many different chemicals with a common action.

Actions and uses

Antihistamines block the effect at specific sites in the body of histamine, a chemical which is released in the body as part of the allergic or inflammatory response and which is therefore partly responsible for the production of inflammation, erythema and pruritis which accompany such reactions. The antihistamine group of drugs have in addition further effects on the autonomic nervous system and

the central nervous system. In clinical practice they are used for the treatment of the following:
1. To suppress generalised minor allergic responses to allergens such as foodstuffs and drugs.
2. To suppress local allergic reactions i.e. inflammatory skin responses to insect stings and bites, contact allergens, urticaria etc.
3. Orally and in eye drops for allergic ocular inflammatory conditions e.g. due to hay fever and allergic rhinitis.
4. As nasal decongestants e.g. in the treatment of allergic rhinitis and hay fever. They are also added to a few proprietary cough preparations because of their decongestant action.
5. In the treatment of nausea and vomiting, particularly motion sickness.
6. As an anti-pruritic agent.
7. They are also used for the treatment of vertigo and the symptoms of vertigo and nausea due to Meniere's disease.

Dosage
See individual drugs.

Nurse monitoring
1. The antihistamines have a sedative effect (except Phenindamine and Terfenadine) and may produce marked drowsiness. In some clinical situations they are actually used for this effect, but where they are used for their other clinical effects, drowsiness may prove a troublesome side effect and the nurse may contribute to patient management by re-emphasising the dangers of driving or using industrial machinery while receiving these drugs.
2. Common side effects include headache, blurred vision, tinnitus, sleep disturbance, gastrointestinal upset and, in susceptible patients, urinary retention.
3. Topical applications of antihistamines may produce skin sensitisation and subsequent eczematous and other eruptions.

ANTI-INFLAMMATORY ANALGESIC DRUGS, NON-STEROIDAL

Actions and uses
This group of drugs relieves pain and reduces inflammation in a variety of diseases affecting the joints, tendons, cartilage and muscle. Thus they are useful in such disorders as rheumatoid arthritis, osteoarthritis, ankylosing spondylitis and gouty arthritis. If given in lower doses for minor painful conditions they are effective analgesics but this practise is to be discouraged as simple analgesics such as Paracetamol are equally effective and do not have the potentially serious side effects of this group of drugs. For convenience the drugs may be classified according to their chemical structure.
1. *Anthranilic acid derivatives*
   Mefenamic acid
2. *Indole acetic acid derivatives*
   Indomethacin
   Sulindac
   Tolmetin
3. *Salicylates*
   Aloxiprin—converted to Aspirin in small intestine
   Aspirin
   Benorylate—converted to Aspirin in blood
   Diflunisal—a long-acting Aspirin-like drug which is less irritant to the gastric mucosa than is Aspirin
   Salsalate—converted to Aspirin in the blood
4. *Phenylacetic acid derivatives*
   Diclofenac
5. *Pyrazoles*
   Azapropazone
6. *Propionic acid derivatives*
   Fenbufen
   Fenoprofen
   Flurbiprofen
   Ibuprofen
   Ketoprofen
   Naproxen
   Suprofen
   Tiaprofenic acid.
7. *Others*
   Piroxicam

Dosage
See individual drugs.

Nurse monitoring

1. As mentioned above this group of drugs are very effective analgesics but they have potentially serious side effects and perhaps the major role to be played by the nurse in management of patients who are in possession of these drugs is to ensure that they are taken in the correct dosage and only for the problems for which they are prescribed.
2. These drugs frequently have gastrointestinal side effects which may range from loss of appetite, nausea, vomiting, and diarrhoea to gastric bleeding which may be either chronic and go unnoticed or be acute and result in haematemesis or melaena. In patients with chronic painful disorders, adequate nutrition is absolutely essential and it is important that the nurse monitors the nutrition of patients on these drugs and where necessary encourages patients to try to overcome any associated anorexia. As a substantial number of patients on these drugs will gradually develop an anaemia, it is important that the nurse observes all patients on these drugs for the clinical signs of anaemia such as pallor, tiredness and dyspnoea on exertion.
3. These drugs are relatively contraindicated in patients with peptic ulceration and they may exacerbate the symptoms of this problem.
4. Asthma may be precipitated in a few patients who are hypersensitive to drugs of this type. This occurs most commonly in the salicylate group but it may also rarely occur with the other groups. An important point to note is that patients who suffer from salicylate-induced asthma may not have their symptoms relieved by changing to one of the other chemical groups.
5. All drugs in this group may cause salt and water retention. This may exacerbate or produce hypertension or cardiac failure. This effect is rarely seen in salicylates except when high dosage is given for the treatment of rheumatic fever.
6. Most anti-inflammatory drugs are metabolised to some extent by the liver and are excreted as metabolites or unmetabolised drugs by the kidney. They will therefore tend to accumulate in patients who have impaired liver or kidney function and be more likely to produce toxic effects.
7. Non-steroidal anti-inflammatory drugs are carried in the blood attached to sites on proteins which circulate in the blood. They have the capacity to displace other drugs from these proteins as the actual active component of any drug is that part which lies free in the plasma rather than that part which is bound to the protein. Any displacement of a drug from the protein will lead to an increased effect. This is especially important with two groups of drugs:
   a. Anticoagulants such as Warfarin. If non-steroidal anti-inflammatory drugs are given to patients who are receiving Warfarin or other anticoagulants, the anticoagulant may be displaced from the proteins and therefore be proportionately more active. This may lead to bleeding and may be especially dangerous if non-steroidal anti-inflammatory drugs' other side effects such as peptic ulceration or gastrointestinal bleeding occur coincidentally.
   b. Oral hypoglycaemics such as Chlorpropamide may also be displaced with resultant increase in effect and this may cause hypoglycaemia.

General notes
See specific drugs.

ANTILYMPHOCYTE IMMUNOGLOBULIN (Pressimmune)

Presentation
Injection—50 mg in 1 ml, 5 ml and 10 ml vials

Actions and uses
Antilymphocyte immunoglobulin is obtained from the blood of horses immunised with human lymphocytes. The immunoglobulin acts as an antibody and inhibits specific immune reactions. Immune reactions are clinically important in two instances:
1. It is immune reactions which lead to the destruction of tissue transplants.
2. Immune reactions appear to be involved in the damage to various tissues of the body caused by auto-immune diseases.

This drug may therefore be used to suppress immune reactions in the above two situations and its advantage is that it suppresses these reactions without reducing the patient's immunity to infection.

Dosage
1. For immunosuppression following organ transplantation: 10–30 mg/kg body weight is given daily by intravenous infusion. Subsequently dosage intervals may be lengthened as the risk of rejection diminishes.
2. In the treatment of auto-immune diseases: 5–15 mg/kg body weight is given daily by intravenous injection.

Nurse monitoring
1. Antilymphocyte immunoglobulin is a foreign protein to the body and therefore allergic reactions including pruritis, urticaria, serum sickness and shock occur in hypersensitive patients. All patients should therefore receive a test dose prior to starting full treatment and after the test dose should be medically supervised for at least an hour. Facilities for administration of intravenous drugs such as adrenaline and corticosteroids should be available as should emergency resuscitation equipment.
2. Adverse effects which may occur during treatment include fever, shivering, nausea, tachycardia and hypotension.
3. Thrombophlebitis may occur after intravenous infusion.
4. Intramuscular injections are painful.
5. Renal damage may occur.

General notes
1. Antilymphocyte immunoglobulin should be stored in a refrigerator.
2. Solutions are prepared by adding the total daily dose to 250–500 ml of 5% dextrose of 0.9% sodium chloride and infused over a period of 2–3 hours.

ASPARAGINASE

Presentation
Injection—10 000 units per vial

Actions and uses
Asparaginase is a cytotoxic drug. It is an enzyme obtained from cultures of a specific type of *E. coli*. It interferes with the synthesis of a specific amino acid required for the growth of malignant cells and therefore reduces the capacity of those cells to both grow and multiply. Its major use is in the induction of remission of acute lymphoblastic leukaemia. It has also been occasionally used in the treatment of acute myeloid leukaemia.

Dosage
It is important to note that a proportion of patients are hypersensitive to the drug and therefore all patients should receive an intradermal test dose of 50 i.u. and the injection site should be observed for three hours for signs of tissue reaction. If tissue reaction occurs this would be a contraindication to using the drug in its standard dosage. The usual initial dose is 200 units/kg body weight daily by slow intravenous injection or infusion over 20–30 minutes. Doses are then increased to a maximum of 1000 i.u./kg according to individual response. It is

recommended that the course of treatment should be continuous as interruption and recommencement of treatment increases the risk of sensitivity reactions.

Nurse monitoring
1. As noted above all patients should receive an intradermal test dose prior to commencing full treatment.
2. Gastrointestinal side effects include anorexia, nausea and vomiting.
3. Suppression of bone marrow function may result in anaemia and increased risk of infection due to suppression of white cell function.
4. In addition to bone marrow suppression which results in thrombocytopenia, levels of fibrinogen and clotting factors are also suppressed by this drug and therefore there is a marked risk of haemorrhage during treatment.
5. Impaired liver function, pancreatitis and hyperglycaemia have also been observed during treatment with this drug.
6. The nurse should be constantly aware that most cytotoxic drugs are irritant to the skin and mucous surfaces, and are in general very toxic. Great care should therefore be exercised when handling these drugs, and in particular spillage or contamination of personnel or the environment must be avoided. If cytotoxic drugs are handled regularly it is theoretically possible that repeated skin contact or inhalation may produce systemic toxic effects and in nurses who have developed hypersensitivity, severe local and general hypersensitivity reactions.

General notes
1. Vials for injection should be stored in a refrigerator.
2. The vials are reconstituted using the accompanying 10 ml sodium chloride 0.9% ampoules.
3. The prepared solution is administered by slow intravenous injection or as a rapid infusion (20–30 minutes) in 0.9% sodium chloride solution.

ASPIRIN

Presentation
Tablets—300 mg

Actions and uses
1. Aspirin relieves pain and reduces inflammation in a variety of diseases affecting the joints, tendons, cartilages and muscles. To produce a significant anti-inflammatory effect in patients with chronic arthropathy very high regular doses are required.
2. Aspirin is an effective analgesic for minor painful disorders such as headache, toothache or muscle strain.
3. Aspirin may be used as an anti-pyretic to lower the temparature of fevered patients.
4. A more recently developed use of Aspirin makes use of its ability to alter the function of platelets and other aspects of blood coagulation. It is given in small doses regularly to prevent transient cerebral ischaemic attacks when these are felt to be likely to be caused by micro-embolisation of platelet thrombi.

Dosage
1. *Adults*: The usual adult anti-inflammatory dose range is 1200 mg to 4 g per day taken in divided doses, often with or after meals in an attempt to reduce gastric irritation.
2. *Children*: Paediatric soluble Aspirin tablets (B.P.C.) are available for administration to children. Each tablet contains 75 mg of Aspirin. Recommended doses are as follows:
1–2 years: one or two tablets not more than four times daily;
3–5 years: three to four tablets not more than three times daily;
6–12 years: four tablets not more than three to four times daily. Aspirin should not be given to children for more than 48 hours unless under medical direction and supervision.

Nurse monitoring
1. The nurse monitoring points described under non-steroid anti-inflammatory analgesic drugs are applicable to Aspirin.
2. Because of the potentially serious complication of metabolic acidosis, Aspirin is completely contraindicated in children under the age of 1, and should be given with great caution to children between the ages of 1 and 7, and as noted above should never be given for more than 48 hours unless under medical supervision. The nurse may play a major role in the prevention of serious metabolic complications which may arise after administration of Aspirin to children under 7 by taking every opportunity to inform parents of the dangers of administering Aspirin in this age group.
3. Toxic effects specific to Aspirin are as follows:
   a. Mild symptoms of intoxication include dizziness, tinnitus, sweating, nausea, vomiting, mental confusion.
   b. More serious signs of toxicity include fever, ketosis, hyperventilation, respiratory alkalosis and metabolic acidosis. This may lead to shock, respiratory failure and coma.
   c. It must be remembered that the early features of toxicity as described above may not occur in children who may present initially with the more serious effects described.
4. Aspirin is readily available in many 'over the counter' preparations. As it has serious potential side effects the nurse should taken every opportunity to advise the patient against taking Aspirin for minor painful complaints and should encourage the use of other drugs such as Paracetamol with less serious side effects.

General notes
1. Aspirin tablets may be stored at room temperature but it is important to remember that they must be kept in a dry atmosphere since in a moist atmosphere the drug may be converted to acetic acid and may therefore be inactive. Drugs which have been inactivated in this way may be detected by their strong 'vinegary' smell.
2. Several forms of proprietary medicines which contain Aspirin included in a wide range of compound (mixed) preparations, many of which are bought over the counter as cold cures.
3. Because of the very high incidence of gastrointestinal upset associated with Aspirin, it is almost always prescribed in soluble form. It is important to remember that the soluble form is not free from such effects.

ASTEMIZOLE (Hismanal)
Presentation
Tablets—10 mg
Actions and uses
Astemizole is an antihistamine and the actions and usses of these drugs in general are described in the antihistamine section. In practice, astemizole is used in the management of hay fever.
Dosage
Adults: 10 mg taken once daily before one of the main meals.
Nurse monitoring
See the section on antihistamines.
General notes
The drug may be stored at room temperature.

ATENOLOL (Tenormin)
Presentation
Tablets—50 mg, 100 mg
Injection—5 mg in 10 ml
Actions and uses
Atenolol is a cardioselective beta-blocking drug and its actions and uses are described in the section on beta-blockers.

Dosage
1. This drug is particularly long acting and single daily doses of 100–200 mg in adults are usually adequate.
2. By injection in cardiac dysrhythmias, 2.5 mg by slow intravenous injection (over 2½ minutes) repeated after 5 minute intervals to a maximum total dose of 10 mg.

Nurse monitoring
1. See beta-adrenoreceptor blocking drugs.
2. Atenolol is a particularly useful drug in patients who have experienced central nervous system side effects from other beta-blockers such as nightmares and hallucinations.

General notes
Atenolol may be stored at room temperature.

AUGMENTIN

(See Note 3, p. 310)
Augmentin is a combination of Amoxycillin and Clavulanic Acid

Presentation
Tablets—each table contains Amoxycillin 250 mg and Clavulanic Acid 125 mg
Suspensions—Amoxycillin 125 mg and Clavulanic Acid 62 mg in 5 ml.
Amoxycillin 125 mg and Clavulanic Acid 31 mg in 5 ml

Actions and uses
The actions and uses of Amoxycillin are described elsewhere; by adding Clavulanic Acid the spectrum of activity of Amoxycillin may be broadened as Clavulanic Acid prevents the breakdown and therefore inactivation of Amoxycillin by Penicillinase (beta-lactamase). This substance is produced by a number of bacteria and effectively renders them penicillin-resistant. Some bacteria therefore resistant to Amoxycillin alone may be effectively treated by Augmentin. In practice this may prove particularly important the treatment of urinary tract athogens such as E. coli and skin and soft tissue infection due to staphylococcus.

Dosage
Doses may be calculated on the basis of the Amoxycillin content and full prescribing instructions are given under Amoxycillin.

Nurse monitoring
1. The nurse monitoring aspects already discussed with Amoxycillin apply to this drug
2. There are currently no reported adverse effects due to the Clavulanic Acid alone.

General notes
Augmentin tablets may be stored at room temperature.

AZAPROPAZONE (Rheumox)

Presentation
Capsules—300 mg
Tablets—600 mg

Actions and uses
See the section on non-steroidal anti-inflammatory analgesic drugs.

Dosage
The initial adult dose is 1200 mg daily taken in two to four divided doses. Once adequate clinical effect has been obtained, the dose is reduced to the minimum that will continue to keep the patient comfortable.

Nurse monitoring
See the section on anti-inflammatory analgesic drugs, non-steroidal.

General notes
Azapropazone capsules may be stored at room temperature.

AZATADINE (Optimine)

Presentation
Tablets—1 mg
Syrup—0.5 mg in 5 ml

Actions and uses
Azatadine is an antihistamine. The actions and uses of antihistamines in general are described in the antihistamine section. Azatadine is used specifically:
1. To suppress generalised minor allergic responses to allergens such as foodstuffs and drugs.

2. To suppress local allergic reactions i.e. inflammatory skin responses to insect stings and bites, contact allergens, urticaria etc.
3. Orally for other allergic conditions e.g. hay fever and allergic rhinitis.

Dosage
1. *Adults*: 1–2 mg b.d.
2. *Children*: 6–12 years—1 mg b.d.

Nurse monitoring
See the section on antihistamines.

General notes
The drug may be stored at room temperature.

AZATHIOPRINE (Imuran)

Presentation
Tablets—50 mg
Injection—Vials containing 50 mg

Actions and uses
Azathioprine is slowly converted in the body to its active derivative 6-Mercaptopurine. It has the following actions:
1. It suppresses the immune response after organ or tissue transplantation and therefore prevents tissue rejection and enhances the survival and function of transplanted organs.
2. It is also used in a number of other diseases where it appears to alter the disease process producing an improvement in symptoms. Examples of such diseases are rheumatoid arthirtis, systemic lupus erythematosus and Crohn's disease.

Dosage
1. For immunosuppression after organ transplantation: The recommended dose is 1–4 mg/kg body weight daily (average 2.4 mg/kg).
2. For the treatment of the other diseases mentioned above: It is usually given in a dose range of 1–2.5 mg/kg.
3. It may be given by intravenous injection at the above doses for short periods when oral treatment is unsuitable.
4. The combination of Azathioprine with a corticosteroid drug usually permits the use of lower doses of both drugs while maintaining their clinical effect.

Nurse monitoring
1. Azathioprine commonly causes gastrointestinal upset and symptoms include anorexia, nausea, vomiting and diarrhoea.
2. It depresses the bone marrow and seems particularly to effect white cell function leading to an increased risk of infection. Patients suffering from acute infection therefore should never be given the drug. Infections by bacteria, fungi, protozoa and viruses which do not normally occur in healthy adults may occur in patients on this drug.
3. It should be used with caution in patients who have existing liver disease and cases of hepatitis and biliary stasis have been reported. Despite this it is worth noting that it is actually used in the treatment of active chronic hepatitis.
4. The drug has been shown to cause fetal abnormality if taken either during pregnancy, or by the father prior to conception. It is important therefore to encourage patients to take adequate contraceptive measures.
5. Serious toxic effects will occur when the drug tends to accumulate in the body. This will occur in two instances:
   a. In patients with reduced renal function
   b. In patients who are also taking Allopurinol which inhibits the body's capacity to metabolise Azathioprine. In such cases the dose of Azathioprine should be reduced accordingly.

General notes
1. Azathioprine tablets and injection should be stored at room temperature.
2. Injection solutions are prepared by adding not less than 5 ml Water for Injection to each 50 mg vial.
3. Solutions are alkaline and very

irritant to the venous tract. They should be injected slowly, preferably via the drip tubing of a running 5% dextrose or 0.9% sodium chloride infusion.
4. Any unused solution should be discarded immediately.

AZLOCILLIN (Securopen)
(See Note 3, p. 310)
Presentation
Injection—0.5 g, 1.0 g, 2.0 g vials and 5 g infusion pack
Actions and uses
Azlocillin is a member of the Penicillin group of antibiotics. It has a much wider spectrum of activity than the parent drug, Benzylpencillin. Its indications are for the treatment of bacterial infection in any tissue of the body when the organism has been shown to be sensitive to it. It is of particular interest to note that this drug is useful in the treatment of serious infections due to pseudomonas species which are frequently resistant to other antibacterial drugs.
Dosage
1. *Adults*: 2–5 g every 8 hours according to the severity of the infection.
2. *Children*: for premature infants and children under 3 kg—
50 mg/kg body weight every 12 hours
Under 3 months: 0.15–0.25 g every 8 hours
3 months to 1 year: 0.25–0.5 g every 8 hours
1 year to 2 years: 0.5 g every 8 hours
2 years to 6 years: 0.5–1 g every 8 hours
6 years and over: 1–3 g every 8 hours
N.B. Doses below 2 g are administered by intravenous bolus injection. Higher doses should be given by rapid intravenous infusion over 20–30 minutes. Solutions for injection should be prepared in a concentration of 10% in Water for Injections.

Nurse monitoring
See Benzylpenicillin.
General notes
1. The drug may be stored at room temperature.
2. 10% solution for injection should be prepared immediately before use and any remaining solution discarded.

B

BAMETHAN (Vasculit)
Presentation
Tablets—12.5 mg
Actions and uses
The actions and uses of this drug are identical to those described for Nicofuranose (q.v.).
Dosage
Adults: 25 mg four times day.
Nurse monitoring
1. The Nurse monitoring points described for Nicofuranose apply to this drug.
2. The drug should be used with great caution in patients with angina pectoris or recent myocardial infarction.

General notes
The drug may be stored at room temperature.

BARBITURATES
Amylobarbitone
Butobarbitone
Cyclobarbitone
Heptabarbitone
Methohexitone
Methylphenobarbitone
Pentobarbitone
Phenobarbitone
Thiopentone

Actions and uses
Barbiturates are drugs which depress the function of the brain. This leads to a number of potential uses:
1. To induce sleep
2. To produce day time sedation
3. As anaesthetics
4. As anticonvulsants.

The very potent short-acting drugs are used as intravenous anaesthetics. Intermediate acting barbiturates readily produce sleep when taken as single night time doses. Phenobarbitone is specially useful as an anticonvulsant. As it has a cumulative action it is not recommended for production of sleep.

Dosage
See individual drugs.

Nurse monitoring
1. Perhaps the most important point to make about barbiturates is that prolonged use can cause physical dependence and addiction. Obviously when used as an anticonvulsant Phenobarbitone is an acceptable form of treatment but there are now available alternative drugs for the induction of sleep and it is not recommended that patients receive barbiturates for this purpose. As many patients receive sleeping tablets on repeat prescriptions there may be a significant number of patients in the community who still receive barbiturates for this purpose. The nurse may play an important role by helping to identify these patients and bringing them to the notice of the doctor.
2. It is extremely dangerous suddenly to stop barbiturate treatment in any patient who has been on such treatment for a prolonged period of time. Epileptic fits and convulsions may be precipitated. The nurse may play an important role by ensuring that patients are aware of this danger.

3. Doses of barbiturates given at night to produce sleep, although effective for this purpose, often lead to 'hang-over' symptoms and confusion the following day particularly in elderly patients. The nurse may play a useful role in identifying this adverse effect.
4. Barbiturate drugs depress respiratory, neurological and cardiovascular function. This is particularly important in the following instances:
   a. Patients with severe respiratory disease may have their respiratory function further depressed by administration of barbiturates. This may lead to death.
   b. Depression of C.N.S. function by barbiturates may be accentuated by the coincident ingestion of alcohol. All patients must be warned of the dangers of taking alcohol with barbiturates.
5. Gastrointestinal upset frequently occurs with oral administration.
6. When given intravenously severe depression of respiration, hypotension, coughing, sneezing and laryngeal spasm may occur.
7. The accidental injection of barbiturate drugs into arteries has caused arterial spasm with resultant gangrene and loss of the affected limb.

General notes
See specific drugs.

BECLAMIDE (Nydrane)

Presentation
Tablets—500 mg

Actions and uses
1. The actions and uses of anticonvulsant drugs in gneral are discussed in the section dealing with anticonvulsant drugs.
2. This drug is particularly useful for the treatment of behavioural disorders in epileptic or non-epileptic patients, particularly when instability is marked or aggressiveness is a feature.

Dosage
1. For the treatment of epilepsy: N.B. Individual dosage requirements vary greatly. The following doses are given as a guide only.
   a. *Adults*: Initially 3–4 g in total per day is taken in divided doses. Treatment is then cautiously and slowly monitored to patients needs. It is important to note that the therapeutic effect of this drug may take up to four weeks to occur.
   b. *Children*:
   Under 5 years—500 mg to 1 g daily in divided doses.
   5–10 years—1500 mg daily in divided doses.
2. For the treatment of behavioural disorders:
   a. *Adults*: Initially 3–4 g per day in total given in divided doses and then adjusted according to patient response.
   b. *Children*:
   Less than 5 years—500 mg to 1 g per day in divided doses.
   5–10 years—1500 mg per day in divided doses.

Nurse monitoring
1. The Nurse monitoring aspects of anticonvulsant drugs in general are discussed in the section dealing with anticonvulsant drugs.
2. As this drug takes up to four weeks to produce its therapeutic effect other anti-epileptic treatment should not be reduced until this period has elapsed.
3. Side effects which are uncommon include dizziness, nervousness, gastrointestinal upset, skin rash and leucopenia.
4. This drug should not be given to pregnant patients.

General notes
The drug should be stored at room temperature.

BECLOMETHASONE (Becotide, Propaderm, Beconase)

Presentation
Inhalation—metered aerosol 50 μg per dose

Inhalation suspension—50 μg in 1 ml
'Rotacaps'—100 and 200 μg
Nasal spray—50 μg per metered dose
Cream—0.025%, 0.5%
Ointment—0.025%

Actions and uses
Beclomethasone is a corticosteroid drug (see the section on corticosteroids) used primarily in three situations:
1. It is administered topically for the treatment of inflammatory skin conditions such as psoriasis, eczema and dermatitis.
2. It is administered by inhalation for the management of asthma.
3. It is instilled nasally in the management of allergic rhinitis and hay fever.

Dosage
1. Topical application should be applied sparingly twice daily.
2. By inhalation:
   a. *Adults*: on average 100 μg (two puffs) three or four times daily. Up to 800 μg may be given in severe cases. Alternatively 100 μg may be administered by nebuliser 2-5 times a day.
   b. *Children*: usually receive half the adult dose and the maximum daily dose by inhalation recommended is 500 μg. It is worth noting that capsules containing dry powder (rotacaps) may be more acceptable to younger patients.
3. For nasal instillation one metered dose (50 μg) is instilled four times daily.

Nurse monitoring
See the section on corticosteroids. It is worth noting that whatever the route of administration, sufficient of this drug may be absorbed to product the systemic effects described in the section mentioned above.

General notes
1. Preparations containing Beclomethasone may be stored at room temperature.
2. In common with other pressurised containers, metered aerosols and nasal sprays should not be punctured or incinerated after use.
3. If necessary Beclomethasone cream may be diluted with Cetomacrogol cream, formula A, or the ointment with white soft paraffin.

BENDROFLUAZIDE (Neo-Naclex)

Presentation
Tablets—2.5 mg, 5 mg

Actions and uses
See the section on thiazide and related diuretics.

Dosage
1. *Adults*: The daily adult dose range is 2.5-10 mg which may be taken as a single morning dose since the duration of action of Bendrofluazide is approximately 24 hours.
2. *Children*:
   Up to 5 years: 1.25 mg
   5 years plus: 2.5 mg.

Nurse monitoring
See the section on thiazide and related diuretics.

General notes
Bendrofluazide tablets may be stored at room temperature.

BENORYLATE (Benoral)

Presentation
Tablets—750 mg
Suspension—4 g in 10 ml

Actions and uses
1. See the section on Aspirin.
2. Benorylate is converted in the blood to Aspirin and Paracetamol. It may therefore occasionally be used successfully in patients who are unable to tolerate Aspirin due to its gastric irritant effect.

Dosage
1. *Adults*: The average adult dosage is 1.5 g (tablets) three times a day or 4 g (10 ml suspension) twice daily.
2. *Children*
   Up to 1 year: 25 mg/kg body weight up to four times dialy 1-2 years: 250 mg up to four times daily

2–6 years: 500 mg up to three times daily
6–12 years: 500 mg up to four times daily.
It must be remembered that as this compound is converted to Aspirin it should be used with great care in children and should really only be given to children under the age of one, under strict medical supervision.

Nurse monitoring
1. The Nurse monitoring notes for Aspirin (q.v.) are applicable to this drug.
2. It is also converted to Paracetamol; the Nurse monitoring notes for Paracetamol (q.v.) are also applicable.

General notes
Benorylate tablets and suspension may be stored at room temperature.

BENPERIDOL (Anquil)

Presentation
Tablets—0.25 mg

Actions and uses
Benperidol is a neuroleptic drug which has many of the actions and uses described for Haloperidol. It has a particular use in the management of patients displaying unusual sexual behavioural disturbances.

Dosage
Adults: The standard dose is 0.25–1.5 mg daily, though up to 9 mg daily has been used in schizophrenia.

Nurse monitoring
See the section on Haloperidol.

General notes
The drug may be stored at room temperature.

BENZATHINE PENCILLIN (Penidural)

(See Note 3, p. 310)

Presentation
Syrup—225 mg in 5 ml (equivalent to Benzylpenicillin 300 000 units in 5 ml)
Paediatric drops—Approximately 115 mg in 1 ml (equivalent to Benzylpenicillin 150 000 units)
Calibrated dropper delivers 100 000 units
Injection—225 mg in 1 ml (equivalent to Benzylpenicillin 300 000 units)

Actions and uses
Benzathine Penicillin has identical actions and uses to those described for Benzylpenicillin (q.v.). It is used either alone or in combination with Benzypenicillin and Procaine Pencillin G and its advantage is that it has a prolonged duration of action, as it is only slowly released from the sites of intramuscular injections. The indications for its use are identical to those described for Benzylpenicillin.

Dosage
1. *Adults*:
   a. Oral: 10 ml syrup (equivalent to 600 000 units of Benzylpenicillin) three to four times per day.
   b. Parenteral: 4 ml (equivalent to 1.2 million units of Benzylpenicillin) repeated after 5–7 days if necessary.
2. *Children*:
   a. Oral: 5 ml syrup (equivalent to 300 000 units of Benzylpenicillin) three to four times per day.
   b. Parenteral: 1–2 ml (equivalent to 300 000–600 000 units of Benzylpenicillin) repeated after 5–7 days if necessary.
3. *Infants*: Orally, one dropper full equivalent to 100 000 units of Benzylpenicillin) 3–4 times per day.

Nurse monitoring
See the section on Benzylpenicillin.

General notes
1. The oral preparation may be stored at room temperature.
2. Preparations for injection should be stored in a refrigerator.

BENZHEXOL (Artane)

Presentation
Tablets—2 mg and 5 mg
Capsules—5 mg sustained release
Syrup—5 mg in 5 ml

Actions and uses
Benzhexol has a number of actions known as 'anticholinergic effects' including the potential to relax muscle and abolish rigidity and tremor. This makes it useful for the treatment of Parkinson's disease and it is often given to psychiatric patients treated with phenothiazine transquillisers who may develop this as a side effect of their phenothiazine therapy.

Dosage
Adults: 6-15 mg daily in three divided doses or as a single dose using slow release capsules.

Nurse monitoring
1. The drug's anticholinergic actions produce dry mouth, blurred vision, constipation and urinary retention.
2. Further common adverse effects include dizziness, nervousness and nausea.
3. Mental confusion and agitation are less common problems.
4. The drug should be used with caution in patients with:
   a. Glaucoma
   b. Gastrointestinal obstruction
   c. Prostatism

General notes
The drug may be stored at room temperature.

BENZODIAZEPINES AND RELATED DRUGS

Chlordiazepoxide
Clobazam
Clonazepam
Diazepam
Flurazepam
Lorazepam
Medazepam
Nitrazepam
Oxazepam
Potassium clorazepate
Temazepam
Triazolam

Actions and uses
Benzodiazepines are sedative drugs. They have this effect by their action on a specific area in the brain known as the limbic system. This area of the brain is thought to be concerned with the control of emotion. The advantage that benzodiazepines have over other central nervous system sedative drugs such as barbiturates, is that they do not have a general depressant effect on cerebral function and therefore are not as dangerous. As well as their sedative effect certain of this drug group have other uses. These are as follows:
1. Nitrazepam, Triazolam and Temazepam have a marked sedative effect and may be taken at night to induce sleep.
2. Clonazepam has a specific anticonvulsant action and is taken orally in the treatment of epilepsies.
3. Chlordiazepoxide has a specific indication for the control of delirium tremens in alcoholic patients.
4. Diazepam is particularly useful for intramuscular or intravenous administration as it provides sufficient sedation to relieve either acute anxiety or to allow minor practical procedures such as dental surgery or endoscopy. Diazepam is also useful in the treatment of status epilepticus and tetanus when it may be given by the intramuscular or intravenous route.

Dosage
See individual drugs.

Nurse monitoring
1. When given during the day for their sedative and anxiolytic action the sedative effect may occasionally be excessive leading to drowsiness and may be accompanied by an inability to walk properly without staggering. These effects are seen particularly when alcohol is taken in addition to the drugs. Patients must therefore be encouraged not to consume alcohol while taking these drugs and in addition they should be warned about the potential dangers of excess sedation when driving or operating machinery.

2. The drugs of this group which are given at night as hypnotics can produce effects lasting into the following day which are known as hang-over effects. These are symptoms of drowsiness, lethargy and headache and may, especially in elderly patients when high dosage has been given, cause frank confusion. Patients themselves may not notice effects of over-sedation and nurses can play an important role in detecting such effects.
3. Occasionally when these drugs are given an unusual or paradoxical reaction may occur and the patient may become agitated, excited and may even experience hallucinations.
4. Drugs of the benzodiazepine group, even when taken in massive overdosage orally, rarely produce profound neurological depression. This makes them preferable to barbiturates. However, it must be stressed that when given intravenously for short-term sedation they may still cause respiratory depression and therefore should never be given intravenously unless facilities for resuscitation are available.
5. These drugs are not recommended for regular use in pregnancy.
6. Nursing mothers should be warned that if they take benzodiazepines while breast feeding the drug will be excreted in their milk and may lead to marked sedation of their children.
7. Side effects of this group of drugs include gastrointestinal upset, blurred vision, dry mouth and headache.

General notes
See specific drugs.

BENZTROPINE (Cogentin)

Presentation
Tablets—2 mg
Injection—1 mg in 1 ml

Actions and uses
1. Benztropine is an anticholinergic drug which has actions and uses identical to those described for Benzhexol (q.v.).
2. Benztropine is also used in clinical practice for emergency treatment of acute dystonic reactions such as torticollis and oculogyric crises.

Dosage
1. For the treatment of Parkinsonism: The adult dose is 1–6 mg per day as a single dose at bedtime. The dose may alternatively be divided and given two or three times a day.
2. For the emergency treatment of acute dystonic reactions: 1–2 mg is given by intramuscular or intravenous injection.

Nurse monitoring
The Nurse monitoring aspects of Benzhexol (q.v.) apply to this drug.

General notes
1. The drug may be stored at room temperature.
2. Solution for injection should be protected from light.

BENZYLPENICILLIN (Crystapen G)

(See Note 3, p. 310)
N.B. Also referred to as Penicillin G and available as the potassium or sodium salt.

Presentation
Tablets—250 mg
Syrup — 125 mg in 5 ml
250 mg in 5 ml
Injection—0.5, 1.5 and 10 mega unit vials
Eye drops and ointment—various strengths

Actions and uses
Benzylpenicillin was the first of the penicillin group of antibiotics and has a bacteriocidal action i.e. it kills bacterial cells in the body. It does this by interfering with the synthesis of bacterial cell walls causing them to burst. It has a narrow antibacterial spectrum. The micro-organisms streptococci, pneumococci, meningococci and

gonococci are usually sensitive to this drug. Nowadays staphylococci are only rarely sensitive. It, therefore, has the following clinical uses:
1. In the treatment of infections caused by the above organisms as outlined in Note 3.
2. In the treatment of venereal disease, both syphilis and gonorrhoea.
3. In the treatment of gonococcal infection of the eye in the newborn (ophthalmia neonatorum).

Dosage

N.B. One mega unit is equivalent to one million units or 600 mg of Penicillin.
1. Oral:
   a. *Adults*: 250–500 mg four times a day
   b. *Children*: 125–250 mg four times a day
   c. *Infants*: 62.5–125 mg four times a day

The drug should preferably be given one hour before meals.

2. Parenteral:
   a. *Adults*: 600–1200 mg daily divided into 2–4 doses. The drug may be given by intramuscular or intravenous bolus injection or intravenous infusion. By the intravenous route at least one minute should be taken for each 300 mg injected.
   b. *Children aged one month to 12 years*: 10–20 mg/kg body weight in total in 24 hours, usually divided into four doses.
   c. *Neonates* (less than 1 month): 30 mg/kg per day in total in divided doses, usually twice daily in the first few days of life and then 3–4 times daily.
3. Topical applications (eye drops and ointment): The doses of these vary widely depending on the condition treated.
4. Intra-thecal route: Rarely Benzylpenicillin is given intrathecally for the treatment of bacterial meningitis. Injection of an excessive dose by this route is highly dangerous and in many centres it is now felt that intravenous dosage is quite adequate, and intrathecal therapy unnecessary. Maximum doses recommended are as follows:
   a. *Adults*: 6 mg dissolved in 10 ml of sodium chloride or 10 ml of the patient's CSF. The usual daily dose is 6 mg but on occasions up to 12 mg may be used.
   b. *For infants and children*: 0.1 mg/kg body weight is suitable. The concentration of Pencillin in the injection should not exceed 0.6 mg/ml.
5. Intra-ocular: In certain eye infections ½ to 1 mega unit may be given by subconjunctival injection.

N.B. It is important to note that the above dosages are only an outline and under certain circumstances much higher doses may be given. Examples of this are in bacterial endocarditis in adults where up to 8 mega units may be given parenterally per day and in neonatal meningitis when the systemic dosage may be 60–90 mg/kg per day in total.

Nurse monitoring

1. Penicillins are most noted for their production of adverse effects in patients who are hypersensitive to the drug group. The effects produce may range from skin rash and urticaria to anaphylactic shock. Patients with a history of Penicillin allergy should never be given Penicillin under any circumstance by any route.
2. As allergy to Penicillin can be so dangerous the nurse may play an important role in the management of these patients by ensuring that their allergy once identified is recorded on patients' Kardexes and in their notes, and brought to the attention of the medical staff.
3. Although oral preparations of Penicillin G are available it is important to note that they are not particularly effective.

4. Oral Penicillins may commonly produce mild diarrhoea.
5. If very high doses are given haemolytic anaemia and convulsion may occur.

General notes
1. Preparations containing Benzylpenicillin may be stored at room temperature.
2. Solutions for injection should be prepared as follows:
   a. Intramuscular injection: Add 1.6–2 ml of Water for Injections to each 1 mega unit vial.
   b. Intravenous injection: Dissolve 1 mega unit in 4–10 ml Water for Injection (note that the maximum infusion rate by intravenous bolus injection is 300 mg/minute).
   c. Intravenous infusion: The dose to be given is added to 500 ml of 0.9% sodium chloride or 0.5% dextrose of dextrose/saline mixture and infused over 4–6 hours.
3. Solutions containing Benzylpenicillin should be used immediately as they quickly deteriorate. Intravenous infusions must never be stored for any length of time. However, buffered solutions, once prepared, may last for three days at room temperature or up to two weeks in a refrigerator.

BEPHENIUM (Alcopar)

Presentation
Granules—2.5 g

Actions and uses
This antihelminthic drug is used in the treatment of:
1. Hookworm (ancylostomiasis)
2. Roundworm (ascariasis)
3. Trichostrongyliasis.

Dosage
1. For adults and children over 10 kg body weight: 2.5 g
2. Children under 10 kg body weight: 1.25 g.

Nurse monitoring
1. The required dose should be mixed in water or a sweet liquid and drunk immediately.
2. In the presence of heavy infestation it is recommended that the treatment be repeated after three days.
3. No purgation is necessary.
4. Gastrointestinal upset may occur including nausea, vomiting, abdominal pain and diarrhoea.

General notes
The drug may be stored at room temperature.

BETA-ADRENORECEPTOR BLOCKING DRUGS (Beta-blockers)

Acebutolol
Atenolol
Labetalol
Metoprolol
Nadolol
Oxprenolol
Pindolol
Propranolol
Sotalol
Timolol

Actions and uses
The sympathetic nervous system exerts its effect by acting at specific sites called beta-adrenoreceptor sites. There are two types:
1. $beta_1$ receptors
2. $beta_2$ receptors

Stimulation of $beta_1$ receptors leads to an increase in heart rate and cardiac output. Stimulation of $beta_2$ receptors causes dilation of the small airways in the lung and dilation of small arteries and arterioles. Beta-adrenoreceptor blocking drugs block the effect of the sympathetic nervous system and therefore potentially produce a reduction in heart rate, cardiac output and blood pressure and may also potentially cause bronchoconstriction and vasoconstriction. The group as a whole may be distinguished on the basis of three pharmacological effects:
1. Cardioselectivity
2. Partial agonist activity
3. Membrane stabilising activity.

By far the most important clinical effect is cardioselectivity. Drugs which are non-selective block sympathetic stimulation at both beta$_1$ and beta$_2$ sites and are therefore likely to produce unwanted side effects of bronchospasm and vasoconstriction. Cardioselective drugs tend to block the beta$_1$ (cardiac) sites rather than the beta$_2$ (peripheral) sites and therefore are less likely to cause side effects. In summary, beta blockers may be used for:
1. The prevention of angina pectoris
2. The management of hypertension
3. The control of cardiac dysrhythmias.

Dosage
See individual drugs.

Nurse monitoring
1. Any patient treated with a beta-blocker may develop heart failure and therefore all patients should be observed for the development of symptoms and signs indicative of this problem.
2. Many diabetics recognise the early symptoms of a hypoglycaemic attack by noticing sweating, tremor and tachycardia. They may prevent the development of a full-blown attack by taking sugar. If diabetics are given beta-blockers these early symptoms may not be felt and hypoglycaemic coma may follow. Thus beta-blockers must be used with great caution in diabetic patients. There is some evidence that cardio-selective beta-blockers are less likely to have this effect and therefore if beta-blockers must be used in diabetic patients a cardiocelective preparation should be chosen.
3. As mentioned above, beta-blocking drugs may cause bronchospasm and vasoconstriction. Non-selective beta-blockers are therefore definitely contraindicated in patients with asthma or peripheral vascular disease. Cardioselective beta-blockers are less likely to exacerbate bronchospasm and peripheral vascular disease but patients given these drugs who have these problems must always be carefully observed in case even the cardioselective drugs cause an exacerbation of symptoms.
4. Gastrointestinal side effects of nausea, vomiting and diarrhoea occur commonly and may be reduced if the drug is taken just before meals.
5. Central nervous system effects include dizziness, drowsiness, lassitude, depression, insomnia, nightmares and hallucinations. These effects are more likely to be seen in lipid soluble beta-blockers such as Propranolol and it is worth noting that Atenolol is the least lipid soluble preparation available and therefore may be the preparation of choice in patients who suffer these symptoms severely.
6. Other side effects include skin rashes, pruritis, and flushing.
7. It is important that the nurse remembers that beta-blockers will by definition produce a slow pulse and pulse rates below 50 per minute are not an indication to stop the drug unless symptoms suggest heart failure is present. A useful point to note is that pulse rates of less than 50 per minute are often acceptable as long as they can be shown to rise after exercise.

General notes
See individual drugs.

BETAHISTINE (Serc)

Presentation
Tablets—8 mg

Actions and uses
Betahistine is an antihistamine. The actions and uses of antihistamines in general are described in the section on antihistamines. In clinical practice Betahistine is used in the treatment of vertigo and the symptoms of vertigo and nausea due to Menière's disease.

Dosage
Adults: 8–16 mg taken three times daily.
Nurse monitoring
See the section on antihistamines.
General notes
The drug may be stored at room temperature.

BETAMETHASONE (Betnelan, Betnesol, Bextasol, Betnovate)
Presentation
Tablets—0.5 mg (plain and soluble)
Injection—4 mg in 1 ml
Inhaler—100 μg per dose
Ointment, cream and application—0.1% (also combined with antibiotic)
Rectal—ointment 0.05% and suppositories 0.5 mg
Eye, ear and nose drops—0.1%
Eye ointment—0.1%
Actions and uses
See the section on corticosteroids.
Dosage
Doses vary considerably with the nature and severity of the illness being treated and it is not therefore appropriate to quote specific instances.
Nurse monitoring
See the section on corticosteroids.
General notes
1. Preparations containing Betamethasone may be stored at room temperature.
2. The injection solution should be protected from light and as with other pressurised inhalers, aerosols should never be punctured or incinerated after use.
3. Intravenous injections are given slowly over 30 seconds to one minute.
4. If given by intravenous infusion, normal saline or 5% dextrose solutions can be used as diluents.

BETHANECOL (Myotonine)
Presentation
Tablets—10 mg and 25 mg
Injection—5 mg in 1 ml
Actions and uses
Many functions of the body including the rate at which the heart beats, the cardiac output, the amount of respiratory secretion, the degree of muscle tone in the bronchi (airway), the movement of the gut wall and the function of the bladder are controlled by the autonomic nervous system. This system is divided into two parts known as the sympathetic and parasympathetic systems. Their interrelation is a complex process and is beyond the bounds of this text. Bethanecol stimulates the parasympathetic segment of the autonomic nervous system. Its useful effects are as follows:
1. It may effect the contraction of bladder muscle and the bladder sphincters promoting micturition. It is used where normal control of bladder function has been lost.
2. It stimulates gastric persistaltic waves and has been used in the management of various gastrointestinal disorders including post-operative abdominal distension and megacolon.

Dosage
1. Orally: 5–30 mg three or four times daily.
2. Subcutaneously: for acute retention of urine—5 mg or 10 mg.

Nurse monitoring
1. The other effects of stimulating the parasympathetic section of the autonomic nervous system are in fact this drug's side effects. They include:
   a. Reduction of heart rate and cardiac output
   b. Peripheral vasodilation
   c. An increase in respiratory secretions and constriction of the bronchi.
2. The drug should be used with great care in patients who have suffered from asthma, chronic obstructive lung disease, or those with urinary or gastrointestinal obstruction.
3. The drug should never be given

to patients who have heart disease.
4. If this drug is given to a patient who has normal sensation to the bladder but has difficulty with passing water, if micturition does not occur severe discomfort will be produced and facilities for catheterisation should be available.

General notes
The drug may be stored at room temperature.

BETHANIDINE (Esbatal)

Presentation
Tablets—10 mg, 50 mg

Actions and uses
See the section on Guanethidine.

Dosage
1. Initially adults are commenced on 10 mg three times a day with increments of 5–10 mg three times daily as required until effective control of hypertension is achieved. Up to 200 mg per day may be necessary in total.
2. Children's doses are:
   Less than 1 year: 2.5 mg.
   1–6 years: 5 mg.
   7 years plus: 5–10 mg.
   These doses are taken three times a day. Children's doses likewise may be increased about 20 times these values to achieve the required effect.

Nurse monitoring
See the section on Guanethidine.

General notes
Bethanidine tablets may be stored at room temperature.

BISACODYL (Dulcolax)

Presentation
Tablets—5 mg
Suppositories—5 mg and 10 mg

Actions and uses
The general actions of laxatives are discussed in the section on laxatives. Bisacodyl is a member of group 1, i.e. it has an irritant action on the gut wall. It is used for the treatment of constipation.

Dosage
1. *Adults*: 10 mg orally at night or one 10 mg suppository inserted each morning.
2. *Children*: one 5 mg suppository inserted each morning.

Nurse monitoring
Its irritant effect on the gut wall may lead to cramping abdominal pain, otherwise there are no specific problems with this drug.

General notes
1. Preparations containing Bisacodyl may be stored at room temperature.
2. It is important that suppositories are not stored in a warm area e.g. above or near a radiator, since they will readily melt.

BLEOMYCIN

Presentation
Injection—ampoules containing 5 and 15 mg

Actions and uses
Bleomycin is a cytotoxic drug derived from a family of antibiotics which have been found to have this action. It has a mode of action similar to that of Actinomycin (q.v.). It is used in the treatment of the following conditions:
1. Squamous cell carcinomas, i.e. in the mouth, nose, throat and oesophagus
2. Hodgkin's disease and other lymphomas
3. Testicular teratoma
4. Bleomycin has also been used in melanoma, carcinoma of the thyroid, lung and bladder.

Dosage
Bleomycin may be used alone but it is usually given in combination with other cytotoxic drugs. It may be administered by various routes including intramuscular, intravenous, intra-arterial, intrapleural or intraperitoneal injection. It has also been injected directly into tumours.
1. *Adult doses*: These vary widely according to the age of the

patient, the route used and the type of tumour being treated. It is usually given by intravenous or intramuscular injection and twice weekly doses of 30 mg for five weeks are used.
2. Doses for children are calculated upon body surface area.

Nurse monitoring
1. It is interesting and important to note that Bleomycin in contrast to most other cytotoxics has little or no harmful effect on the bone marrow.
2. Gastrointestinal symptoms such as anorexia, nausea and vomiting may occur during treatment and stomatitis often occurs.
3. Because the drug is irritant, local reactions and thrombophlebitis
4. Most patients develop skin lesions after receiving full courses. These skin lesions include hyperkeratosis, impaired nail formation, reddening and peeling of the skin and alopecia.
5. Interstitial pneumonia may develop during treatment and if the drug is continued fatal pulmonary fibrosis may result. This effect limits the total dose given to any one patient to 300 mg at a maximum.
6. If patients are known to have impaired renal function reduced dosages are used.
7. It is important to note that when Bleomycin is to be given intramuscularly injections may be prepared using a 0.1% lignocaine solution. Local pain may be considerably reduced by this action.
8. The nurse should be constantly aware that cytotoxic drugs are highly dangerous and therefore must be handled with great care. Spillage and contamination of the skin of the patient or nurse may lead to a degree of absorption of the drug which, if chronically repeated, may cause damage and the skin may also be sensitised to the drug making it, in some cases, impossible for the nurse to continue working with the drug.

General notes
1. Bleomycin injection may be stored at room temperature. It is stable for up to 3 years and an expiry date is printed on the label of individual ampoules.
2. Any solution remaining after injection should be immediately discarded.
3. Recommended diluent is 0.9% sodium chloride.
4. Bleomycin solutions should not be mixed with other drugs, except where lignocaine is added for intramuscular injection.

BRETYLIUM TOSYLATE (Bretylate)
Presentation
Injection—100 mg in 2 ml
Actions and uses
Bretylium tosylate has a suppressant effect on the heart muscle and its conducting tissues and can be used to treat abnormal ventricular dysrhythmias. It is rarely used as a first choice nowadays, but it is sometimes used when patients have proved resistant to other drugs such as Lignocaine, Mexiletine, Disopyramide or beta-blockers.
Dosage
The drug is given intramuscularly. Intravenous injection confers no advantage and may produce more serious side effects. The adult dosage is 5 mg/kg body weight given at intervals of 6–8 hours.
Nurse monitoring
1. The nurse will virtually never see this drug used outwith coronary care or other intensive care units and even in these specialist units it will be used only rarely, if at all.
2. The patient should be in the supine position during treatment as the drug produces hypotension.
3. The development of nausea or vomiting is an indication to reduce the dosage or withdraw the drug altogether.

General notes
Bretylium tosylate injection should be stored in a refrigerator.

BROMELAINS (Ananase Forte)

Presentation
Tablets each containing Bromelain concentrate equivalent to 100 000 rorer units of activity.

Actions and uses
This enzyme formulation is thought to reduce inflammatory oedema associated with:
1. Soft tissue injury
2. Cellulitis
3. Furunculosis
4. Skin ulceration of varicose or decubitus or diabetic aetiology.

Dosage
For adults: 1 tablet four times a day orally. Children's dosages should be at the discretion of the prescribing physician.

Nurse monitoring
1. This drug should never be given to patients who are known to be allergic to pineapple or products or products of pineapple.
2. The drug should be used with great caution in patients with abnormalities of the blood clotting system such as haemophilia, or with severe hepatic or renal disease.
3. The drug should be used with great caution in patients already receiving anticoagulant therapy as this drug may increase the anticoagulant effect.
4. Side effects occur rarely and include sensitivity reactions such as skin rash, nausea, vomiting, diarrhoea and menorrhagia.

General notes
The drug may be stored at room temperature.

BROMHEXINE (Bisolvon)

Presentation
Tablets—8 mg
Elixir—4 mg in 5 ml
Injection—4 mg in 2 ml

Actions and uses
Bromhexine stimulates the mucous glands of the respiratory tract to produce a water, less vicous mucus and also breaks down thick immobile mucus in the respiratory tract. This action facilitates the removal of mucus and therefore makes the drug useful in the treatment of asthma, bronchitis, bronchiectasis and sinusitis.

Dosage
1. *Adults*:
   a. Orally:—8–16 mg three or four times daily
   b. By slow intravenous or deep intramuscular injection—8–24 mg daily
   c. By intravenous infusion—4–20 mg may be added to 250–500 ml of 5% dextrose or 4–40 mg to 250–500 ml of normal saline. The maximum daily dosage by intravenous infusion is the same as other parenteral routes, i.e. 24 mg per day.
2. *Children*:
   Less than 5 years: 4 mg twice daily
   5–10 years: 4 mg four times daily
   N.B. Injection routes are not recommend for children.

Nurse monitoring
1. Occasional gastrointestinal upset may occur. The drug is not recommended in patients with peptic uleration.
2. Changes in liver function tests have occasionally been reported.

General notes
1. Preparation containing Bromhexine may be stored at room temperature.
2. Elixir and solution for injection should be protected from light.

BROMOCRIPTINE (Parlodel)

Presentation
Tablets—2.5 mg
Capsules—10 mg

Actions and uses
Bromocriptine inhibits the release of the hormones prolactin and growth hormone normally produced in the pituitary gland which lies within the brain. This makes it useful in clinical practice in a number of situations:
1. For the treatment of acromegaly

(a disease caused by excess secretion of growth hormone, usually by a tumour of the pituitary associated with excessive growth of facial bones, hands and feet, headache, sweating, hypertension, heart disease and chest disease).
2. For the inhibition of puerperal lactation.
3. For the treatment of infertility in females when this is found to be associated with an excess production of prolactin.
4. The drug is used for the treatment of galactorrhoea (production of milk by the breast) when this is shown to be due to an excess production of prolactin.
5. Since Bromocriptine exerts its action by stimulating receptor sites which respond to the natural substance, dopamine, i.e. it exerts a dopaminergic action, this effect in a specific area of the brain (the extrapyramidal system) which co-ordinates movement produces benefit in symptoms associated with Parkinson's disease. Parkinson's disease is characterised by a lack of dopamine in the brain.

Dosage
1. For the treatment of acromegaly: The dosage is adjusted according to response, monitored both clinically and by measuring blood levels of growth hormone. It is worth noting that acromegalics require fairly high doses for effective treatment.
2. For the inhibition of puerperal lactation: 2.5 mg twice daily.
3. For the treatment of infertility: Inititally 2.5 mg once or twice a day is given and the dose is gradually increased until menstruation or pregnancy is achieved.
4. For the treatment of galactorrhoea: Initially 2.5 mg once or twice a day with gradual increments in the dose until galactorrhoea ceases.
5. In the treatment of Parkinson's disease (usually in conjunction with Levodopa): A daily dose ranging from 10-100 mg may be used depending upon the balance between patient response and the occurrence of unwanted side effects. Daily doses are achieved by the use of gradual dosage increments following an initial low dose until the optimum is reached in the individual.

Nurse monitoring
1. Perhaps the most important problem with this drug is that it produces nausea. This can be be minimised by commencing with a very low dose and building up the dose slowly and by starting therapy on a once daily basis at night. However, despite this nausea remains a major problem.
2. Other less common side effects include: postural hypotension, dizziness, headache, vomiting and constipation.
3. Rare side effects include drowsiness, confusion, agitation, hallucination, dyskinesia, dry mouth and leg cramps.
4. Note that side effects are considerably more likely to occur with high doses such as those used in the treatment of Parkinson's disease.

General notes
The drug may be stored at room temperature.

BROMPHENIRAMINE (Dimotane)

Presentation
Tablets — 4 mg
12 mg (slow release)
Elixir—2 mg in 5 ml

Actions and uses
Brompheniramine is an antihistamine. The actions and uses of antihistamines in general are discussed in the antihistamine section. Brompheniramine is specifically used:
1. To suppress generalised minor allergic responses to allergens such as foodstuffs and drugs.
2. Orally for allergic conditions e.g. hay fever and allergic rhinitis.

3. As a nasal decongestant e.g. in the treatment of allergic rhinitis and hay fever. It is also added to a few proprietary cough preparations because of its decongestant action.

Dosage
1. *Adults*:
   a. Standard tablets: 4–8 mg four hourly.
   b. Slow release tablets: 12–24 mg twice a day.
2. *Children*:
   Less than 3 years: 1 ml syrup/kg per day.
   3–6 years: one-quarter of adult dose.
   6–12 years: one-half of adult dose.

Nurse monitoring
See the antihistamines section.

General notes
The drug may be stored at room temperature.

BUMETANIDE (Burinex)

Presentation
Tablets—1 mg, 5 mg
Injection — 1 mg in 4 ml
6.25 mg in 25 ml

Actions and uses
Bumetanide has a mode of action and uses identical to those described under Frusemide (q.v.).

Dosage
Bumetanide is 40 times more potent than Frusemide i.e. 1 mg Bumetanide produces the same effect as 40 mg of Frusemide. Recommended doses are therefore 1/40th of those discussed under Frusemide.

Nurse monitoring
The Nurse monitoring notes for thiazide diuretics are applicable to Bumetanide. It should be noted that problems with transient deafness do not seem to occur with Bumetanide as they do with Frusemide.

General notes
Bumetanide tablets and injection are stored at room temperature. The injection solution is sensitive to light and is therefore packed in amber coloured ampoules. Unlike Frusemide, Bumetanide is stable in dextrose solutions and dextrose 5% injection may be used as a diluent before infusion. The standard dose by intravenous infusion is 2–5 mg in 500 ml of diluent given over a period of 30–60 minutes.

BUPIVACAINE (Marcain)

Presentation
Injection — Plain 0.25% and 0.5%
With adrenaline 0.25% and 0.5%

Actions and uses
This potent local anaesthetic drug has a much longer duration of action than Lignocaine. It is used in minor surgical and obstetric procedures to produce extradural block, digital block, nerve plexus block and pudendal block.

Dosage
Individual doses vary considerably with the type of procedure and the patient response. It is recommended that the maximum dosage in any 4-hour period should be 2 mg/kg body weight.

Nurse monitoring
1. The Nurse monitoring aspects of the local anaesthetic, Lignocaine (q.v.) apply to this drug.

General notes
The drug may be stored at room temperature.

BUPRENORPHINE (Temgesic)

Presentation
Injection — 0.3 mg in 1 ml
0.6 mg in 2 ml
Tablets, sublingual—0.2 mg

Actions and uses
This narcotic analgesic drug has a moderate analgesic action and is not subject to the legal requirements of 'controlled drugs'. It is used for the treatment of conditions associated with moderate to severe pain.

Dosage
1. By injection: The drug is recommended for the treatment of adults only in dosages of

0.3–0.6 mg every 6–8 hours by intramuscular or slow intravenous injection.
2. Oral: In adults only in a dose of 0.2–0.4 mg dissolved under the tongue every 6–8 hours or as required for pain.

Nurse monitoring
1. The problem of addiction with continued use has not yet been encountered with this drug.
2. The drug is not subject to the legal requirements of 'controlled drugs'.
3. Constipation and suppression of cough may occur.
4. With excessive dosage there is a risk of sedation and respiratory depression.

General notes
1. The drug may be stored at room temperature.
2. The drug should be protected from light.

BUSULPHAN (Myleran)

Presentation
Tablets—0.5 mg, 2 mg

Actions and uses
Busulphan is a cytotoxic drug which is converted in the body to a highly reactive product which in turn binds irreversibly to substances in cells which are essential for cell growth and division. The process of growth and division is therefore blocked by this action. Rapidly dividing cells such as tumour cells and cells of the bone marrow are more likely to be affected by this drug than slowly dividing cells. In practice Busulphan has the following uses:
1. It is used in the treatment of chronic myeloid leukaemia.
2. It is used in the treatment of primary polycythaemia.

Dosage
The average adult dose is 2–4 mg daily taken for a period of 6 months when an optimum response is usually achieved. If treatment is stopped at this stage relapse often occurs 6–18 months later. Patients are therefore usually continued on maintenance doses ranging from 0.5–3 mg per day and with maintenance therapy the disease may be controlled for longer periods of time i.e. two years or more. This regime is not used in the treatment of children.

Nurse monitoring
1. Excessive bone marrow depression may occur and thrombocytopenia with resultant haemorrhage is particularly common. Anaemia and infection due to suppression of white cell production also occur.
2. If patients are given this drug for several years pulmonary fibrosis may develop. This may present as progressive breathlessness on exertion or may be detected on routine X-ray examination. If this side effect is noticed at an early stage and the drug is stopped then stoppage of the drug and a course of steroid therapy may reverse the process. If the effect is not recognised progressive irreversible fibrosis with respiratory failure and death will follow. It is important, therefore, that all staff involved in the care of patients on this treatment should observe the patient for development of such symptoms.
3. Other side effects include skin pigmentation which may be extensive and especially affects light exposed areas, pressure areas, skin creases, axillae and nipples. Amenorrhoea, testicular atrophy and gynaecomastia may also occur.
4. Adrenal gland insufficiency (Addison's disease) has been reported as a rare complication of this treatment.
5. The nurse should be constantly aware that most cytotoxic drugs are irritant to the skin and mucous surfaces, and are in general very toxic. Great care should therefore be exercised when handling these drugs, and in particular spillage or contamination of personnel or the environment must be avoided. If cytotoxic drugs are handled regularly it is

theoretically possible that repeated skin contact or inhalation may produce systemic toxic effects and in nurses who have developed hypersensitivity, severe local and general hypersensitivity reactions.
General notes
Busulphan may be stored at room temperature.

BUTOBARBITONE (Soneryl)
Presentation
Tablets—100 mg
Actions and uses
Butobarbitone is a barbiturate drug (q.v.). Its main use is as a hypnotic drug but occasionally it is used as a day-time sedative.
Dosage
1. For hypnosis: 100–200 mg on retiring.
2. For day-time sedation: 100 mg twice daily.

Nurse monitoring
See the section on barbiturate drugs.

General notes
Butobarbitone tablets may be stored at room temperature.

BUTRIPTYLINE (Evadyne)
Presentation
Tablets—25 mg, 50 mg
Actions and uses
Butriptyline is a tricyclic antidepressant drug. Its actions and uses are described in the section on tricyclic antidepressant drugs.
Dosage
The average oral dosage for the treatment of depression is 25 mg three times a day. It may be increased if required to a maximum of 150 mg per day in total.
Nurse monitoring
See the section on tricyclic antidepressants.
General notes
Butriptyline tablets may be stored at room temperature.

C

CALCIFEROL (Sterogyl)

Calciferol is a mixture of Ergocalciferol and Cholecalciferol

Presentation
Tablets — 10 000 units/tablet
50 000 units/tablet
Oral solution—3000 units in 1 ml and 400 000 units/ml (Sterogyl)
Injection—300 000 units in 1 ml

Actions and uses
The actions and uses for Calciferol are identical to those described in the section for Vitamin D.

Dosage
1. For the treatment of Vitamin D deficiency states (q.v.): Initially 500–5000 units of Calciferol per day depending on the severity of the deficiency state and the age of the patient. The dose should thereafter be carefully monitored by regular estimation of blood calcium and assessment of clinical improvement and should be tailored to suit the needs of the individual patient.
2. For the treatment of resistant rickets and hypoparathyroidism: Much higher doses of between 50 000 to 150 000 units per day are necessary.

Nurse monitoring
The Nurse monitoring notes on Vitamin D (q.v.) are applicable to this drug.

General notes
The drug may be stored at room temperature.

CALCITRIOL (Rocaltrol)

This drug is also known as One-25 Dihydroxycholecalciferol.

Presentation
Capsules—0.25 μg and 0.5 μg

Actions and Uses
The actions and uses of Calcitriol are identical to those described in the section for Vitamin D.

Dosage
For the treatment of renal osteodystrophy:
1. In adults and children over 20 kg body weight the initial dose recommended is 1 μg with subsequent dosage adjusted according to clinical and biochemical response.
2. Children under 20 kg body weight: 0.05 μg/kg per day with subsequent adjustments in dosage according to clinical and biochemical response.

Nurse monitoring
The Nurse monitoring aspects of this drug are identical to those described for Vitamin D in general (q.v.)

General notes
The drug may be stored at room temperature.

CAPREOMYCIN (Capastat)

Presentation
Injection—1 mega unit (equivalent to 1 g) vials

Actions and uses
Capreomycin is a drug which has been found to be useful in the treatment of tuberculosis due to the organism *Mycobacterium tuberculosis*. It is, however, because of its severe side effects (see below) reserved for use in patients who either cannot tolerate more commonly used drugs or where

culture tests indicate that the organism has become resistant to the more commonly used drugs.

Dosage
Adults: 1 mega unit (1 g) daily by intramuscular injection.

Nurse monitoring
1. Patients undergoing treatment for tuberculosis receive their drugs for considerable periods of time. The nurse may play an important role in reminding patients that their drug therapy must be taken regularly for as long as recommended by medical staff, whether or not they themselves feel that they have recovered.
2. This drug is associated with a number of potentially serious side effects and its use is limited to the situations described above.
3. Painful hardening of the skin at injection sites is common and therefore frequent variation of injection site is recommended.
4. Widespread metabolic disturbance may occur involving protein, calcium and potassium metabolism in the body.
5. Progressive damage to the liver and kidney may occur.
6. Severe neurological side effects including vertigo, tinnitus and deafness (which may be occasionally irreversible) may occur.
7. Hypersensitivity reactions including skin rash, fever, eosinophilia may occur.
8. The drug should be used with caution in patients with reduced renal or liver function or where other drugs which are known to be potentially ototoxic (i.e. aminoglycoside antibiotics (q.v.)) are to be used.
9. It is usually recommended that liver function, renal function, blood calcium, potassium levels and auditory function be regularly monitored during treatment.

General notes
1. Vials of Capreomycin should be stored in a cool place, preferably a refrigerator.
2. The injections are prepared by the addition of 2 ml sodium chloride 0.9%.

CAPTOPRIL (Capoten)

Presentation
Tablets—25 mg, 50 mg, 100 mg

Actions and uses
Captopril is a drug which has an antihypertensive action. It achieves this by blocking the effects of an enzyme which would otherwise produce in the body the chemical angiotensin, a potent vasoconstricting substance which may produce an increase in blood pressure. (Because of this action it is often termed an angiotensin-1-converting enzyme inhibitor.) The drug is useful in the management of severe hypertension when other more standard therapy regimes have failed.

Dosage
Adults:
  a. Initial therapy—at initiation of Captopril therapy low doses (i.e. 5 mg) should be administered initially and gradually built up until the blood pressure is controlled
  b. Maintenance treatment should be altered according to the effect on the patient's blood pressure and usually lies in the range of 25 to 150 mg three times a day.

Children: Proportionately small doses should be given as initial treatment and the maintenance dose falls within the range 1–6 mg per kilogram body weight in total daily, usually given in 3 divided doses.

Nurse monitoring
1. Within a few hours of the initial dose of Captopril a sudden precipitous fall in blood pressure may occur (especially when patients have previously been treated with diuretics). This exaggerated hypotensive effect may persist for up to 24 hours. Patients should be carefully monitored therefore during the

first 24 hours of treatment.
2. With this drug, the concentration of potassium in the blood may rise, particularly if patients are also receiving potassium-sparing diuretics or have an element of renal failure. A high blood potassium (hyperkalaemia) may cause dangerous cardiac dysrhythmias.
3. Common side effects include pruiritic skin rash, altered taste, stomatitis, oral ulceration, gastric irritation and abnormal liver function tests.
4. Rare side effects include paraesthesia, cough and bronchospasm, neutropenia and agranulocytosis.
5. There have been some reports of the drug causing both proteinuria and changes in renal function.
6. Since the drug is mainly excreted unchanged in the kidney, reduced dosages are indicated in patients with impaired renal function.

General notes
Captopril tablets may be stored at room temperature.

CARBAMAZEPINE (Tegretol)
Presentation
Tablets—100 mg, 200 mg and 400 mg
Syrup—100 mg in 5 ml

Actions and uses
Carbamazepine has two main uses:
1. It is an anticonvulsant drug and the actions and uses of anticonvulsants in general are described in the section on anticonvulsants.
2. It has been found to be an effective analgesic for treating the pain associated with trigeminal neuralgia.

Dosage
1. For the treatment of epilepsy: It is advised that a gradually increasing dosage regime is used and this should be adjusted to suit the needs of the individual patient.
    a. *Adults*: Initially 100–200 mg once or twice daily followed by a slow increase until the best response is obtained. This usually occurs when the patient is receiving 800–1200 mg in total per day but in some instances 1600 mg daily may be necessary.
    b. *Children*:
    Less than 1 year: 100–200 mg per day given in divided doses.
    1–5 years: 200–400 mg per day given in divided doses.
    5–10 years: 400–600 mg per day in total given in divided doses.
    10–15 years: 600–1000 mg per day given in divided doses.
    The above doses are maintenance doses. Initial doses should be considerably smaller.
2. For the treatment of trigeminal neuralgia: The individual dosage requirements of Carbamazepine vary considerably depending on the age and weight of the patient. An initial dose of 100 mg per day is recommended. Under normal circumstances, 200 mg 3–4 times daily is sufficient to maintain a pain-free state and in rare instances a total dose of 1600 mg per day must be necessary.

Nurse monitoring
1. The Nurse monitoring aspects of anticonvulsant drugs in general are discussed in the section on anticonvulsants.
2. Drowsiness and dizziness are common at the start of treatment especially if the initial dose is high or is subsequently increased too quickly.
3. Dry mouth, diarrhoea, nausea and vomiting are common side effects.
4. Unusual side effects include skin rash, light-sensitive dermatitis, jaundice, leucopenia and aplastic anaemia.

General notes
The drug may be stored at room temperature.

CARBENICILLIN (Pyopen)

(See Note 3, p. 310)

Presentation
Injection—Vials containing 1 g, 5 g and 5 g infusion pack.

Actions and uses
Carbenicillin is a member of the Penicillin group of antibiotics which has been found to be particularly useful against pseudomonas aeruginosa and proteus species. These two groups of organisms are particularly resistant to most antibiotics. Carbenicillin therefore is used for the treatment of bacteraemia, septicaemia, endocarditis, meningitis, infected burns and infected wounds when they are caused by these organisms.

Dosage
Carbenicillin is given by slow intravenous injection (over 3–4 minutes) or by rapid intravenous infusion (over 30–40 minutes using the special infusion pack) or by the intramuscular route. Dose ranges are as follows:
1. *Adults*:
   a. Intramuscular: 1–2 g four to six hourly.
   b. Intravenous bolus or intravenous infusion: 5 g four to six hourly.
2. *Children*:
   a. Intramuscularly: 50–100 mg/kg body weight in total daily given in 4–6 divided doses.
   b. Intravenously: 250–400 mg/kg body weight in total daily given in 4–6 divided doses.

Nurse monitoring
1. The Nurse monitoring notes for all penicillins as described under Benzylpenicillin (q.v.) apply to Carbenicillin.
2. It is important to note that Carbenicillin is used for the treatment of severe infections by organisms normally resistant to most other antibiotics. It is important therefore to ensure that the dosage given is adequate and appropriate for the patient and condition under treatment. Treatment with lower dosage may lead to failure to eradicate the infection and acquisition of resistance to the drug by the organism. Dosages should never be lower than those recommended except in the situation where the patient under treatment has impaired renal function.

General notes
1. Carbenicillin injection should be stored in a cool place, preferably a refrigerator.
2. To prepare injections or infusion:
   a. For intramuscular use: add 2 ml Water for Injection to each 1 g vial.
   b. For intravenous use: dilute initially by adding 5 ml to each vial and after dissolution further dilute to 20 ml prior to administration.
   c. Intravenous infusions are prepared by mixing the contents of each vial with the 50 ml of diluent provided. This may be further diluted in 0.9% sodium chloride, 5% dextrose or dextrose/saline mixtures.

CARBENOXOLONE (Biogastrone, Duogastrone, Pyrogastrone)

Presentation
Tablets—50 mg
Capsules—50 mg (positioned-release)
Also combined Carbenoxolone and antacid tablets.

Actions and uses
Carbenoxolone is effective in healing peptic ulcers. It is postulated to do this by the following mechanisms:
1. It increases mucus production which in turn protects gastric mucosa from damage.
2. It reduces the back diffusion of hydrogen ions from the stomach contents into the muçosa, again protecting the mucosa from damage.
3. It increases the life span of gastric epithelial cells. The drug is taken as conventional tablets for the treatment of gastric ulcer.

When treating duodenal ulcers, positioned-release capsules must be used. In general it is thought that ulcers will heal after 4–6 weeks treatment.

Dosage
Gastric ulcer: 100 mg three times daily after meals for one week, followed by 50 mg three times daily until the ulcer has healed.
Duodenal ulcer: 50 mg four times daily, 15–30 minutes before meals.

Nurse monitoring
1. The principal problem with Carbenoxolone is that it causes sodium and water retention with consequent oedema, hypertension and hypokalaemia. It must therefore be used with great caution in patients with hypertension, heart disease, renal or liver dysfunction.
2. It should be remembered that hypokalaemia is particularly dangerous in patients taking Digoxin or other cardiac glycosides and this constitutes a relative contraindication for the coincident use of these two drugs.

General notes
Preparations containing Carbenoxolone may be stored at room temperature. Positioned-release capsules (for the treatment of duodenal ulcer) must be swallowed whole; these capsules are specially designed so that they resist degradation in the stomach and liberate the drug in the duodenum.

CARBIMAZOLE (Neo-Mercazole)

Presentation
Tablets—5 mg

Actions and uses
Carbimazole inhibits the production of thyroxine by the thyroid gland. This action is shared by its active metabolite, Methimazole. Both these drugs are therefore termed anti-thyroid drugs and are used in the treatment of thyrotoxicosis. They may be used on their own for prolonged periods in the treatment of this disease or they may be given for a short period in thyrotoxic patients prior to surgery.

Dosage
1. *Adults*: Initially a high dose is used in order to render the patient euthyroid (i.e. to produce a normal thyroid function). 30–60 mg is usually given for the first month. After this the dose is gradually reduced to maintain the patient in a clinically and biochemically euthyroid state. The total daily dosage is usually taken in three divided doses.
2. *Children*: An average daily dose for children is 5 mg three times per day initially reducing to doses as determined by the clinical and biochemical state of the patient.

Nurse monitoring
1. A rare but extremely important adverse effect of this drug is the production of bone marrow depression. Depression of white cell function leads to an increased liability to infection and this side effect often manifests itself as a throat infection. All patients receiving this drug should therefore be warned to report immediately the development of a sore throat and the drug should be stopped while blood tests are performed. The nurse may play an important role by emphasising the importance of reporting this development to the patient.
2. Other side effects include nausea, headache, arthralgia, gastrointestinal upset, skin rash and uncommonly hair loss.
3. If Carbimazole is given to a pregnant patient adverse effects on the thyroid function of the developing fetus may occur. It is therefore particularly important to achieve the correct dosage in pregnant patients.
4. As the drug is actively secreted in breast milk mothers receiving this drug should be advised not to breast feed.

General notes
Tablets containing Carbimazole may be stored at room temperature.

CARFECILLIN (Uticillin)

(See Note 3, p. 310)
Presentation
Tablets—500 mg
Actions and uses
After absorption from the gut this drug is converted in the body to the active drug, Carbenicillin (q.v.). It is therefore equivalent to giving Carbenicillin orally. It is used primarily to treat infections of the urinary tract i.e. cystitis, pyelonephritis, when they are caused by sensitive micro-organisms, in particular *E. coli*, proteus species, *Streptococcus faecalis* and occasionally *Pseudomonas aeruginosa*
Dosage
1. *Adults*: 500 mg–1 g three times a day.
2. *Children*: The dose range is 30–60 mg/kg body weight in total per day divided into three doses.

Nurse monitoring
See the section on Benzylpenicillin.
General notes
Carfecillin tablets may be stored at room temperature.

CEFACLOR (Distaclor)

(See Note 3, p. 310)
Presentation
Capsules—250 mg
Syrup — 125 mg in 5 ml
        250 mg in 5 ml
Actions and uses
This drug is a member of the cephalosporin group of antibiotics and its actions and uses are described in the section dealing with the group. Cefaclor is a 1st Generation cephalosporin. It may be given orally.
Dosage
1. *Adults*: 250 mg to 500 mg 8-hourly
2. *Children*: 20 mg/kg body weight daily in total given in three divided doses.

Nurse monitoring
See the section on cephalosporins.
General notes
1. The drug may be stored at room temperature.
2. Once prepared the syrup should be refrigerated and used within 14 days.

CEFADROXIL (Baxan)

(See Note 3, p. 310)
Presentation
Capsules—500 mg
Suspension — 125 mg in 5 ml
             250 mg in 5 ml
             500 mg in 5 ml
Actions and uses
This drug is a member of the cephalosporin group of antibiotics and its actions and uses are described in the section dealing with the group. Cefadroxil is a 1st Generation cephalosporin.
Dosage
1. *Adults*: 1 g twice daily (or once daily for urinary tract infection).
2. *Children*:
   Under 1 year old: 25 mg/kg body weight in total daily in 2 divided doses.
   1–6 years old: 125–250 mg twice daily
   over 6 years old: 250–500 mg twice daily.

Nurse monitoring
See the section on cephalosporins.
General notes
1. The drug may be stored at room temperature.
2. Once prepared the suspension is stable if stored at room temperature for 7 days (or 14 days if refrigerated).

CEFAMANDOLE (Kefadol)

(See Note 3, p. 310)
Presentation
Injection — 500 mg and 1 g in 10 ml vials
            2 g in 100 ml vials
Actions and uses
This drug is a member of the cephalosporin group of antibiotics and its action and uses are described in the section on cephalosporins. Cefamandole is a 2nd Generation cephalosporin.

Dosage

1. *Adults*: The dose range is 500 mg–2 g 4 to 8-hourly by intravenous injection or deep intramuscular injection. Intravenous bolus injections are given slowly over 3–5 minutes or alternatively by infusing in 0.9% sodium chloride, 5% dextrose or dextrose/saline mixtures.
2. *Children*: The dose range is 50–100 mg/kg body weight in total daily given either 4–8 hourly by deep intramuscular injection or intravenous bolus injection or intravenous infusion.

Nurse monitoring

See the section on cephalosporins.

General notes

1. The drug should be stored at room temperature.
2. After reconstitution vials should be stored in a refrigerator and must be discarded if unused after 96 hours.
3. Prolonged storage at room temperature will generate carbon dioxide gas within the vial and create increased pressure.
4. The drug should be reconstituted as follows:
   a. For intramuscular injection add 3 ml Water for Injection or 0.9% sodium chloride to each 1 g.
   b. For intravenous injection, after reconstitution the drug should be diluted to 10 ml and given over a period of 3–5 minutes.
   c. If given by continuous intravenous infusion, the drug may be diluted in any common infusion solution and administered over the appropriate time.

CEFOTAXIME (Claforan)

(*See Note 3, p. 310*)

Presentation

Injection—500 mg, 1 g and 2 g vials

Actions and uses

This drug is a member of the cephalosporin group of antibiotics and its action and uses are described in the section on cephalosporins. Cefotaxime is a 3rd Generation cephalosporin.

Dosage

1. Adults: 2–12 g daily in total in 2, 3 or 4 divided doses depending upon the nature and severity of infection. May be administered by intramuscular and intravenous injection or by intravenous infusion.
2. Children: 100–200 mg/kg body weight in total daily in 2–4 divided doses.

Nurse monitoring

See the section on cephalosporins.

General notes

1. The drug should be stored at room temperature.
2. It should be reconstituted as follows:
   a. For intravenous or intramuscular injection, add 2 ml Water for Injections to 500 mg vial, 4 ml to 1 g vial and 10 ml to 2 g vial. Lignocaine 1% may be used in place of Water for Injections if pain on injection is a problem.
   b. For intravenous infusion, dissolve in 100 ml sodium chloride 0.9%, dextrose 5% or dextrose/saline mixtures and administer over 20–60 minutes.
3. After reconstitution, intramuscular and intravenous injections should be administered immediately and any drug remaining should be discarded. Solutions for infusion should be discarded after 24 hours.

CEFSULODIN (Monaspor)

(*See Note 3, p. 310*)

Presentation

Injection—500 mg and 1 g vials

Actions and uses

This drug is a member of the cephalosporin group of antibiotics and its actions and uses are described in the section on cephalosporins. Cefsulodin is a 3rd Generation cephalosporin.

Dosage
1. *Adults*: 1–4 g daily in 2–4 divided doses, administered by intramuscular and intravenous injection or by intravenous infusion.
2. *Children*: 20–50 mg/kg body weight in 2–4 divided doses.

Nurse monitoring
See the section on cephalosporins.

General notes
1. The drug should be stored at room temperature.
2. It should be reconstituted as follows:
   a. For intramuscular injection, add 3 ml of 0.5% lignocaine injection to each vial (500 mg or 1 g).
   b. For intravenous injection, add 5 ml to 500 mg vial or 10 ml to 1 g vial of Water for Injections.
   c. For intravenous infusion, dissolve in 100 ml sodium chloride 0.9% dextrose 5% or dextrose/saline mixtures and administer over 30–60 minutes.
3. Intramuscular and intravenous injections should be prepared immediately before administration. Infusions should be used within 12 hours if stored at room temperature or 24 hours if refrigerated.

CEFTAZIDIME (Fortum)

(*See Note 3, p. 310*)

Presentation
Injection—500 mg, 1 g and 2 g vials

Actions and uses
This drug is a member of the cephalosporin group of antibiotics and its actions and uses are described in the section on cephalosporins. Ceftazidime is a 3rd Generation cephalosporin.

Dosage
1. *Adults*: 1–6 g daily in 2 or 3 divided doses, administered by intramuscular and intravenous injection or by intravenous infusion.
2. *Children*: 30–100 mg/kg body weight in 2 or 3 divided doses.

Nurse monitoring
See the section on cephalosporins.

General notes
1. The drug should be stored at room temperature.
2. It should be reconstituted as follows:
   a. For intramuscular injection, add 1.5 ml to 500 mg and 3 ml to 1 g vial of Water for Injections or sodium chloride 0.9% injection.
   b. For intravenous injection, add 5 ml diluent to 500 mg vial and 10 ml to 1 g and 2 g vials.
   c. For intravenous infusion, dissolve in 50 ml sodium chloride 0.9%, dextrose 5% or dextrose/saline mixtures and administer over 20–30 minutes.
3. Carbon dioxide gas is formed during the mixing of ceftazidime injection creating an increase in the internal pressure of the vial.
4. Prepared solutions for injection may be stored for up to 18 hours at room temperature if not immediately used.

CEFTIZOXIME (Cefizox)

(*See Note 3, p. 310*)

Presentation
Injection—500 mg, 1 g and 2 g vials

Actions and uses
This drug is a member of the cephalosporin group of antibiotics and its actions and uses are described in the section on cephalosporins. Ceftizoxime is a 3rd Generation cephalosporin.

Dosage
1. *Adults*: 1–9 g daily in 2 or 3 divided doses, administered in intramuscular or intravenous injection or intravenous infusion.
2. *Children*: 30–150 mg/kg body weight daily in 2–4 divided doses.

Nurse monitoring
See the section on cephalosporins.

General notes
1. The drug should be stored at room temperature.
2. It should be reconstituted as follows:
   a. For intramuscular and intravenous injections, add 2 ml to 500 mg vial, 3 ml to 1 g vial and 6 ml to 2 g vial of Water for Injections.
   b. If intramuscular injections are very painful, the injection may be prepared using 0.5% lignocaine injection.
   c. Intravenous infusions are prepared in 50–100 ml sodium chloride 0.9%, dextrose 5% or dextrose/saline mixtures and administered over 20–30 minutes.
   d. Solutions for injection or infusion should be used within 8 hours of preparation if stored at room temperature.

CEFOXITIN (Mefoxin)
(See Note 3, p. 310)
Presentation
Injection—1 g and 2 g vials
Actions and uses
This drug is a member of the cephalosporin group of antibiotics and its action and uses are described in the section on cephalosporins. Cefoxitin is a 2nd Generation cephalosporin.
Dosage
1. *Adults*: 1–2 g may be given every 8 hours by intramuscular or intravenous bolus injection or intravenous infusion in all common infusion fluids.
2. *Children*: 80–160 mg/kg body weight in total daily given in four or six divided doses.

N.B. The intramuscular injection may be reconstituted with 0.5% or 1% Lignocaine to reduce pain at the injection site.
Nurse monitoring
See the section on cephalosporins.
General notes
1. The drug should be stored in a refrigerator.
2. Reconstituted solutions for injection must be used within 24 hours if kept at room temperature or one week if refrigerated.
3. To prepare an injection:
   a. For intramuscular use: add 2 ml diluent to each 1 g vial.
   b. For intravenous use: add 10 ml diluent to each 1 g vial.
4. Intravenous injections should be given slowly over 3–5 minutes.

CEFUROXIME (Zinacef)
(See Note 3, p. 310)
Presentation
250 mg, 750 mg and 1.5 g vials
Actions and uses
This drug is a member of the cephalosporin group of antibiotics and its actions and uses are described in the section on cephalosporins. Cefuroxime is a 2nd Generation cephalosporin.
Dosage
1. *Adults*: The dose range is 750 mg–1.5 g three times daily by intramuscular or intravenous bolus injection or rapid i.v. infusion over 30 minutes. The i.v. infusion may be given in most common infusion fluids.
2. *Children*: The dose range varies from 30–100 mg/kg body weight per day in total given in three or four divided doses.
Nurse monitoring
See the section on cephalosporins.
General notes
1. The drug should be stored in a refrigerator and protected from light.
2. After reconstitution solutions may be kept for 5 hours at room temperature or 48 hours if refrigerated.
3. To prepare injections:
   a. For intramuscular use add 1 ml of Water for Injection to the 250 mg vial or 3 ml to the 750 mg vial.
   b. For intravenous use each 250 mg should be diluted in 2 ml of Water for Injection.

CEPHALEXIN (Ceporex, Keflex)

(See Note 3, p. 296)

Presentation
Tablets—250 mg, 500 mg
Capsules—250 mg, 500 mg
Syrup — 125 mg in 5 ml
         250 mg in 5 ml
         500 mg in 5 ml

Actions and uses
This drug is a member of the cephalosporin group of antibiotics and its actions and uses are described in the section dealing with the group. Cephalexin is a 1st Generation cephalosporin. It may be given orally.

Dosage
1. *Adults*: 1–4 g in total per day given in divided doses either 6 hourly or 12 hourly.
2. *Children*: 25–50 mg/kg body weight in total is given each day in divided doses either 6 hourly or 12 hourly. For severe infections up to 100 mg/kg in total daily given in four divided doses has been used.

Nurse monitoring
See the section on cephalosporins.

General notes
1. The drug may be stored at room temperature.
2. The syrup should be used within 10 days of preparation.

CEPHALORIDINE (Ceporin)

(See Note 3, p. 310)

Presentation
Injection — 250 mg, 500 mg and 1 g vials

Actions and uses
This drug is a member of the cephalosporin group of antibiotics and its actions and uses are described in the section on cephalosporins. It is only active when given by injection.

Dosage
1. *Adults*:
   a. By deep subcutaneous, intramuscular or intravenous bolus injection a maximum of 6 g is given daily in 2–4 divided doses.
   b. Rapid intravenous infusions of doses equivalent to the above may be given over 30–60 minutes.
   c. Where appropriate the drug may be given by alternative routes as follows:
      (i) Intrathecally the maximum daily dose for adults is 50 mg. It should be diluted in 2–10 ml of normal saline or the patient's own CSF.
      (ii) Intrapleurally 250 mg may be instilled into the pleural cavity.
      (iii) Subconjunctivally 50 mg dissolved in 0.5 ml of Water for Injection may be administered where appropriate.
2. *Children*:
   a. By deep subcutaneous, intramuscular or intravenous bolus injection 15–60 mg/kg body weight in total each day may be given in divided doses.
   b. Intravenous infusions may be given over 30–60 minutes in the same dose as described above
   c. Intrathecal dosage for children is 12–25 mg.
3. In neonates 30 mg/kg may be given daily 12-hourly.

Nurse monitoring
1. The Nurse monitoring notes for cephalosporins (q.v.) apply to this drug.
2. It is especially important to note that Cephaloridine is more likely than the other cephalosporins to cause renal damage and it is recommended that blood levels be measured during treatment to ensure that toxic levels are not reached.

General notes
1. The vials may be stored at room temperature.
2. Once prepared the vials should be used within 24 hours
3. If left standing the vials may become cloudy. This indicates that the drug has precipitated from solution and such vials require shaking and warming in the hand to achieve resolution.

CEPHALOSPORINS

A group of antibiotics which includes:

Cefaclor	Cefuroxime
Cefadroxil	Cephalexin
Cefamandole	Cephaloridine
Cefotaxime	Cephalothin
Cefoxitin	Cephazolin
Cefsulodin	Cephradine
Ceftazidime	Latamoxef
Ceftizoxime	

Actions and uses

The cephalosporin group of antibiotics have a bactericidal action i.e. they kill organisms present in body tissues. They have a wide spectrum of activity which resembles that of Ampicillin and other broad spectrum penicillins, although a few important differences exist between different cephalosporins. This has led to the classification of these drugs into 3 distinct categories termed 1st, 2nd and 3rd generations.

1. 1st Generation cephalosporins are usually effective against Gram-positive micro-organisms (streptococcus, staphylococcus and clostridia) and some Gram-negative micro-organisms (*Neisseria meningitidis* and *Neisseria gonorrhoea*). However Enterobacteria, Proteus (with the exception of *P.mirabalis*), *Haemophillus influenzae* and the coliforms (*E.coli, Ps. aeruginosa* and Klebsiella) are generally unaffected by these drugs. Some organisms rapidly develop resistance to 1st Generation cephalosporins by producing a cephalosporin inactivating substance called beta-lactamase.
2. 2nd Generation cephalosporins have a similar spectrum to 1st Generation drugs but, in addition, they are less liable to inactivation by beta-lactamase and are therefore often effective against bacteria which have developed resistance to 1st Generation drugs. They also extend the spectrum to include activity against *Haemophillus influenzae* and Enterobacteria.
3. 3rd Generation cephalosporins further extend the spectrum of the cephalosporin group by their action against *Pseudomonas aeruginosa* and they may be particularly useful for the prevention and treatment of infections due to this micro-organism.

The cephalosporins, in addition to their use in the treatment of infections produced by the above, are also used for the prophylactic prevention of post-operative infection after gynaecological, abdominal, neurological and orthopaedic surgery and in patients treated with anti-cancer drugs who have a diminished (natural) immunity to infection with a host of pathogenic micro-organisms.

Dosage

See individual drugs.

Nurse monitoring

1. Allergy is the most common problem with these drugs. This may be:
   a. Immediate, comprising of variable reactions ranging from itch and rash to bronchospasm and anaphylactic shock.
   b. Skin rash, fever and lymphadenopathy may develop after several days of treatment.

   It is important to note that patients already sensitive to Penicillin have a higher risk of developing sensitivity to cephalosporins than do patients who are not allergic to Penicillin.
2. It is important to note that intravenous administration of cephalosporins may produce irritation and thrombophlebitis.
3. Intramuscular injections are painful.
4. Cephaloridine is particularly noted for its ability to cause renal damage, especially at higher doses. Other cephalosporins have a lesser risk of causing this problem. The risk of renal damage is especially high if other nephrotoxic drugs such as Gentamicin, Kanamycin, Tobramycin or Amikacin are given at the same time.

5. All cephalosporin drugs may accumulate if renal function is impaired and this may lead to toxicity. Reduced doses should therefore be given to patients with renal disease.

General notes
See specific drugs.

CEPHALOTHIN (Keflin)

(See Note 3, p. 310)

Presentation
Injection—1 g and 4 g vials

Actions and uses
This drug is a member of the cephalosporin group of antibiotics and its actions and uses are described in the section dealing with the group. Cephalothin is a 1st Generation cephalosporin.

Dosage
1. *Adults*: 1 g 4–6 hourly to a maximum of 12 g per day by intravenous injection or infusion.
2. *Children*: 80–160 mg/kg body weight in total daily given in divided doses either 4 or 6 hourly.

Nurse monitoring
See the section on cephalosporins

General notes
1. The drug may be stored at room temperature.
2. After reconstitution solution in vials may precipitate and become cloudy. Vigorous shaking and warming in the palm of the hand is necessary to achieve resolution.
3. Reconstituted solutions may be kept for 48 hours but i.v. infusions must be given within 24 hours of preparation.
4. a. For direct intravenous administration a solution containing 1 g of Cephalothin in 5 ml of diluent may be slowly injected directly into a vein over a period of 3–5 minutes.
   b. For intermittent intravenous infusion the drug may be diluted by adding 40 ml of Water for Injection or 5% dextrose or normal saline.
   c. For continuous intravenous infusion 4 g of Cephalothin may be (after reconstitution with water) diluted in 500 ml of normal saline or 5% dextrose and given over the appropriate period.

CEPHAZOLIN (Kefzol)

(See Note 3, p. 310)

Presentation
Injection—500 mg and 1 g vials

Actions and uses
This drug is a member of the cephalosporin group of antibiotics and its actions and uses are described in the section dealing with the group. Cephazolin is a 1st Generation cephalosporin.

Dosage
The drug may be given by intramuscular and intravenous bolus injections or intravenous infusions in the following doses:
1. *Adults*: dosage ranges from 500 mg 12 hourly to 1 g 6–8 hourly depending on the nature and severity of the infection.
2. *Children*: dosage ranges from 25 mg–50 mg/kg body weight in total daily usually given in three or four divided doses.

Nurse monitoring
See section on cephalosporins.

General notes
1. The drug may be stored at room temperature.
2. This drug should not be mixed with other antibiotics in the same syringe or infusion fluid.
3. To reconstitute vials add 2–4 ml of Water for Injection to each vial.
4. Intravenous infusions may be given in sodium chloride 0.9%, dextrose 5% or dextrose saline mixtures. After reconstitution 500 mg or 1 g of the drug may be diluted in 50–500 ml of any of these solutions.
5. For intravenous bolus injection the drug should be diluted after reconstitution to at least 10 ml with Water for Injection and it

should be given over 3–5 minutes.
6. Once reconstituted vials of injection should be used within 24 hours if kept at room temperature or 96 hours if refrigerated.

CEPHRADINE (Velosef)

(*See Note 3, p. 310*)
Presentation
Capsules—250 mg, 500 mg
Syrup — 125 mg in 5 ml
　　　　　 250 mg in 5 ml
Injection—250 mg, 500 mg and 1 g vials
Actions and uses
This drug is a member of the cephalosporin group of antibiotics and its actions and uses are described in the section dealing with the group. Cephradine is a 1st Generation cephalosporin.
Dosage
1. *Adults*: 2–4 g daily in total is given in four divided doses orally or by intramuscular or intravenous injection or by intravenous infusion.
2. *Children*: 25–50 mg/kg body weight per day in total is given in four divided doses orally. If the parenteral route is necessary the total daily dosage is higher and lies in the range of 50–100 mg/kg body weight per day in total.

Nurse monitoring
See the section on cephalosporins.
General notes
1. The drug should be stored at room temperature.
2. Syrup should be used within 7 days if kept at room temperature or 14 days if refrigerated following reconstitution.
3. Reconstitution of injections:
   a. For intramuscular injections add 1.2 ml Water for Injection to 250 mg of powder, 2 ml to 500 mg and 4 ml to 1 g.
   b. For intravenous injections add 5 ml Water for Injection to 250 mg and 500 mg vials and 10 ml Water for Injection to 1 g vials.
   c. For intravenous infusions the drug should be dissolved in 10 ml of Water for Injection prior to dilution in the appropriate infusion solution.

Cephradine may be added to isotonic (normal) sodium chloride, 5% dextrose solution or one-sixth molar sodium lactate solution. When mixed in this way it will be potent for up to 8 hours.
N.B. After adding water all vials must be shaken thoroughly for several minutes to ensure the powder is dissolved. After injections are prepared in the above manner, for intramuscular or intravenous bolus injection they should be used within 2 hours.

CHENODEOXYCHOLIC ACID (Chendol)

Presentation
Capsules—125 mg
Actions and uses
This drug is a naturally occurring bile acid which, after oral administration, increases the bile acid pool and thus the amount of dissolved cholesterol and phospholipid. In addition, it is likely that the output of cholesterol secreted into the bile is reduced. The net result is to prevent the precipitation of cholesterol from solution and therefore the formation of cholesterol gallstones; existing cholesterol stones will gradually redissolve, possibly obviating the need for surgical removal.
Dosage
Adults: Usually 10–15 mg/kg body weight daily in divided doses or as a single dose at bedtime. Treatment courses are determined by the size of stones e.g. a few months for small gallstones with as long as 2 years for large stones.
Nurse monitoring
1. It is important to note that Chenodeoxycholic Acid therapy is not a suitable treatment for all patients with gallstones and that the nature and size of the stones

are important. Those for whom treatment is unsuitable are:
a. Patients with radio-opaque stones.
b. Those with non-functioning gallbladders.
c. Pregnant patients or female patients contemplating pregnancy.
d. Patients with chronic liver disease of inflammatory bowel disease.
2. The only side effects of treatment are diarrhoea and pruritis which commonly occur. The incidence of diarrhoea is reduced following a dosage reduction.
3. Abnormal liver function tests and liver damage occurred during administration of this drug.

General notes
Chenodeoxycholic Acid capsules should be stored at room temperature in well-sealed containers.

CHLORAL HYDRATE (Noctec)

Presentation
Capsules—500 mg
Mixture—500 mg in 5 ml
Paediatric Elixir—200 mg in 5 ml

Actions and uses
Chloral Hydrate is a general central nervous system depressant. It has been in clinical use for many years and has maintained its popularity as a sleep-inducing agent despite the development of many newer hypnotic drugs during this period. In particular, the drug has found widespread popularity in young and elderly patients who generally tolerate it well. The sedative action of Chloral Hydrate is partly due to Trichloroethanol, a metabolite to which it is converted in the body.

Dosage
Adults: 500 mg–2 g taken on retiring.
Children: 30–50 mg/kg body weight as a single dose.

Nurse monitoring
1. Chloral Hydrate administration may be associated with a degree of nausea and gastrointestinal upset and patients should be advised to take their dosages well diluted with water, fruit juices or beverages to minimise the irritant effect on the gut mucosa.
2. Skin rashes occasionally occur and contact of liquid Chloral Hydrate with skin can produce skin irritation; if this occurs the area of contact should be thoroughly washed.
3. Chloral Hydrate capsules must never be bitten since they contain concentrated liquid drug which can produce severe irritation if liberated in the mouth.
4. Despite its irritant effect, Chloral Hydrate is generally well tolerated. In patients who suffer troublesome gastrointestinal upsets, a more palatable alternative is available (see Triclofos).

General notes
Chloral Hydrate capsules and mixtures may be stored at room temperature. Once diluted, liquid doses must be taken immediately. Mixture and Elixir are relatively unstable and require to be freshly prepared for each prescription: these should not be kept by patients for longer than 2 weeks from time of issue.

CHLORAMBUCIL (Leukeran)

Presentation
Tablets—2 mg, 5 mg

Actions and uses
Chlorambucil is a member of the nitrogen mustard group. It damages cells by irreversibly binding important constituents which are necessary for cellular growth and reproduction. The drug has been shown in practice to be particularly active against lymphoid tissues and appears to destroy not only proliferating cells but also mature circulating lymphocytes. This makes it particularly useful in the treatment

of lympho-proliferative disorders. Its main uses are as follows:
1. Lympho-proliferative disorders such as chronic lymphatic leukaemia and the lymphomas.
2. It is the drug of choice for the rare condition of Waldenstrom's microglobulinaemia.
3. It has been used in the treatment of carcinoma of the breast, lung and ovary.
4. It has an immunosuppressant action and may be used in the management of some auto-immune diseases such as rheumatoid arthritis, and systemic lupus erythematosus. It is worth noting that it is used only in severe cases of rheumatoid arthritis which have proved rapidly progressive and resistant to treatment with alternative regimes.

Dosage
1. As a cytotoxic drug:
   a. Initial dosage for adults and children is 0.1–0.2 mg/kg body weight and it is taken for up to 6 weeks at this dosage.
   b. Once remission is obtained continuous maintenance therapy is with 0.03–0.1 mg/kg body weight daily.
   It has been found that short, interrupted courses appear to be safer and are usually preferred.
2. The dosage when used as an immunosuppressive is as follows: high doses of the order 200–300 μg/kg per day.

Nurse monitoring
1. Chlorambucil exerts a depressant effect on the bone marrow and may cause leucopenia, thrombocytopenia and anaemia. Patients may therefore suffer from severe and life-threatening infection or may develop severe haemorrhage. Patients who are given the drug for a considerable period of time may develop irreversible bone marrow damage leading to fatal aplastic anaemia.
2. Nausea and vomiting are uncommon at the usual dose levels but may occur with higher doses.
3. Skin – rash, alopecia and liver damage are occasional complications.
4. As the drug affects dividing cells it redcuces sperm formation and may affect the growing fetus.
5. The nurse should be constantly aware that most cytotoxic drugs are irritant to the skin and mucous surfaces, and are in general very toxic. Great care should therefore be exercised when handling these drugs, and in particular spillage or contamination of personnel or the environment must be avoided. If cytotoxic drugs are handled regularly it is theoretically possible that repeated skin contact or inhalation may produce systemic toxic effects and in nurses who have developed hypersensitivity, severe local and general hypersensitivity reactions.

General notes
Tablets may be stored at room temperature.

CHLORAMPHENICOL (Chloromycetin)
(See Note 3, p. 310)

Presentation
Capsules—250 mg
Suspension—125 mg in 5 ml
Injection—1 g and 1.2 g vials
Eye ointment—1%
Eye drops—0.5%
Ear drops—10%

Actions and uses
Chloramphenicol is an antibiotic which has a bacteriostatic action i.e. it inhibits further growth and replication of bacteria. Its mechanism of action is by inhibiting protein synthesis in cells and therefore preventing their growth. It is a highly effective antibiotic. Because of its possible severe toxicity its use is restricted to certain serious infections where it is

known to be superior to other antibiotics. These are:
1. Typhoid fever
2. Meningitis due to *Haemophilus influenzae*.

Topical applications of the drug are not associated with its more serious side effects and it is used widely for the treatment of infections of the eye and external ear.

Dosage
1. Oral:
   a. *Adults*: 500–750 mg four times a day.
   b. *Children*: 50 mg/kg daily in total usually taken in four divided doses.
2. By intramuscular or intravenous infection:
   a. *Adults*: up to 1 g 6-hourly.
   b. *Children*: 50 mg/kg daily usually divided into four or six doses. For serious infections in children, twice the above dosage may occasionally be used.
   c. *Premature and newborn infants*: 25 mg/kg in total per day in four divided doses.
3. Eye drops 0.5% or eye ointment 1%: A small quantity of ointment or two eye drops in the affected eye every one to three hours until the eye has been free of visible signs of infection for 48 hours is recommended.
4. For ear drops: 1–3 drops every three to four hours is recommended.

Nurse monitoring
1. The reason that this highly effective antibiotic is now recommended for restricted use only is that it has a number of serious and potentially fatal side effects. These are as follows:
   a. The drug may depress bone marrow function. This may be detected by serially examining the blood and usually reversion to normality will follow stoppage of treatment.
   b. An irreversible aplastic anaemia with depression of formation of all types of blood cells leaving the patient anaemic and at risk of severe haemorrhage and infection may occur independently from the above effect. Although this side effect is more common when the drug is used in high dosage and for prolonged periods, the fact that it is irreversible and leads to certain death makes it a strong contraindication to the general use of this drug for mild infections.
   c. A syndrome known as 'grey baby syndrome' may occur in babies. Babies' livers cannot metabolise Chloramphenicol as well as adults and as a result high concentrations of Chloramphenicol itself occur in the blood. This leads to circulatory collapse with shock, respiratory difficulty, cyanosis, vomiting, refusal to suckle and passage of loose green stools. If this syndrome is not recognised the child may die.
2. Other side effects which may occur with this drug include nausea, vomiting, an unpleasant taste in the mouth, abdominal pain and diarrhoea and optic neuritis. The latter side effect is very rare.

General notes
The drug may be stored at room temperature.

CHLORDIAZEPOXIDE (Librium)

Presentation
Tablets—5 mg, 10 mg, 25 mg
Capsules—5 mg, 10 mg
Injection—100 mg in 2 ml

Actions and uses
Chlordiazepoxide is a member of the benzodiazepine group (q.v.). Its principal use is in the treatment of anxiety but it has been found to be particularly useful in addition for the control of symptoms associated with acute withdrawal of alcohol in chronic alcoholism (delirium tremens).

Dosage
1. For treatment of anxiety:
   a. Adults receive a total of up to 30 mg daily in divided doses. Up to 100 mg may very occasionally be required.
   b. Children receive doses in the range of 5–20 mg per day in total usually given in divided doses.
2. For the control of delirium tremens or for the rapid relief of acute anxiety of phobia: 50–100 mg by intramuscular injection maybe administered. The injection may be repeated at intervals of 2–4 hours.

Nurse monitoring
1. For general notes see the section on benzodiazepines.
2. It is essential that the nurse notes that Chlordiazepoxide injection may be given by the deep intramuscular route but should never be given intravenously.

General notes
1. Preparations containing Chloridiazepoxide may be stored at room temperature.
2. When preparing solution for injection the special solvent provided in the container must be used.
3. When reconstituted injections should be carefully examined for signs of haziness which indicate drug breakdown.
4. Chloridiazepoxide injection solutions must never be diluted or mixed with any other drug in the same syringe.

CHLORMETHIAZOLE (Heminevrin)

Presentation
Capsules—192 mg
Syrup—250 mg in 5 ml (as edisylate)
Injection—0.8% solution for intravenous infusion

Actions and uses
Chlormethiazole is a central nervous system depressant which has several uses in clinical practice.

1. It is a general sedative and hypnotic drug which alleviates acute restlessness and anxiety (particularly delirium tremens in alcohol withdrawal) and induces sleep.
2. It possesses anticonvulsant activity and is administered by intravenous infusion in acute convulsive states e.g. status epilepticus, pre-eclampsia.

Dosage
1. Oral
   a. For sedative effects: Adult dose is 1 capsule (or 5 ml syrup) three times daily.
   b. For hypnotic effects: Adult dose is 2 capsules (or 10 ml syrup) at night.
   c. For delirium tremens: Adult dose is up to 12 capsules in total daily given in 3–4 divided doses.
2. Intravenous infusion—*Adults*: dose range is 4–20 ml/minute of 0.8% Chlormethiazole infusion depending upon indication and severity.

Nurse monitoring
1. It is important that the nurse fully understands the apparent major differences in the strengths of Chlormethiazole capsules and syrup since confusion when substituting one dosage form for another can lead to overdosage or underdosage. Capsules contain 192 mg Chlormethiazole (base) while the syrup contains 250 mg Chlormethiasole edisylate/5 ml. The difference in weight is due to the inactive edisylate group and is irrelevant to the clinical effect. Therefore when substituting capsules for syrup or vice versa, note that 1 capsule is equivalent to 5 ml syrup.
2. It should be noted that Chlormethiazole administration is commonly associated with nasal congestion and irritation and occasionally conjunctival irritation about 15–30 minutes after a dose is administered. If these effects are severe or prevent sleep, alternative treatment may be necessary. A less common

but equally important side effect is severe headache.
3. Chlormethiazole is often used as a hypnotic in elderly subjects because it is generally well tolerated and is short-acting. However, it should be stressed that occasionally a prolonged 'hangover' effect lasting into the following day is noted which can impair mobility and awareness in elderly patients.
4. Intravenous administration may produce a fall in blood pressure and depression of respiration, particularly if given rapidly, and it may be necessary to monitor patients accordingly.
5. Irritation at the intravenous site may be noted as superficial thrombophlebitis.
6. Since Chlormethiazole is a depressant of the central nervous system, concurrent use of other CNS depressant drugs (including alcohol) will produce excessive sedation.

General notes
Chlormethiazole capsules and syrup may be stored at room temperature. The solution for intravenous infusion, however, should be stored in a refrigerator.

CHLOROQUINE (Nivaquine, Avloclor)

Presentation
Tablets—200 mg (as sulphate), 250 mg (as phosphate)
Syrup—50 mg in 5 ml.

Actions and uses
Chloroquine is a drug which was originally used for the treatment of malaria. Recently is has been found to be effective in a number of situations which are as follows:
1. Malaria
2. Amoebic hepatitis
3. Systemic lupus erythematosus (although it is only really useful for the control of skin lesions in this disease)
4. Rheumatoid arthritis.

Dosage
1. Malaria:
   a. Acute attacks:
      i. *Adults*: An initial dose of 600 mg is given followed by 300 mg 6–8 hours later and then 300 mg on each of two following days.
      ii. *Children*:
         Age 1–4: 150 mg by mouth followed 6 hours later by 75 mg and then 75 mg daily for two days.
         Age 5–8: 300 mg followed 6 hours later by 150 mg then 150 mg for two days.
   b. *Cerebral malaria:*
      i. *Adults*: An intramuscular or intravenous injection of 200–300 mg is given initially followed by 200 mg at intervals of 6 hours up to a total of 800 mg during the first 24 hour.
      ii. Children are treated with an initial injection of 5 mg/kg body weight intramuscularly repeated once 6 hours later if necessary.
   c. For the suppression of malaria:
      i. *Adults*: 300–600 mg is given weekly during exposure to risk and for 4–8 weeks thereafter
      ii. *Children*: Weekly doses of 5 mg/kg body weight are given for the same duration of time.
2. Hepatic amoebiasis:
   a. *Adults*: 300 mg of Chloroquine base is given orally twice daily for two days and then once a day for a further 2–3 weeks.
   b. *Children*: The dosage is 6 mg/kg body weight twice daily for two days initially and then 6 mg/kg daily for 2–3 weeks.
3. Rheumatoid arthritis: Control of symptoms is achieved by treatment for 2–3 months with doses of between 75–300 mg of Chloroquine base daily.
4. Discoid lupus erythematosus: The usual initial dose is 150 mg of Chloroquine base twice or thrice daily reducing to a

maintenance dose of 150 mg or less daily.

Nurse monitoring
1. Chloroquine is generally well tolerated when given in antimalarial doses and toxic effects are rarely seen.
2. The higher prolonged doses given for treatment of rheumatoid arthritis and lupus erythematosus are associated with side effects and it is in the early detection of these side effects that the nurse's major role lies in the management of patients on these drugs. Pruritis is commonly found. Headache, and gastrointestinal upset occur less frequently. Rarely the bone marrow may be suppressed inducing blood dyscrasias such as agranulocytosis, thrombocytopenia and neutropenia. Other rare side effects include altered skin pigmentation and muscle weakness.
3. The major problem with prolonged or high dosage treatment with Chloroquine is damage to the retina which may result in permanent visual impairment. Patients should therefore be regularly assessed by measurement of visual acuity and other means and the drug should, if possible, be stopped should this side effect develop.
4. The drug should be used with great caution, in patients with liver disease, psoriasis, gastrointestinal, neurological or blood disorders.

General notes
Chloroquine tablets may be stored at room temperature. The syrup must be protected from light.

CHLOROTHIAZIDE (Saluric)

Presentation
Tablets—500 mg

Actions and uses
See the section on thiazide and related diuretics.

Dosage
1. *Adults*: The daily adult dose range is 500 mg–1 g (1000 mg) twice daily. The duration of action of Chlorothiazide is approximately 12 hours.
2. *Children*:
Up to 1 year—125 mg.
1–7 years—250 mg.
7 years plus—500 mg.
The above doses are taken as a single daily dose. Premature infants require much lower doses e.g. 62.5 mg.

Nurse monitoring
See the section on thiazide and related diuretics.

General notes
Chlorothiazide tablets may be stored at room temperature.

CHLORPHENIRAMINE (Piriton)

Presentation
Tablets—4 mg, 8 mg and 12 mg (slow release)
Syrup—2 mg in 5 ml
Injection—10 mg/ml

Actions and uses
Chlorpheniramine is an antihistamine. The actions and uses of antihistamines in general are described in the section on antihistamines. In clinical practice Chlorpheniramine is used:
1. To suppress generalised minor allergic responses to allergens such as foodstuffs and drugs.
2. To suppress local allergic reactions i.e. inflammatory skin responses to insect stings and bites, contact allergens, urticaria etc.
3. Orally for allergic conditions e.g. hay fever and allergic rhinitis.

Dosage
1. *Adults*:
   a. Orally: Standard preparation: 4 mg three to four times daily. Slow release preparation: 8–12 mg twice per day.
   b. By intravenous, intramuscular or subcutaneous injection: 10–20 mg
2. *Children*:

Standard preparation (tablets or syrup):
Less than one year (syrup recommended) 1 mg (2.5 ml) twice per day.
One to 5 years (syrup recommended) 1–2 mg (2.5–5 ml) three times daily.
6 to 12 years (tablets or syrup) 2–4 mg three times daily.

Nurse monitoring
See the section on antihistamines.

General notes
The drug may be stored at room temperature.

CHLORPROMAZINE (Largactil)

Presentation Tablets—10 mg, 25 mg, 50 mg, 100 mg
Syrup—25 mg in 5 ml
Suspension—100 mg in 5 ml
Injection — 25 mg in 1 ml
50 mg in 2 ml
Suppositories—100 mg

Actions and uses
1. Chlorpromazine is a phenothiazine drug and its actions and uses are described in the section on phenothiazine drugs.
2. The drug has a particular use in the control of intractable hiccoughs.
3. It is used in rare circumstances when the induction of hypothermia is desirable.
4. It is used in obstetric practice for the treatment of pre-eclampsia and eclampsia.

Dosage
1. *Adults*: The dosage varies widely with individual patients. As a rough guide the following regimes are suggested:
    a. Oral: 25 mg three times is an average dose, although in some cases total dosage may be increased up to 1 g per day if necessary.
    b. Intramuscularly: 25–50 mg is administered and repeated at 6–8 hourly intervals as required.
    c. Intravenously: The drug should be diluted with at least 10 times its own volume of normal saline and given extremely slowly. It is worth pointing out that only very rarely should this drug be given intravenously and only under strict medical supervision.
    d. Rectally: One 100 mg suppository is given and repeated at intervals of 6–8 hours if necessary. By the rectal route the onset of action is slower and the duration of effect more prolonged.
2. *Children*:
Under the age of 5 the oral dose is 5–10 mg three times daily. Over the age of 5 one-third to one-half of the adult dosages are recommended.

Nurse monitoring
See the section on phenothiazine drugs.

General notes
1. Preparations containing Chlorpromazine may be stored at room temperature.
2. Syrup, suspension and solution for injections should be protected from light.
3. Injection solutions may develop a pink or yellow discolouration and if this is noted the solution should be discarded.

CHLORPROPAMIDE (Diabinese, Melitase)

Presentation
Tablets—100 mg, 250 mg

Actions and uses
See the section on hypoglycaemic drugs, oral (1).

Dosage
50–500 mg as a single morning dose.

Nurse monitoring
See the section on hypoglycaemic drugs, oral (1).

General notes
Tablets may be stored at room temperature.

CHLORTETRACYCLINE (Aureomycin)

(See Note 3, p. 310)

Presentation
Capsules—250 mg
Ointment and cream—3%
Eye ointment—1%

Actions and uses
See the section on tetracycline.

Dosage
The adult oral dose is 250 mg four times a day.

Nurse monitoring
See the section on tetracyclines.

General notes
The drug may be stored at room temperature.

CHLORTHALIDONE (Hygroton)

Presentation
Tablets—50 mg, 100 mg

Actions and uses
See the section on thiazide and related diuretics.

Dosage
The usual adult dose range is 50–100 mg daily or on alternate days. Single daily doses are sufficient because of the very long action of Chlorthalidone (48 hours or more).

Nurse monitoring
See the section on thiazide and related diuretics.

General notes
Chlorthalidone tablets may be stored at room temperature.

CHOLESTYRAMINE (Questran)

Presentation
Sachets—4 g

Actions and uses
Cholestyramine is an anionic ion exchange resin with the following actions:
1. It binds bile acids present in the gut and therefore increases faecal excretion of bile acids: this in turn causes an increase in cholesterol and lipid metabolism.
2. It reduces the rate of fat absorption from the gut, it therefore has the following uses in clinical practice:
    i. To reduce plasma cholesterol in patients with hypercholesterolaemia.
    ii. To relieve pruritus associated with elevated plasma bile acid levels in patients with cholestatic jaundice.
    iii. To treat diarrhoea associated with vagotomy and other gastrointestinal surgery or radiotherapy which is effective because bile acids when they are bound to cholestyramine do not have the laxative effect that they would have if they were free in the gut.

Dosage
1. For the treatment of hypercholesterolaemia the usual dose is of the order 3–6 sachets (12–24 g) daily, taken as a single dose or in up to 4 divided doses.
2. For the treatment of pruritus—1 or 2 sachets (4–8 g) daily.
3. For the treatment of diarrhoea as for hypercholesterolaemia.
4. For the treatment of children (aged 6–12 years): The initial dose (which may be modified according to the response) is determined by the formula:
Body weight in lb × adult dose

Nurse monitoring
Cholestyramine is a particularly unpleasant preparation for patients to consume. This unpleasantness may be alleviated by encouraging patients to mix it with water, fruit juice, soup or soft fruit.
1. It is important for the nurse to note that cholestyramine may also bind and inactivate other drugs in the gastrointestinal tract and it is advisable to take any other medication 30 minutes to 1 hour before any dose of cholestyramine.
2. The drug interferes with fat absorption and therefore may reduce absorption of the fat soluble vitamins A, D and K. A

description of deficiency syndromes associated with these vitamins are described under each vitamin in the text. When a vitamin deficiency is identified, parenteral vitamin supplementation may be required.
3. The most frequent side effects associated with this treatment are gastrointestinal upsets and constipation. As the drug is not absorbed, systemic toxicity does not occur.

General notes
Cholestyramine sachets may be stored at room temperature.

CHOLINE MAGNESIUM TRISALICYLATE (Trilisate)

Presentation
  Tablets—500 mg (as salicylate)
Actions and uses
  See the section on anti-inflammatory analgesic drugs, non-steroidal.
Dosage
  Adults: 1–1.5 g taken twice daily.
Nurse monitoring
  See the section on anti-inflammatory analgesic drugs, non-steroidal.
General notes
  Choline Magnesium Trisalicylate tablets may be stored at room temperature.

CHOLINE THEOPHYLLINATE (Choledyl)

Presentation
  Tablets—100 mg, 200 mg
  Syrup—62.5 mg in 5 ml
Actions and uses
  This drug is chemically related to Aminophylline whose actions and uses are described in the section on Aminophylline. It is used in the management of bronchospasm associated with asthma and other conditions such as chronic bronchitis.
Dosage
  1. *Adults*: 400–1600 mg daily in four divided doses.
  2. *Children*:
     3–6 years: 62.5–125 mg three times per day.
     Over 6 years: 100 mg three to four times a per day.
Nurse monitoring
  The Nurse monitoring aspects for Aminophylline (q.v.) apply to this drug.
General notes
  1. This drug may be stored at room temperature.
  2. The drug should be protected from light.
  3. The commercial syrup contains a high quantity of sugar and this should be taken into account when treating diabetic patients, or when treating patients who are intolerant of disaccharide.

CHYMOTRYPSIN (Chymar, Zonulysin)

Presentation
  Chymar lyophilised—Each vial contains 5000 USP Chymotrypsin units
  Chymar aqueous—5 ml vial, 5000 USP Chymotrypsin units per ml
  The lyophilised form is normally administered as a single injection. The aqueous form is formulated as a multi-dose vial.
Actions and uses
  1. This enzyme compound is thought to be useful in the reduction of inflammatory oedema associated with accidental injury, dentistry, eye conditions, genito-urinary and respiratory diseases and obstetric and gynaecological conditions.
  2. In ophthalmic surgery sterile Chymotrypsin solution has a specialised use in that it may be administered during cataract surgery.
Dosage
  1. For either the lyophilised or aqueous form: 5000 units one to three times daily until clinical improvement is obtained. The number of injections should thereafter be reduced as patient response permits.

2. For administration during cataract surgery: A 1 in 5000 or 1 in 10 000 solution in sterile saline is supplied.

Nurse monitoring
1. Local reactions to the injection are rare but may include pain, erythema, local oedema and urticaria.
2. Rarely a generalised anaphylactic reaction may occur.

General notes
1. The preparation should be stored in a cool atmosphere away from direct sunlight.
2. After reconstitution of the lyophilised form with 1 ml of normal saline, the solution may be used within 48 hours or if refrigerated within seven days.
3. Lyophilised Chymar has a shelf-life of more than 5 years. Aqueous Chymar has a shelf-life of two years (aqueous Chymar should never be frozen).

CIMETIDINE (Tagamet)

Presentation
Tablets—200 mg, 400 mg
Syrup—200 mg in 5 ml
Injection—200 mg in 2 ml

Actions and uses
Cimetidine acts on specific sites in the stomach and reduces the production of gastric acid and the enzyme pepsin. As the sites are called H_2-receptors, the drug is known as an H_2-receptor antagonist. It has been most successfully used in the treatment of duodenal ulceration and Zollinger-Ellison syndrome. It is also used commonly for the treatment of gastric ulcers and less commonly for the treatment of reflux oesophagitis.

Dosage
1. Oral: It is now generally accepted that once an ulcer is diagnosed Cimetidine, if chosen as the treatment for this condition, should be administered in the dosage of 200 mg three times a day and 400 mg at bedtime. Some ulcers, however, will heal with a dosage of 400 mg twice daily. The patient should be treated for 4–8 weeks at this dosage. The drug is then continued for one year at a dose of 400 mg at night. The effect of prolonged nocturnal treatment is to reduce the effect of recurrence of incidence of symptoms.
2. Parenterally: On occasions it is deemed necessary to give this drug parenterally and the recommended dosage is 200 mg by intravenous bolus or 200 mg over two hours by infusion repeated at 4–6 hourly intervals. The maximum rate of infusion should not normally exceed 150 mg/hour for 2 mg/kg body weight per hour). By continuous intravenous infusion the normal rate is 75 mg/hour.
3. For the treatment of Zollinger-Ellison syndrome which is characterised by severe peptic ulceration caused by the action of gastrin produced by a tumour in the pancreas—much higher doses of up to 2 g per day in total may be required.

Nurse monitoring
1. The drug is popular with patients as it leads to rapid resolution of symptoms. The nurse may play an important role in encouraging patients only to take the dosage prescribed and not to commence new courses without prior medical consultation.
2. The drug may interfere with anticoagulant control in patients on Warfarin and therefore patients should be closely monitored and dosages adjusted accordingly.
3. As the drug is excreted by the kidney, reduced doses are required for patients with impaired renal function.
4. Many side effects have been described including diarrhoea, altered liver function tests, bradycardia, mental confusion, hallucinations, breast tenderness, gynaecomastia and galactorrhoea.

General notes
1. Preparations containing Cimetidine may be stored at room temperature.
2. When added to intravenous infusion fluids, 5% Dextrose, normal saline or dextrose/saline mixtures should be used.

CINNARIZINE (Stugeron)

Presentation
Tablets—15 mg
Capsules—75 mg

Actions and uses
Cinnarazine is an antihistamine. The actions and uses of antihistamines in general are described in the section on antihistamines. In clinical practice Cinnarazine is used
1. In the treatment of nausea and vomiting, particularly motion sickness.
2. In the treatment of vertigo and the symptoms of vertigo and nausea due to Menière's disease.
3. To improve blood flow to ischaemic tissues (due to its vasodilator action) in peripheral vascular disease.

Dosage
1. Nausea/vomiting and Menière's disease:
   a. *Adults*: 30 mg initially, then 15–30 mg every 8 hours.
   b. *Children*: Half the adult dose
2. As a vasodilator: 75 mg every 8 hours for adults only.

Nurse monitoring
See the section on antihistamines.

General notes
The drug may be stored at room temperature.

CISPLATIN (Neoplatin)

Presentation
Injection—10 mg, 50 mg vials

Actions and uses
Cisplatin is a cytotoxic drug which appears to interfere with cellular reproduction. Since tumour cells reproduce at a rapid rate they are particularly sensitive to the effects of this drug. It has been used in the treatment of cancer of the testes, ovaries, bladder, head and neck cervix, prostate, oesophagus and lung.

Dosage
1. When used as a sole anti-tumour agent the recommended dose for adults and children is 50–75 mg/m^2 body surface area as a single intravenous infusion every 3–4 weeks. An alternative regime is to give 15–20 mg/m^2 by intravenous infusion daily for five days every 3–4 weeks.
2. When used in combination with other cytotoxic drugs low doses may be given.
3. In practise it has been found that repeated courses are often necessary.

Nurse monitoring
1. Cisplatin is particularly toxic to the kidney and a progressive fall in renal function may occur. As this effect is dose related it must be shown by laboratory testing that renal function has returned to normal before repeat courses are given. Regular 24 hour urine collections for creatinine clearance are therefore obtained.
2. Almost all patients treated with this drug suffer from anorexia, nausea and vomiting.
3. Bone marrow suppression may occur leading to anaemia, haemorrhage due to thrombocytopenia and infection due to suppression of white cell function.
4. Other adverse effects include tinnitus, hearing loss, peripheral neuropathy, abnormal liver function and abnormal cardiac function.
5. Anaphylactic reaction characterised by facial oedema, wheezing, tachycardia and hypotension may occur within minutes of drug administration.
6. In common with all cytotoxic drugs there are potential risks to normal fetal development if treatment is given during pregnancy.

General notes
1. Cisplatin vials may be stored at room temperature.
2. They should be reconstituted with 10 ml or 50 ml of Water for Injections to provide a solution containing 1 mg in 1 ml.
3. The drug is diluted in 2 litres of dextrose/saline mixture and infused over a 6–8 hour period.
4. Prepared solutions should be kept at room temperature and are stable for up to 24 hours.
5. Refrigeration will produce precipitation from solution and is therefore not advised.

CLEMASTINE (Tavegil)
Presentation
Tablets—1 mg
Elixir—0.5 mg in 5 ml
Actions and uses
Clemastine is an antihistamine. The actions and uses of antihistamines in general are described in the section on antihistamines. Clemastine is used in clinical practice:
1. To suppress generalised minor allergic responses to allergens such as foodstuffs and drugs.
2. To suppress local allergic reactions i.e. inflammatory skin responses to insect stings and bites, contact allergens, urticaria etc.

Dosage
Adults: 1 mg twice daily.
Nurse monitoring
See the section on antihistamines.
General notes
The drug may be stored at room temperature.

CLINDAMYCIN (Dalacin-C)
(*See Note 3, p. 310*)
Presentation
Capsules—75 mg, 150 mg
Syrup—75 mg in 5 ml
Injection—150 mg in 1 ml
Actions and uses
The actions and uses of Clindamycin are identical to Lincomycin (q.v.). Clindamycin is in general better absorbed from the gut than Lincomycin.

Dosage
1. *Adults*:
   a. Orally: 150–300 mg 6-hourly.
   b. Intramuscular injection: 600 mg–2.7 g daily in total, in two, three or four divided doses.
   c. Intravenously the dosages are identical for intramuscular injection. The drug should be rapidly infused over 10 minutes to one hour.
2. *Children*:
   a. Orally:
      Less than 1 year: 37.5 mg 8-hourly.
      1–3 years: 37.5 mg 6-hourly.
      4–7 years: 75 mg 6-hourly.
      Over 7 years: 112.5–150 mg 6-hourly.
   b. Intramuscular dosage for children is 15–40 mg/kg body weight per day in total given in three or four divided doses.
   c. Intravenous dosage is identical to intramuscular dosage.

Nurse monitoring
The Nurse monitoring notes for Clindamycin are identical to those for Lincomycin (q.v.).
General notes
All preparations may be stored at room temperature.

CLOBAZAM (Frisium)
Presentation
Capsule—10 mg
Actions and uses
Clobazam is a member of the benzodiazepine group (q.v.) and its principal use is in the treatment of anxiety.
Dosage
1. *Adults*: 10 mg two or three times daily.
2. *Children*: Children over the age of three should receive half the adult dose.
3. In hospitalised patients with severe anxiety states maximum doses of 60 mg per day in total have been given.

Nurse monitoring
See the section on benzodiazepines.
General notes
1. Clobazam capsules may be stored at room temperature.
2. The capsules should be protected from light.

CLOBETASOL (Dermovate)

Presentation
Ointment and cream—0.05%
Scalp application—0.05%
Actions and uses
Clobetasol is a very potent topical corticosteroid (q.v.) which is applied topically for the treatment of inflammatory skin conditions e.g. psoriasis, eczema, dermatitis etc.
Dosage
Cream, ointment and scalp application are applied sparingly once or twice daily to the affected area.
Nurse monitoring
Although applied topically, significant amounts of this drug may be absorbed to produce some or all of the side effects described in the section on corticosteroids.
General notes
Ointment, cream and scalp application containing Clobetasol may be stored at room temperature.

CLOBETASONE (Eumovate)

Presentation
Ointment and cream—0.05%
Actions and uses
A moderately potent corticosteroid (q.v.) which is applied topically for the treatment of inflammatory skin conditions e.g. psoriasis, eczema, dermatitis etc.
Dosage
Apply sparingly to the affected area up to four times daily.
Nurse monitoring
Although applied topically, significant amounts of this drug may be absorbed to produce some or all of the side effects described in the section on corticosteroids.

General notes
Ointment and cream containing Clobestasone may be stored at room temperature.

CLOFIBRATE (Atromid-S)

Presentation
Capsules—500 mg
Actions and uses
Clofibrate has a number of complex and as yet not clearly defined actions on body metabolism. Its overall effect is to reduce blood cholesterol. It may be used to reduce the cholesterol level in the blood of patients who have a familial predisposition to high blood cholesterol and who tend to develop ischaemic heart disease early in life.
Dosage
The recommended dose for adults and children is 20–30 mg/kg body weight given in two or three divided doses.
Nurse monitoring
1. This drug may produce side effects of nausea, abdominal pain and diarrhoea.
2. One of the mechanisms by which Clofibrate reduces blood cholesterol is to raise the level of cholesterol in the bile and prolonged use may be associated with the development of gall stones.
3. If patients have liver disease associated with impaired liver function they should not receive this drug.

General notes
Clofibrate capsules may be stored at room temperature.

CLOMIPHENE (Clomid)

Presentation
Tablets—50 mg
Actions and uses
In the normal female during each menstrual cycle the growth of a follicle, ovulation and the development of the endometrium is stimulated by two hormones from

the pituitary known as luteinizing hormone (LH) and follicle stimulating hormone (FSH). Late in the menstrual cycle, sufficient oestrogen is produced during the menstrual process for these pituitary hormones to be inhibited and by this process a regular cycle of menstruation is produced. Clomiphene blocks the inhibitory action of oestrogens on the pituitary and therefore stimulates further production of the pituitary hormones. This action is useful in the treatment of infertility when it has been shown that ovulation is not taking place, as the stimulation of pituitary hormones may induce ovulation.

Dosage
50 mg daily for five days with subsequent courses for up to six cycles until pregnancy occurs.

Nurse monitoring
1. Because of its mechanism of action Clomiphene is likely to lead to the stimulation of the development of more than one ovum and multiple pregnancies may occur. This risk is usually explained to patients prior to commencing treatment.
2. As Clomiphene stimulates the ovaries and produces ovarian enlargement its administration is contraindicated should the patient be known to have an ovarian cyst.
3. Common side effects include hot flushes and abdominal pain and distension.
4. Less common side effects include blurring of vision, ocular damage, fatigue, dizziness, headache, nausea, vomiting, breast tenderness, heavy periods, urinary frequency and very rarely loss of hair.
5. Abnormalities in liver function have occurred when patients receive this drug.

General notes
1. The drug may be stored at room temperature.
2. Tablets should be protected from moisture, light and excessive heat.

CLOMIPRAMINE (Anafranil)
Presentation
Capsules—10 mg, 25 mg, 50 mg
Syrup—25 mg in 5 ml
Injection—25 mg in 2 ml
Tablets—75 mg, slow release

Actions and uses
Clomipramine is a tricyclic antidepressant drug. Its actions and uses are described in the section on tricyclic antidepressants.

Dosage
For the treatment of depression the following regimes may be used:
1. By the oral route: 30–50 mg per day may be taken in three divided doses. Alternatively the entire daily dose may be taken on retiring or as a single dose using 75 mg slow release tablets.
2. Where injections are necessary e.g. for the treatment of uncooperative patients or at the beginning of therapy when a more rapid effect is required: 25 mg by intramuscular injection may be given up to six times daily.

Nurse monitoring
See the section on tricyclic antidepressant drugs.

General notes
1. Preparations containing Clomipramine must be stored at room temperature.
2. Solutions for injection and syrup must be protected from light.

CLONAZEPAM (Rivotril)
Presentation
Tablets—0.5 mg, 2 mg
Injection—1 mg in 1 ml

Actions and uses
Clonazepam is a benzodiazepine drug (q.v.) which has a marked anticonvulsant action. It is used in all forms of epilepsy particularly of the petit mal variety. It may be given prophylactically by the oral route to prevent epilepsy and by slow intravenous injection for the treatment of status epilepticus.

Dosage

1. Oral prophylactic doses are as follows:
   a. *Adults*: 4–8 mg orally daily in three or four divided doses.
   b. *Children*:
      Up to 1 year: 0.5–1 mg
      1–5 years: 1–3 mg
      5–12 years: 3–6 mg
      The above doses are total dosages and should be administered in three or four divided doses daily.
2. For the treatment of status epilepticus: A slow intravenous injection is administered over a period of 30 seconds. More rapid injections produce hypotension and apnoea. Recommended doses are 1 mg for adults and 0.5 mg in infants and children.

Nurse monitoring

1. See the section on benzodiazepines for general Nurse monitoring points on this drug.
2. A particular adverse effect with this drug is increased salivation and bronchial hypersecretion. This produces 'drooling' and may prove troublesome in patients with obstructive airways disease.
3. In common with anticonvulsant drug therapy in general, Clonazepam should never be abruptly withdrawn but should instead be replaced with an alternative medication after gradual reduction in dose.

General notes

1. Preparations containing Clonazepam may be stored at room temperature.
2. The injection should be protected from light.
3. The injection consists of a dry powder in a vial with 1 ml of solvent. For reconstitution the solvent is Water for Injections. It should be added immediately before use. If necessary the injection can be diluted in an intravenous infusion containing sodium chloride or dextrose.
4. Any injection which is not used must be immediately discarded.
5. Intravenous infusions must be used within 12 hours.

CLONIDINE (Catapres, Dixarit)

Presentation
Tablets—25 μg, 0.1 mg, 0.3 mg
Injection—0.15 mg in 1 ml

Actions and uses

1. Clonidine reduces the blood pressure in two ways:
   a. It reduces the sympathetic nerve activity stimulated by centres in the brain
   b. It affects the peripheral blood vessels altering their response to vasoconstrictor substances.
2. Small doses of Clonidine have been found to be effective in the prophylaxis of migraine.
3. The drug has also been used to treat menopausal vascular flushes. Again very small doses are used (see below).

Dosage

1. In the treatment of hypertension the recommended adult dosage is as follows:
   a. 0.15–0.3 mg may be given by slow intravenous injection. The effects lasts for several hours and may be repeated up to a maximum dosage of 0.75 mg in 24 hours.
   b. The initial oral dose is 50–100 μg three times daily increasing as required to a maintenance range of between 0.3 and 1.2 mg three times per day.
2. For the prophylaxis of migraine and the treatment of menopausal vascular flushes a dose range of 50–150 μg per day is recommended.

Nurse monitoring

1. There is no doubt that the most important fact to remember about this drug is that if it is stopped suddenly serious rebound hypertension may occur within 24 hours. Therefore the drug should never be stopped suddenly unless the patient is under constant medical supervision.
2. Clonidine may worsen symptoms of depression and therefore is relatively contraindicated in depressed patients.

3. Recognised side effects include bradycardia, headache, sleep disturbances, nausea, constipation and impotence in males. Facial pallor has also been noted.
4. Dry mouth, sedation and postural hypotension commonly occur during the early stages of treatment.
5. Rarely a Raynaud's type phenomenon with cyanosis, pallor and paraesthesia of the extremities may develop rapidly at the commencement of treatment.

General notes
Clonidine tablets and injection may be stored at room temperature. For ease of administration the injection solution can be diluted with 5% dextrose and 0.9% sodium chloride injection.

CLOPENTHIXOL (Clopixol)

Presentation
Tablets—10 mg, 25 mg
Injection — 200 mg in 1 ml ampoules as decanoate
2 g in 10 ml vials as decanoate

Actions and uses
Clopenthixol is a member of a group of neuroleptic drugs which are used for their tranquillising or calming effect in patients with severe behavioural disorders. It therefore shares many of the actions and uses described for phenothiazines.

Dosage
Adults
1. By the oral route, initially 20–30 mg daily in divided doses with maintenance dosages in the range 20–50 mg daily. Up to 150 mg daily may be required to control severe cases.
2. Clopenthixol decanoate injection produces a long-acting (depot) effect and doses of 200–400 mg by the intramuscular route may be administered at 2–4 week intervals.

Nurse monitoring
See the section on phenothiazines

General notes
Clopenthixol tablets and injections should be stored at room temperature.

CLOTRIMAZOLE (Canesten)

Presentation
Cream—1%
Powder—1%
Topical spray—1%
Pessaries—100 mg and 200 mg

Actions and uses
This drug has a broad spectrum of action against many fungi and also exhibits activity against trichomonas, staphylococcus, streptococcus and bacteroides. It has a wide range of uses including:
1. All fungal skin infections due to dermatophytes, yeasts, moulds and other fungi including trichophyton species, candida, ringworm (tinea) infections, athletes foot, paronychia, pityriasis versicolor, erythrasma, intertrigo, fungal nappy rash, candida vulvitis and balanitis. It should be noted that the drug is not recommended as a sole treatment for pure trichomoniasis.

Dosage
1. Cream, powder or spray: To be thinly and evenly applied to the affected area two or three times daily and rubbed in gently. Treatment should be continued for at least one month or for at least two weeks after the disappearance of all signs of infection.
2. Pessaries: Two tablets should be inserted daily preferably at night for three consecutive days. Alternatively one pessary may be inserted for six days.

Nurse monitoring
1. Rarely patients may experience local mild burning or irritation immediately after applying the preparation.

General notes
Preparations may be stored at room temperature.

CLOXACILLIN (Orbenin)

(See Note 3, p. 310)

Presentation
Capsules—250 mg, 500 mg
Syrup—125 mg in 5 ml
Injection—vials containing 250 mg and 500 mg

Actions and uses
Cloxacillin is a member of the Penicillin group of antibiotics and has actions and uses similar to those described for Benzylpenicillin (q.v.). In practice, however, it has a distinct advantage over Benzylpenicillin in that it is often effective against infections due to *Staphylococcus aureus* which are resistant to Benzylpenicillin. The drug is well absorbed after oral administration.

Dosage
1. *Adults*:
   a. Orally: 500 mg four times a day
   b. Intravenous and intramuscular: 250–500 mg 4 to 6-hourly.
   c. Intra-articular and intrapleural: 500 mg is given once daily.
2. *Children*:
   Less than 2 years: one-quarter of the adult dose.
   Over 2 years: one-half of the adult dose.

Nurse monitoring
See the section on Benzylpenicillin.

General notes
1. Preparations containing Cloxacillin may be stored at room temperature.
2. Once reconstituted injection solutions must be used immediately.
3. Once reconstituted the syrup should be used within seven days.
4. Injections are prepared as follows:
   a. For intramuscular injection the vials should be diluted with 1.5–2 ml of Water for Injection.
   b. For intravenous injection: 1 g should be dissolved in 20 ml of Water for Injection and given either directly over 3–4 minutes or added to 0.9% sodium chloride, 5% dextrose or dextrose/saline mixtures and infused over 4–6 hours.
   c. For intra-articular or intrapleural injection: The vials should be diluted with 5–10 ml Water for Injection.

CODEINE PHOSPHATE

Presentation
Tablets—15 mg, 30 mg and 60 mg
Linctus—15 mg in 5 ml
Syrup—25 mg in 5 ml

Actions and uses
Codeine phosphate is a member of the narcotic group of analgesics. It has, however, a very mild analgesic action. It has the following uses:
1. As a mild analgesic, usually in combination with Aspirin in Codeine compound tablets (Codis).
2. It may be used for the treatment of diarrhoea when it has a constipating effect.
3. It may be used as a cough suppressant.

Dosage
1. For mild analgesia: In combination with Aspirin adults should receive two Codeine compound tablets 4–6 hourly.
2. For constipating action:
   a. Adults should receive 15–60 mg three or four times a day.
   b. *Children*:
      Less than 1 year old: It is not recommended that such children receive this drug.
      1–7 years: 1.25–2.5 ml of the linctus (15 mg in 5 ml) three or four times a day.
3. As a cough suppressant: 2.5–10 ml of syrup or 5–10 ml of linctus three to four times daily.

Nurse monitoring
1. The drug has none of the severe problems associated with narcotic analgesics (q.v.), but if used as a mild analgesic constipation may be a problem.

General notes
The drug may be stored at room temperature.

COLCHICINE
Presentation
Tablets—250 µg, 500 µg
Actions and uses
Colchicine interferes with the uptake of uric acid crystals by white cells in gouty joints. The result of this is that inflammation is reduced and symptoms of pain are relieved. Its only use is in the treatment of acute gout.
Dosage
Adults: An initial dose of 1 mg is given followed by subsequent doses of 500 µg every two hours until relief of pain is obtained or vomiting or diarrhoea occur. At that stage dosage should be reduced to a maximum of 3 mg in every subsequent 24 hours.
Nurse monitoring
1. Although Colchicine is a very effective drug its use is limited by the frequent occurrence of side effects such as nausea, abdominal pain and diarrhoea. Indeed these side effects may necessitate withdrawal of treatment.
2. High dosage may cause skin rashes, renal damage and alopecia has followed prolonged use.
3. It is recommended that Colchicine be used with caution in elderly patients with heart disease and in patients with kidney or gastrointestinal disease.
4. It is worth noting that fatalities have occurred after overdosage of Colchicine with doses as low as 7 mg and therefore any patient accidentally or purposefully ingesting excess doses of this drug must be referred to a hospital urgently for treatment.
General notes
Colchicine tablets may be stored at room temperature. They should be protected from light.

CONTRACEPTIVES, ORAL

Oestrogen   *Progestogen*
Ethinyloestradiol + Norethisterone
(*Trade names*: Anovlar 21, Brevinor, Gynovlar 21, Loestrin, Minovlar, Minovlar ED, Norimin, Norlestrin, Orlest 21, Ovysmen)
Ethinyloestradiol + Norgestrel
(*Trade names*: Eugynon 30, Ovran, Ovran 30, Microgynon, 30, Ovranette)
Ethinyloestradiol + Lynoestrenol
(*Trade name*: Minilyn)
Ethinyloestradio + Ethynodiol
(*Trade name*: Conova 30, Ovulen 50)
Mestranol + Norethisterone
(*Trade name*: Norinyl 1, Norinyl 1/28, Ortho-Novin, 1/50)
Ethynodiol only
(*Trade name*: Femulen)
Norgestrel only
(*Trade name*: Microval, Norgeston, Neogest)
Norethisterone only
(*Trade name*: Micronor, Noriday)

Oral contraceptives act by a number of mechanisms:
1. They act on an area of the brain called the hypothalamus which normally releases substances which in turn cause another area of the brain called the pituitary to release substances known as gonadotrophins. These gonadotrophins stimulate ovulation. Oral contraceptives halt this action.
2. Oral contraceptives affect the endometrium (the lining of the uterus) making the implantation of an ovum less likely and therefore reducing the chances of successful pregnancy.
3. The cervical mucus is made more viscous and therefore spermatozoa have greater difficulty in reaching the uterus and fertilising the ovum.

Oral contraceptives may be made up of two main types of hormones:
1. Oestrogens which principally inhibit ovulation.
2. Progestrogens which also inhibit ovulation but have in addition an

effect on the cervical mucus. For the most part combinations of both oestrogens and progestrogen are used as they are thought to be more reliable. Recently it has been found that the dose of oestrogen required for successful contraception is lower than was previously thought necessary. These two hormmones may be combined for the purposes of contraception in two different ways:
1. The combination of both drugs may be started on the fifth day after the start of menstruation and continued for twenty days. No further drugs are taken until the fifth day of the next episode of bleeding.
2. Oestrogen only may be given for 15-21 days with progestrogen being added to the last 5-10 days of the 21 day course.

It is important in addition to note that some contraceptive pills are now being produced which contain progestogens only.

Dosage
1. For combination tablets: One tablet is taken daily for 21 days starting on the fifth day of menstruation. To assist patients who have difficulty remembering when to stop and start treatment, many contraceptives come in packs of 28 days, 7 of these being dummy tablets.
2. Progestogen-only tablets are taken every day without break during the cycle.

Nurse monitoring
The taking of the contraceptive pill has, because of considerable publicity given to it in the national press, created many anxieties in women's minds. In addition various situations arise in which women may wonder whether it is appropriate either to commence or continue such treatment. Nurses may find themselves being asked about such situations and therefore the Nurse monitoring section on these drugs will be based on the type of question which the nurse may have to answer.
1. Are there any women who should not take the pill? It is recommended that the pill be avoided in certain groups of patients and these are as follows:
   a. Patients with cardiovascular disease including hypertension, previous stroke, angina pectoris, myocardial infarction or venous thrombosis.
   b. Patients with liver disease (some authorities believe that the contraceptive pill may be given to patients with liver disease if their liver function tests are normal).
   c. Any patient who has or has in the past had breast cancer or cancer of gynaecological origin.
   d. It is felt that patients who have or have had hypertension, facial nerve palsy or migraine may be at risk of cerebral thrombosis and therefore they should be discouraged from using the contraceptive pill.
2. How soon after having a baby can I start the pill? It is advisable to wait for the first period to occur prior to commencing the contraceptive pill. It is important, however, to ensure that alternative precautions are taken as even if a patient is breast feeding, there is a risk of pregnancy.
3. Can I breast feed when taking the pill? There is very little risk to the suckling infant from the low doses of oestrogen and progestrogen in the contraceptive pill and therefore it is not contraindicated from the point of view of the infant. However, there may be a reduction in milk production after recommencing the pill and this may lead to failure of breast feeding.
4. What must I do if I forget a dose?
   a. If a combined preparation is being taken, the dose may be taken up to 12 hours

after the usual time safely. After 12 hours there is a definite risk and if three days or more has elapsed then the course should be completed missing out the tablets which have been omitted but alternative precautions to avoid pregnancy must be used.
  b. With the progestogen only pills, missing a dose by even 3 hours or more may be important and additional precautions are advised until at least 14 consecutive days treatment have again been taken.
5. If I stop the pill to become pregnant how long should I wait before attempting to become pregnant? It is best to wait until at least one true period has occurred after stopping the pill. This allows calculation of dates and assessment of maturity and development of the fetus to be performed more accurately.
6. Will the pill damage my baby if I do become pregnant? Although there is a theoretical risk that the baby might be damaged, in practice there is no evidence that any damage occurs.
7. How long can I take the pill for? Provided no severe side effects occur, and regular checks are made at visits to a general practitioner or family planning clinic, the pill may be continued for as long as the patient desires. More specific advice on this point should be sought from the patient's own general practitioner or family planning clinic.
8. What do I do if I require an operation? A combined preparation should be stopped six weeks prior to operation. Progestogen only pills may be continued. If surgery is necessary at short notice the doctor or surgeon involved should be informed that the patient is on the pill.
9. Will my periods be regular when I take the pill? It is important to point out that the bleeding which occurs is not actually a period but episodes of bleeding will tend to occur regularly if the combined preparations are used. A beneficial effect is that bleeding may become lighter and pain encountered with periods may be abolished. If progestogen only pills are used, irregularities in the menstrual cycle and therefore irregular bleeding may occur in the early months of treatment and occasionally periods may be missed altogether.
10. Can other drugs I take interfere with the pill? A number of drugs including antibiotics (particularly Rifampicin), Ergotamine, barbiturates, anticonvulsants, Aminocaproic Acid, tranquillisers, corticosteroids, antihistamines, Phenylbutazone and Oxyphenbutazone have been thought to have a theoretical risk of reducing the effectiveness of oral contraceptives. The evidence is more firm for barbiturates, anticonvulsants and Rifampicin. Alternative means of contraception should be used if these drugs are taken in short courses and if they are to be taken for more prolonged courses this problem should be discussed further with the patient's medical practitioner.
11. Side effects with the contraceptive pill are common and these may be divided into two major groups:
  a. Those arising just after the commencement of the contraceptive pill for the first time. These are largely due to the oestrogen and include nausea, vomiting, breast discomfort, fluid retention, depression, headache, lethargy, abdominal discomfort, vaginal discharge,

cervical erosions and a syndrome of general irritability.
b. Actual side effects include depression, altered sexual drive, jaundice, salt and water retention, hypertension, altered glucose tolerance, thrombophlebitis and thrombo-embolism.
12. The results of many biochemical tests may be altered in patients taking the pill and in order to avert unnecessary worry for the patient and unnecessary use of health service resources, nurses may play an important role in encouraging patients always to tell medical staff at consultation that they are using the oral contraceptive.

CORTICOSTEROIDS

The following corticosteroids are in current clinical use:

Aldosterone	Fluocinolone
Beclomethasone	Fluocinonide
Betamethasone	Fluocortolone
Clobetasol	Fluprednylidene
Clobetasone	Flurandrenolone
Cortisone	Halcinonide
Desonide	Hydrocortisone
Dexamethasone	Methylprednisolone
Difluocortolone	Prednisolone
Fluclorolone	Prednisone
Fludrocortisone	Triamcinolone

Actions and uses

Corticosteroids are a group of mainly synthetic subtances which are derived from a hormone, Hydrocortisone, which is produced in the body by the cortex of the adrenal glands. All these drugs have two major effects which are described as glucocorticoid and mineralocorticoid. The glucocorticoid activity is responsible for the anti-inflammatory action of corticosteroids which makes the drug useful in a wide range of diseases including rheumatoid disease, connective tissue disease, inflammatory bowel disease, allergic conditions, asthma and inflammatory skin conditions such as eczema, dermatitis and psoriasis. The mineralocorticoid activity has little usefulness clinically and is responsible for a number of side effects including salt and water retention. Corticosteroids are used both systemically and topically in the form of tablets, injections, ointments, creams, eye drops, enemas and suppositories.

Dosage

For dosage and route of administration see individual drugs.

Nurse monitoring

1. Corticosteroids produce many side effects, especially if given in high dose or for prolonged periods of time. By far the most important side effect is suppression of the ability of the adrenal gland of the body to produce Hydrocortisone. This means that any patient who is either on steroids or has recently been on prolonged or high doses of steroid will be unable to produce steroids in response to any stress such as infection or injury. As a consequence they may demonstrate more severe reactions to such stresses and on occasion this may result in a fatal outcome. The nurse's primary role in the management of patients on corticosteroids, therefore, is to bear in mind that any patient who is on, or who has recently been on corticosteroids will, if they suffer injury or infection or require an operation, need to have their dosage at least doubled during such stress period. In addition, any patient who has been on prolonged courses of corticosteroids should never have their drug stopped suddenly for any reason.
2. Patients who have been on steroids for a long period develop what is known as 'Cushingoid' symptoms. This includes a moon face, obesity, purple striae and acne.

3. The electrolyte disturbances associated with corticosteroid treatment include:
   a. Salt and water retention with hypertension.
   b. Hypokalaemia with resultant muscle weakness
   c. Altered glucose metabolism with the possible precipitation of diabetes
   d. Altered calcium/phosphorus balance producing osteoporosis and a tendency towards bone fracture.
4. Depression and psychosis are occasionally associated with steroid treatment.
5. Gastric upset and occasionally peptic ulceration may be associated with steroid treatment.
6. Wound healing may be delayed significantly. This is especially important in patients who have to undergo an operation while on steroid treatment.
7. Corneal ulceration and cataract formation may occur.
8. There is an increased risk of infection by bacteria, viruses and fungi, such as oral candidiasis, when patients are treated with steroids.
9. It is important to note that the above effects can occur with prolonged or high dosage of steroids administered by any route including topical application to the skin.
10. It is also extremely important to note that corticosteroids should not be given to patients who have active infection such as chickenpox, poliomyelitis, tuberculosis and infection due to Herpes virus.

CORTISONE (Cortelan, Cortistab, Cortisyl)

Presentation
Tablets—5 mg, 25 mg
Injection—25 mg in 1 ml

Actions and uses
Cortisone is a corticosteroid drug and has actions and uses as described in the section on corticosteroids. It is converted in the body to the active component Hydrocortisone. As this conversion varies greatly between patients it is usually preferable to administer Hydrocortisone itself as this enables medical staff to more accurately predict the active amount of drug being received.

Dosage
Dosages vary widely depending on the type of illness, severity of the disease, and the route of administration. It is therefore impossible to outline dosage regimes in this text.

Nurse monitoring
See the section on corticosteroids.

General notes
Tablets containing cortisone may be stored at room temperature.

CO-TRIMOXAZOLE (Septrin, Bactrim)

(See Note 3, p. 310)
Co-Trimoxazole is a combination of a sulphonamide (sulphamethoxazole) and Trimethoprim

Presentation
Tablets—
  400 mg Sulphamethoxazole + 80 mg Trimethoprim
  800 mg Sulphamethoxazole + 160 mg Trimethoprim
  100 mg Sulphamethoxazole + 20 mg Trimethoprim (Paediatric)
Suspension—
  400 mg Sulphamethoxasole + 80 mg Trimethoprim in 5 ml
  200 mg Sulphamethoxazole + 40 mg Trimethoprim in 5 ml (Paediatric)
Injection—
  800 mg Sulphamethoxazole + 160 mg Trimethoprim in 3 ml (intramuscular)
  400 mg Sulphamethoxazole + 80 mg Trimethoprim in 5 ml (for intravenous infusion)

Actions and uses
Sulphonamide drugs and Trimethoprim when used alone are bacteriostatic i.e. they prevent further growth and division of

bacteria. It has been found that the combined use of these two substances is preferable for two reasons:
1. The combination of the two substances is bactericidal in action i.e. bacteria present are killed rather than simply inhibited from further growth and division.
2. The combination of the two different mechanisms of action makes it more difficult for bacteria to develop resistance to the drug.

The organisms against which Co-trimoxazole is effective include haemophilus, proteus, escherichia, neisseria, salmonella, shigella, *Streptococcus pyogenes* and staphylococcus. It should be noted that infections with pseudomonas organisms are usually not successfully treated with this compound. In clinical practice the drug is widely used in treatment of chest and urinary tract infections and for the prophylaxis of urinary tract infections.

Dosage
1. Oral:
   a. Adults should receive 800 mg of Sulphamethoxazole and 160 mg of Trimethoprim twice daily.
   b. Children should receive the following doses:
      Less than 1 year: 20 mg of Sulphamethoxazole and 4 mg of Trimethoprim per kg twice daily.
      1–7 years: one-quarter of the adult dose.
      Over 7 years: one-half of the adult dose.
2. Parenteral administration:
   a. Adults should receive 1 ampoule (3 ml) twice daily.
   b. Children over 6 should receive half the adult dose. It is not recommended that the intramuscular preparation be used in younger children due to the inadequacy of muscle mass in which to inject the preparation.
3. By the intravenous route adults should receive 2 ampoules (10 ml) twice daily. Each ampoule (5 ml) should be diluted to 125 ml immediately prior to infusion. A number of solutions may be used for dilution including 5 and 10% dextrose, 5% laevulose, 0.9% sodium chloride, dextran 40, dextran 70, Ringer's solution and sodium chloride 0.18% and dextrose 4% injection.
4. The intravenous doses for children are as follows:
   6 weeks to 6 months of age: 1.25 ml diluted appropriately twice per day.
   6 months to six years: 2.5 ml diluted appropriately twice daily.
   6 years to 12 years: 5 ml diluted appropriately twice per day.
   Over 12 years: adult doses are recommended.

N.B. Reduced doses are used for patients with renal disease.

Nurse monitoring
1. The Nurse monitoring notes on sulphonamides (q.v.) and Trimethoprim (q.v.) are applicable to this drug.
2. It is worth noting that the risk of macrocytic (megaloblastic) anaemia with this drug is only really important with prolonged full dose therapy and can be prevented by giving folinic acid, although if macrocytic anaemia develops it is preferable to use an alternative antibiotic.

General notes
1. Oral preparations may be stored at room temperature.
2. As noted above intravenous infusion ampoules should be diluted immediately before use and if not used immediately should be disposed of.
3. No other substances should be added to intravenous infusions of Co-trimoxazole.
4. Intravenous infusions should be administered slowly with each dose being given over approximately 1–1½ hours.

CYANOCOBALAMIN—VITAMIN B[12] (Hepacon, Cytamen, Cytacon)

Presentation
Tablets—50 µg per tablet
Injection — 250 µg in 1 ml
            1000 µg in 1 ml
Oral liquid—35 µg in 5 ml

Actions and uses
Cyanocobalamin (Vitamin B[12]) is indicated for the treatment of megaloblastic anaemia where this has been shown to be due to a deficiency of Vitamin B[12] by the appropriate laboratory test. Deficiency of Vitamin B[12] occurs either where there is a deficiency in the gut of a substance (intrinsic factor) normally produced by the stomach which is essential for the absorption of Vitamin B[12], this condition being known as pernicious anaemia, or it may be due to other forms of malabsorption. More rarely Vitamin B[12] deficiency may be seen in people who have a strict vegetarian diet.

Dosage
1. Parenterally:
   a. For the treatment of pernicious anaemia: Initially 250–1000 µg intramuscularly on alternate days for two weeks and then 1000 µg monthly
   b. For the prophylaxis of megaloblastic anaemia due to gastrectomy, malabsorption syndrome or strict vegetarianism: 250–1000 µg monthly.
2. Orally:
   a. *Adults*: 300 µg per day
   b. *Children*: 35–70 µg 2–3 times per day

Nurse monitoring
1. Sensitisation to Vitamin B[12] is extremely rare. It may present as an itching rash and very exceptionally as anaphylactic shock.
2. Cyanocobalamin contains Cyanide. This is contraindicated for use in patients suffering from either tobacco amblyopia or Leber's optic atrophy (optic atrophy and optic neuritis).
3. Hydroxycobalamin is in general to be preferred to Cyanocobalamin as it has a longer duration of action.

General notes
Ampoules should be protected from light.

CYCLANDELATE (Cyclospasmol, Cyclobral)

Presentation
Tablets—400 mg
Capsules—400 mg
Suspension—400 mg in 5 ml

Actions and uses
The actions and uses of this drug are identical to those described for Nicofuranose (q.v.). It has been proposed that this drug may improve blood flow in cerebrovascular disease.

Dosage
Initially 1.2–1.6 g per day in divided doses. Maintenance doses of 400–800 mg daily may be adequate.

Nurse monitoring
1. The side effects of this vasodilator drug include flushing of the skin of the head and neck, dizziness, faintness, postural hypotension and tachycardia.
2. The drug should not be administered to patients who have recently suffered a myocardial infarction or stroke.

General notes
The drug may be stored at room temperature.

CYCLIZINE (Valoid)

Presentation
Tablets—50 mg
Injection—50 mg in 1 ml

Actions and uses
Cyclizine is an antihistamine. The actions and uses of antihistamines in general are described in the section on antihistamines. Cyclizine is used in clinical practice:
1. In the treatment of nausea and vomiting, particularly motion sickness.

Dosage
1. *Adults*: Orally, intramuscularly or intravenously: 50 mg three times daily.
2. *Children*: (1–10 years): Up to 25 mg orally three times per day.

Nurse monitoring
See the section on antihistamines.

General notes
The drug may be stored at room temperature.

CYCLOBARBITONE (Phanodrom)

Presentation
Tablets—200 mg

Actions and uses
Cyclobarbitone is a barbiturate drug (see the section on barbiturates) which is taken at night as a hypnotic.

Dosage
100–200 mg or retiring.

Nurse monitoring
See the section on barbiturate drugs.

General notes
Cyclobarbitone tablets may be stored at room temperature.

CYCLOPENTHIAZIDE (Navidrex)

Presentation
Tablets—0.5 mg

Actions and uses
See the section on thiazide and related diuretics.

Dosage
The daily adult range is 0.25–1.00 mg usually as a single daily dose. The duration of action is 12 hours plus.

Nurse monitoring
See the section on thiazide and related diuretics.

General notes
Cyclopenthiazide tablets may be stored at room temperature.

CYCLOPHOSPHAMIDE (Endoxana)

Presentation
Tablets—10 mg, 50 mg
Injection—100 mg, 200 mg, 500 mg, 1 g

Actions and uses
Cyclophosphamide is a member of the nitrogen mustard group. It is converted by the liver to a number of highly reactive metabolites. These metabolites interfere with the enzyme systems essential for cell growth and therefore diminish tumour growth. It has a wide range of uses which are as follows:
1. It is widely used to good effect in Hodgkin's disease, lymphosarcoma, multiple myeloma, reticulum cell scarcoma, chronic lymphocytic leukaemia and ovarian carcinoma.
2. It has also been used in the treatment of carcinoma of the breast and lung.
3. It is used in a number of non-malignant diseases including rheumatoid arthritis, systemic lupus erythematosus, nephrotic syndrome and other auto-immune diseases.

Dosage
1. As a cytotoxic drug: This depends on the tumour type, the state of the patient and other factors including coincident administration of other cytotoxic drugs. Various regimes are used and include:
   a. 2–6 mg/kg body weight daily by single intravenous injection
   b. 2–6 mg/kg body weight in divided oral doses
   c. 10–15 mg/kg as single intravenous doses at weekly intervals.
   d. 60–80 mg/kg as single intravenous injections at 3–4 weekly intervals.
2. For an immunosupressant effect, daily oral doses of 1.5–3 mg/kg are used.

N.B. All above doses are for adults.

Nurse monitoring
1. Cyclophosphamide may be given orally or intravenously but it is unsuitable for intramuscular use.

2. It is essential that all patients receiving this drug should maintain an adequate fluid intake as this has been shown to reduce the incidence of haemorrhagic cystitis which results from an irritant effect on the bladder surface due to metabolites.
3. Bone marrow suppression is a common side effect of this drug. The white cells are more commonly affected than platelets and therefore infection in patients on this drug may be particularly severe and life threatening.
4. Gastrointestinal toxicity is common with this drug and may present as anorexia, nausea and vomiting.
5. Alopecia is a common side effect and the risk increases as higher doses of the drug are used. As alopecia is a particularly distressing side effect, patients require a good deal of psychological support and should be constantly encouraged by the fact that their hair will return after cessation of treatment, and indeed in some patients the hair will reappear while they are still receiving the drug.
6. Uncommon side effects include liver toxicity, cardiac damage, skin and nail pigmentation, dizziness, diarrhoea, thyroid dysfunction and the syndrome of inappropriate secretion of antidiuretic hormone. Jaundice, colitis, mucosal ulceration, interstitial pulmonary fibrosis and side effects on the clotting mechanism are also seen.
7. Cyclophosphamide enhances the effect of oral anti-diabetic drugs and should therefore be used with caution in diabetics. Any diabetic receiving this drug should be carefully monitored as change in hypoglycaemic therapy may be necessary.
8. The nurse should be constantly aware that most cytotoxic drugs are irritant to the skin and mucous surfaces, and are in general very toxic. Great care should therefore be exercised when handling these drugs, and in particular spillage or contamination of personnel or the environment must be avoided. If cytotoxic drugs are handled regularly it is theoretically possible that repeated skin contact or inhalation may produce systemic toxic effects and in nurses who have developed hypersensitivity, severe local and generaly hypersensitivity reactions.

General notes
1. It is important to note that solutions prepared using Water for Injection should be used within 2 hours.
2. The drug is usually injected directly into the vein over a period of about two minutes or added to the drip tubing of a running 0.9% sodium chloride or 5% dextrose infusion.
3. Cyclophosphamide tablets and vials for injection may be stored at room temperature.

CYCLOSPORIN (Sandimmun)

Presentation
Injection — 50 mg in 1 ml
150 mg in 5 ml
Oral solution—100 mg in 1 ml

Actions and uses
Cyclosporin is an immunosuppressant drug which is used for organ transplantation (involving skin, heart, kidney, pancreas, cornea, bone marrow, etc.) to reduce the likelihood of rejection and graft-versus-host disease. It acts on human t-lymphocytes which undergo a complex change during the development of the normal immune response.

Dosage
These vary considerably depending upon the nature of the organs transplanted, and the manufacturer's literature should be consulted.

Nurse monitoring
1. Intravenous infusions should be

administered in glass, not PVC, containers.
2. Cyclosporin produces a series of side effects which are dose-related i.e. will diminish when dosage is reduced, including; increased growth of body hair (hirsutism), tremor, kidney and liver impairment, gingival hypertrophy and gastrointestinal upsets.
3. Close monitoring of liver and kidney function and of blood level of the drug itself should be carried out.
4. Intravenous infusion may be associated with hypersensitivity reactions, usually to an inactive constituent of the preparation rather than to the drug itself.
5. Cyclosporin given in combination with other drugs which carry a known risk of producing renal damage will increase the possibility of kidney dysfunction.
6. Concurrent administration of Ketoconazole will increase blood levels of Cyclosporin and hence the incidence of side effects.

General notes
1. Cyclosporin oral solution must not be refrigerated since precipitation of the drug will occur.
2. Once opened, the oral solution should be discarded if unused after 2 months.

CYPROHEPTADINE (Periactin)

Presentaion
Tablets—4 mg
Syrup—2 mg in 5 ml

Actions and uses
Cyproheptadine is an antihistamine. The actions and uses of antihistamines in general are discussed in the section on antihistamines. In clinical practice Cyproheptadine is used:
1. To suppress local allergic reactions i.e. inflammatory skin responses to insect stings and bites, contact allergens, urticaria etc.
2. To stimulate the appetite in patients who have problems with eating sufficiently, such as anorexia nervosa sufferers.
3. To counteract the effects of the chemical released in the rare syndrome known as carcinoid syndrome which is characterised by diarrhoea, flushing and skin rash.

Dosage
Adults: 4 mg three times daily.

Nurse monitoring
See the section on antihistamines.

General notes
The drug may be stored at room temperature.

CYPROTERONE ACETATE (Androcur)

Presentation
Tablets—50 mg

Actions and uses
Cyproterone acetate has an anti-androgenic action. The actions of androgens are described in the section on androgens. In clinical practice the drug is used for the following conditions:
1. It may be used to treat hirsutism in the female.
2. It can also be given to treat symptoms of sexual precocity and sexual deviation in the male.

Dosage
1. For hirsutism in females: 50 mg daily for short courses during each menstrual cycle, usually combined with oestrogenic treatment.
2. For deviant sexual behaviour in males: 50 mg twice daily.

Nurse monitoring
1. When administered to male patients:
   a. A reduction in sperm count and therefore fertility usually occurs.
   b. Gynaecomastia (breast enlargement) and tenderness of the breast may occur.
2. When administered to females: Galactorrhoea and breast enlargement may occur.
3. Common symptoms during the

first few weeks of treatment include tiredness, fatigue and lassitude. These symptoms usually disappear after three months of treatment.
4. Weight gain is a common problem with prolonged administration of this drug.
5. This drug should not be given to patients with adrenal dysfunction or diabetes mellitus.
6. Other contraindications to treatment include a history of thrombosis or embolism and a history of depression.
7. With long-term treatment hypochromic anaemia may occur.

General notes
The drug may be stored at room temperature.

CYTARABINE (Alexan, Cytosar) (Also described as Cytosine Arabinoside and Ara-C)

Presentation
Injections—100 mg and 500 mg in Vials with 5 ml ampoules containing solvent or as ready-mixed solutions.

Actions and uses
Cytarabine is a cytotoxic drug which is thought to act by inhibiting an enzyme essential in the synthesis of DNA which in turn is an essential step in the growth and division of any cell. It has two major uses:
1. Its use as a cytotoxic drug has been confined to the treatment of leukaemias, especially acute myeloid leukaemia in adults.
2. As it also exerts an anti-viral action it has been used in the treatment of infections due to Herpes virus.

Dosage
Cytarabine is given by intravenous infusion and intravenous, subcutaneous and intrathecal injections. It is often given in combination with a variety of other cytotoxic agents.
1. For remission in acute myeloid leukaemia:
   a. 2–4 mg/kg body weight daily may be given by rapid intravenous injection
   b. 0.5–1 mg/kg daily may be given by continous injection
   Courses of up to 10 days of either of the above are usually given.
   c. An alternative regime is to administer 3–5 mg/kg on five consecutive days with further five day courses repeated after periods of up to 10 days until an effect is achieved.
   d. A further alternative is to administer very short courses of extremely high dosages, e.g. of the order 2 g per square metre of body surface by intravenous infusion.
2. For maintenance treatment: 1 mg/kg has been given by subcutaneous injection once or twice weekly.
3. In the treatment of leukaemic meningitis intrathecal doses of up to 50 mg have been given on two to three occasions.
4. In the treatment of infection due to Herpes virus 100 mg/m^2 body surface area has been given by intravenous injection daily. An alternative regime is 2–4 mg/kg body weight daily.
5. For the treatment of encephalitis intrathecal doses of 10 mg/m^2 body surface area have been given.

Nurse monitoring
1. When patients are receiving this drug nausea, vomiting, diarrhoea, and oral ulceration frequently occur.
2. A most important side effect of this drug is suppression of bone marrow with resultant increased risk of haemorrhage, anaemia and infection.
3. More rarely skin rashes, pain in the abdomen, chest and joints and neurotoxic and nephrotoxic side effects have been reported.
4. Patients with impaired liver function are at an increased risk of suffering toxic effects.
5. As animal studies on this drug have demonstrated adverse effects on fetal development it is completely contraindicated in pregnancy and any woman

receiving the drug should be encouraged to take adequate contraceptive measures.
6. The nurse should be constantly aware that most cytotoxic drugs are irritant to the skin and mucous surfaces, and are in general very toxic. Great care should therefore be exercised when handling these drugs, and in particular spillage or contamination of personnel or the environment must be avoided. If cytotoxic drugs are handled regularly it is theoretically possible that repeated skin contact or inhalation may produce systemic toxic effects and in nurses who have developed hypersensitivity, severe local and general hypersensitivity reactions.

General notes
1. The injection should be stored in a refrigerator.
2. Reconstituted solutions may be retained for up to 48 hours at room temperature.
3. Any solution in which a slight haze has developed must be immediately discarded.
4. Solutions are prepared by adding the accompanying 5 ml diluent to provide an injection containing 20 mg/ml.
5. Note that intrathecal injections must be prepared by using Water for Injection as the solvent provided contains Benzyl Alcohol and may be irritant if injected into the CSF.
6. Intravenous infusions are given in 0.9% sodium chloride or 5% dextrose solution.

D

DACARBAZINE (DTIC)
Presentation
Injection—100 mg, 200 mg
Actions and uses
Decarbazine is a cytotoxic drug. The precise method of action remains to be discovered. Its most important use is in the treatment of malignant melanoma. It is also used in the treatment of sarcoma and Hodgkin's disease and to a lesser extent in tumours of the colon, ovary, breast, lungs and testis.
Dosage
1. 2–4.5 mg/kg body weight daily may be given by intravenous injection for 10 days, repeated at intervals of four weeks.
2. An alternative regime is to give 250 mg/m^2 daily intravenously for five days and repeat at intervals of three weeks'.
3. Intravenous injections should be given over a period of about one minute.

Nurse monitoring
1. Bone marrow depression producing anaemia, haemorrhage due to thrombocytopenia and infection due to suppression of white cell production may occur in a severe degree.
2. Frequent and distressing side effects include anorexia, nausea and vomiting.
3. Other less common adverse effects include diarrhoea, muscle pain, tiredness, alopecia, facial flushing, paraesthesia, altered liver function.
4. It is extremely important for the nurse to note that Dacarbazine is a very irritant drug and contact with the skin or eyes must be avoided.
5. The nurse should be constantly aware that most cytotoxic drugs are irritant to the skin and mucous surfaces, and are in general very toxic. Great care should therefore be exercised when handling these drugs, and in particular spillage or contamination of personnel or the environment must be avoided. If cytotoxic drugs are handled regularly it is theoretically possible that repeated skin contact or inhalation may produce systemic toxic effects and in nurses who have developed hypersensitivity, severe local and general hypersensitivity reactions.

General notes
1. Dacarbazine injection must be stored in a refrigerator and protected from light.
2. Solutions are prepared by adding 9.9 ml to each 100 mg vial or 19.7 ml to each 200 mg vial using Water for Injection.
3. Prepared solutions are stable for 72 hours under refrigeration.

DANAZOL (Danol)
Presentation
Capsules—100 mg and 200 mg
Actions and uses
This drug inhibits the production of the hormones normally secreted by the pituitary which stimulate function of the ovaries and endometrium of the ovaries during the menstrual cycle.

It is used most commonly in clinical practice for the treatment of endometriosis but it has also been used for the treatment of gynaecomastia, fibrocystic mastitis precocious puberty and pubertal breast hypertrophy.

Dosage
It is important to note that the therapeutic effect of Danazol is controlled by careful dosage adjustment, according to individual response.
For the treatment of endometriosis the usual adult dose range is between 200 and 800 mg daily.
2. For the treatment of precocious puberty in children: 100–400 mg may be given daily according to the child's age and weight.

Nurse monitoring
1. The drug's androgenic properties can produce side effects of acne, oily skin, fluid retention, hirsutism, deepening voice and clitoral hypertrophy.
2. Other side effects include flushing, reduction in breast size, skin rash, anxiety, dizziness, vertigo, headache, nausea and loss of hair.
3. Due to the risk of fluid retention, the drug should be used with great caution in patients with heart disease, kidney disease or epilepsy.
4. If patients have impaired liver function, the dosage required will usually be reduced.

General notes
The drug may be stored at room temperature.

DANTHRON (Dorbanex)

Presentation
Liquid — 25 mg in 5 ml
75 mg in 5 ml
Capsules—25 mg

Actions and uses
The actions and uses of laxative drugs are described in the section on laxatives. Danthron derivatives such as Dorbanex act by the first mechanism of action in that they irritate the bowel wall.

Dosage
25–75 mg taken at bedtime; doses in the lower range are used for children.

Nurse monitoring
1. The irritancy of the drug on the gut wall may produce excessive motility and cramping abdominal pain to the extent of causing quite severe discomfort.
2. When the drug is excreted it may turn the urine a red/pink colour. If both the nurse and patient have knowledge of this potential side effect, potential serious alarm may be allayed.
3. If there is coincident incontinence such as in the elderly or babies, the skin may be irritated by the drug in the urine and therefore unless rapid cleansing of the skin can be guaranteed, the drug should probably be avoided in such cases.

General notes
1. Preparations containing Danthron may be stored at a room temperature.
2. Liquid mixture must be thoroughly shaken before each dose is withdrawn.

DAUNORUBICIN (Cerubidin, Rubidomycin)

Presentation
Injection—20 mg

Actions and uses
This drug is an anthracycline antibiotic and although it has a similar action to Doxorubicin (q.v.) it has a different spectrum of clinical use in that it is of great value in the treatment of acute leukaemia but has little place in the treatment of solid tumours for which Doxorubicin is frequently used.

Dosage
The drug is given by intravenous injection. The usual dosage is 0.5–3 mg/kg body weight. The intervals between injection vary widely according to the treatment schedule being used. The total

number of injections required varies considerably between patients.

Nurse monitoring
The Nurse monitoring notes on Daunorubicin are identical to those for Doxorubicin (q.v.).

General notes
1. Daunorubicin injection should be stored in a cool place and protected from light. It is normally recommended that it be kept under refrigeration.
2. The injection is prepared by dissolving the required dose in 10–20 ml of sodium chloride 0.9% and it is then injected into the tube of a fast running intravenous infusion of normal saline.
3. Any unused solution should be immediately discarded.

DEBRISOQUINE (Declinax)

Presentation
Tablets—10 mg, 20 mg

Actions and uses
See the section on Guanethidine.

Dosage
The initial adult dosage is usually 10 mg once or twice a day. This is built up gradually to a maximum of 60 mg per day in total. In cases of severe hypertension the starting dose may be 20 mg once or twice daily building up to 120 mg per day in total and doses as high as 300 mg have been used.

Nurse monitoring
See the section on Guanethidine.

General notes
Debrisoquine tablets may be stored at room temperature.

DEGLYCYRRHIZINISED LIQUORICE (Caved-S)

Presentation
Tablets—380 mg (also includes antacids)

Actions and uses
Deglycyrrhizinised liquorice is known to have a healing action on peptic ulcers. The mechanism of this healing action is unknown. It has been used to treat both gastric and duodenal ulcers and is usually given in courses of up to 6 weeks in duration.

Dosage
Gastric ulcer: 2 tablets three times daily. Duodenal ulcer: 2 tablets three to six times daily.

Nurse monitoring
Mild diarrhoea occasionally occurs in patients receiving this drug.

General notes
Nil.

DEMETHYLCHLORTETRACYCLINE (Ledermycin)

(See Note 3, p. 310)
Note: May also be referred to as Demeclocycline

Presentation
Tablets—300 mg
Capsules—150 mg
Syrup—75 mg in 5 ml
Oral drops—60 mg in 1 ml

Actions and uses
1. The actions and uses of Demethylchlortetracycline as an antibacterial antibiotic are identical to those described for tetracyclines in general (q.v.).
2. The drug has a peculiar effect on the brain in that it inhibits production of antidiuretic hormone (Vasopressin) by the hypothalamus. This hormone is important in maintaining adequate concentrations of body fluids and under certain rare circumstances an excess of ADH may be produced. This may be treated by administration of Demethylchlortetracycline in the doses described below.

Dosage
1. For the treatment of infection:
   a. *Adults*: 150 mg four times a day or 300 mg twice a day.
   b. *Children*:
   less than 1 year—30 mg/day in total given in two divided doses
   1–5 years: 60–120 mg/day in total given in four divided doses

5–9 years: 120–240 mg/day in total given in two or three divided doses
9–15 years: 270–600 mg in total per day given in four divided doses.
2. For the treatment of inappropriate ADH secretion, 600–1200 mg per day in total is given in divided doses.

Nurse monitoring
1. The general Nurse monitoring notes on tetracyclines (q.v.) are applicable to Demethylchlortetracycline.
2. It is important to note that the incidence of photosensitivity reactions is particularly high with this drug.
3. It is absolutely essential to remember that the drug in syrup should not be diluted for ease of administration.

General notes
The drug may be stored at room temperature.

DESIPRAMINE (Pertofran)

Presentation
Tablets—25 mg

Actions and uses
Desipramine is a tricyclic antidepressant drug. Its actions and uses are described in the section on tricyclic antidepressants.

Dosage
For the treatment of depression 25 mg three or four times per day orally is usually given. This may be increased to a maximum total daily dose of 200 mg if required.

Nurse monitoring
See the section on tricyclic antidepressant drugs.

General notes
Desipramine tablets may be stored at room temperature.

DESONIDE (Tridesilon)

Presentation
Cream and ointment—0.05%

Actions and uses
A potent corticosteroid (q.v.) which is used in the treatment of inflammatory skin conditions e.g. psoriasis, eczema, dermatitis etc.

Dosage
The ointment or cream is applied sparingly to the affected area two to three times daily.

Nurse monitoring
Although applied topically, significant amounts of this drug may be absorbed to produce some or all of the side effects described in the section on corticosteroids.

General notes
1. Desonide cream and ointment should be stored in a cool, dry place.
2. If necessary the cream may be diluted with cetamacrogol (A or B) or aqueous cream B.P.
3. Ointment may be diluted with white soft paraffin B.P.
4. Diluted ointments and creams should be used within two or three months of preparation.

DEXAMETHASONE (Oradexon, Decadron)

Presentation
Tablets—0.5 mg, 0.75 mg, 2 mg
Injection—5 mg in 1 ml, 8 mg in 2 ml, 100 mg in 5 ml

Actions and uses
See the section on corticosteroids.

Dosage
Doses vary considerably with the nature and severity of the illness being treated and it is not therefore appropriate to quote specific instances.

Nurse monitoring
See the section on corticosteroids.

General notes
1. Preparations containing Dexamethasone may be stored at room temperature but should be protected from light.
2. Intravenous infusions are prepared by adding Dexamethasone injection to saline or dextrose solution. They must be discarded if unused after 24 hours.

DEXTROMORAMIDE (Palfium)

Presentation
Tablets—5 mg and 10 mg
Injection — 5 mg in 1 ml
10 mg in 1 ml
Suppositories—10 mg

Actions and uses
Dextromoramide is a narcotic analgesic and its general actions and uses are described in the section on narcotic analgesics.

Dosage
For adults:
1. Orally or by subcutaneous or intramuscular injection: 5 mg repeated 4–6 hourly according to the patient's response.
2. Rectally: a 10 mg suppository should be administered 4–6 hourly according to patient response.

Nurse monitoring
See the section on narcotic analgesic drugs.

General notes
1. The drug should be stored in a locked (controlled drug) cupboard.
2. The drug should be stored at room temperature.

DEXTROPROPOXYPHENE (Doloxene, Depronal SA, Distalgesic)

Presentation
Capsules—65 mg
N.B. Dextropropoxyphene is also included in a few preparations with salicylate or paracetamol. Distalgesic is the best example of this.

Actions and uses
Dextropropoxyphene is a derivative of the narcotic analgesic group of drugs. It has a much milder analgesic effect than other members of the group and it is used for the treatment of mild or moderately painful conditions such as headache or musculoskeletal pain.

Dosage
Adults: two tablets 4–6 hourly when required for pain. If slow release capsules of the pure drug are used, the dosage is 150 mg 8 to 12 hourly.

Nurse monitoring
1. The incidence of problems with addition due to prolonged use of Dextropropoxyphene is not as great as with other stronger members of the narcotic analgesic group of drugs but it is worth noting that some degree of dependence may occur in some cases.
2. The drug is not subject to the legal requirements of 'controlled drugs' such as Morphine.
3. Dextropropoxyphene enhances the effect of Warfarin and may lead ot an increased bleeding tendency in patients receiving this drug. Warfarin dosage should be carefully monitored when Dextropropoxyphene is introduced.
4. The drug is associated with few if any side effects. However, a major problem which should probably severely restrict the general use of Dextropropoxyphene is that if it is taken in overdose it can cause profound respiratory depression. This has led to a number of fatalities.

General notes
The drug may be stored at room temperature.

DIAMORPHINE (Heroin)

Presentation
Diamorphine is available in a variety of preparations including injections and mixtures containing various strengths and often in combination with other drugs.

Actions and uses
Diamorphine is a narcotic analgesic and its general actions and uses are described in the section on narcotic analgesics.

Dosage
Dosage varies widely depending on the condition under treatment and the individual's response to the drug. Initial doses (given as a guideline only) would be 5–10 mg by subcutaneous, intramuscular or intravenous routes, repeated 4–6 hourly as required according to the patient's response and increased

appropriately as tolerance (q.v.) develops.
Nurse monitoring
See the section on narcotic analgesics.
General notes
1. The drug should be stored in a locked (controlled drug) cupboard.
2. The drug should be stored at room temperature.

DIAZEPAM (Diazemuls, Stesolid, Valium)

Presentation
Tablets—2 mg, 5 mg, 10 mg
Capsules—2 mg, 5 mg
Syrup—2 mg in 5 ml
Injection—10 mg in 2 ml, 20 mg in 4 ml
Rectal solution—5 mg and 10 mg
Suppositories—5 mg and 10 mg

Actions and uses
Diazepam is a member of the benzodiazepine group (q.v.) and of this group it has perhaps the widest application:
1. It may be taken orally during the day for the treatment of anxiety.
2. In large doses it may be taken as an hypnotic.
3. It may be administered intravenously or intramuscularly for the control of acute muscle spasm in such conditions as tetanus or status epilepticus.
4. It may be given orally for the relief of muscle spasm associated with chronic neurological abnormalities such as cerebral palsy and disseminated sclerosis.
5. It may be given intravenously for sedation immediately prior to minor surgical, dental and investigative procedures.
6. It may be administered by the rectal route as an alternative to the oral or injectable routes. Suppositories are often useful prophylaxis if used during febrile illness in patients with a history of febrile convulsions, and rectal solution is an alternative to injections in the control of convulsions.

Dosage
1. For the treatment of anxiety: 6–30 mg may be given daily either by the oral or intramuscular route.
2. For the treatment of insomnia: A single dose ranging from 5–30 mg may be taken on retiring.
3. a. In tetanus 0.1–0.3 mg/kg body weight by intravenous injection of 1–4 hours.
   b. In status epilepticus an initial dose of 0.15–0.25 mg/kg body weight may be given by the intravascular or intravenous route. A second dose may be given 30 minutes to one hour later. Occasionally continuous intravenous infusions of 3–10 mg/kg body weight for 24 hours may be required.
4. For the control of muscle spasm associated with chronic neurological disorders: Dosages are adjusted on an individual basis to try to obtain the best relief from spasm without inducing excess sedation.
5. When given intravenously for sedation prior to dental, surgical or investigative procedures doses of between 5 and 15 mg are given. It must be emphasised that the intravenous administration of Diazepam in such circumstances is not entirely safe and facilities for resuscitation must always be available as respiratory arrest may occur.
6. By the rectal route: 5 mg or 10 mg as suppository or rectal solution.

Nurse monitoring
1. For general notes see the section on benzodiazepines.
2. During intravenous injection (where 5 mg/minute is a reasonable infusion rate) the patient becomes drowsy and develops slurred speech. This is generally an indication that the optimum dose has been administered. Patients who have received intravenous Diazepam should remain under observation

for at least an hour after the procedure has been completed as they may be quite markedly sedated.
3. As emphasised above, there is always the danger of respiratory arrest with intravenous administration of Diazepam.
4. The injection solution is irritant and may cause redness around the injection site and thrombophlebitis for a period after administration. It should be noted that for this reason the intravenous use of 'Diazemuls' which contains Diazepam in a fat emulsion is preferred. The fat emulsion provides a protective coating along the vein tract and hence reduces the irritant effect.

General notes
1. Preparations containing Diazepam may be stored at room temperature.
2. The injection solution should never be mixed with other drugs in the same syringe.
3. If at all possible injection solution should be administered undiluted. However, when intravenous infusion is necessary, it may be added to normal saline or 5% dextrose. When such infusions are prepared they should be used within 6 hours and if some solution remains it should be discarded and replaced with a fresh solution.

DIAZOXIDE (Eudemine)

Presentation
   Injection—300 mg in 20 ml
Actions and uses
   Diazoxide is a potent vasodilator drug, its effect being mainly on the arterioles. When given intravenously it produces a rapid fall in blood pressure and it has been widely used in the treatment of hypertensive crises. It has tended to be replaced by other drugs which allow more effective control of blood pressure.
Dosage
   The drug is only effective intravenously and as it is rapidly inactivated it must be given rapidly i.e. in less than 30 seconds. Patients should be living flat during administration. The duration of action is usually 4–6 hours. It may be given as required up to four times in 24 hours.

Nurse monitoring
1. As mentioned above the drug effect is so rapid and profound that patients should be supine during administration. Even so hypotension not rapidly reversible is not uncommon.
2. Pain may commonly be felt at the injection site.
3. Repeated dosage may produce the following effects:
   a. Hyperglycaemia: Thus the urine should be tested for glucose. Treatment with oral hypoglycaemic drugs may be necessary.
   b. Salt and water retention: Thus a careful check for symptoms of heart failure must be made.
   c. Hyperuricaemia: Actual joint pain is rarely noted.
4. There have been reports that when the drug is used in hypertensive crises in labouring patients, delivery may be delayed unless oxytocin is concurrently administered.
5. Long-term dosage is usually not recommended because of the following effects: Hyperglycaemia, salt and water retention, hypertrichosis, skin rash, leucopenia, thrombocytopenia, extrapyramidial effects, hyperuricaemia.

General notes
   Diazoxide injection may be tstored at room temperature. It must be given undiluted and never mixed with other drugs.

DICHLORALPHENAZONE (Welldorm)

Presentation
   Tablets—650 mg
   Elixir—225 mg in 5 ml
Actions and uses
   Dichloralphenazone is an hypnotic drug which is taken to induce sleep.

Dosage
1. *Adults*: 1300 mg–1950 mg on retiring.
2. *Children*:
   Less than 1 year— 112.5–225 mg.
   1–5 years—225–450 mg.
   6–12 years—450–900 mg.

Nurse monitoring
1. Patients receiving this drug commonly suffer what is known as a hang-over effect. Symptoms are of tiredness and drowsiness the day after administration of the drug and headache is a common feature. There is no way of dealing with this problem other than to change to a shorter acting hypnotic.
2. Dichloralphenazone can affect patients' requirements for anticoagulants such as Warfarin and patients should be closely observed and have their clotting times frequently checked. During commencement of the drug Warfarin dosage may require to be increased to maintain its effect and when the drug is stopped the dose may require to be decreased to avoid the possibility of bleeding.
3. Other side effects which occur with this drug include skin rashes, nausea and vomiting.
4. In patients with the rare disease of acute intermittent porphyria this drug may precipitate acute symptoms and is therefore contraindicated.

General notes
1. Preparations containing Dichloralphenazone may be stored at room temperature.
2. The elixir should be stored in well sealed bottles and away from direct sunlight.
3. If necessary it may be diluted with syrup for ease of administration.

DICHLOROPHEN (Antiphen)

Presentation
Tablets—500 mg

Actions and uses
This antihelminthic drug is used for the treatment, both in the United Kingdom and tropical countries, of human tapeworm infestations caused by *Taenia saginata*. It is also used for infections caused by *Hymenolepis nana* and *Diphyllobothrium latum* (fish tapeworm).

Dosage
1. *Adults*: Either
   a. 18 tablets in a single dose
   b. 12 tablets on each of two successive days
   c. 4–6 tablets three times in 24 hours.
2. *Children*: Either
   a. 4–8 tablets on each of two successive days
   b. 2–4 tablets three times in 24 hours.

Nurse monitoring
1. Preliminary starvation or additional purgation are not necessary for efficacy, but best results are usually obtained if the drug is given in the morning on an empty stomach.
2. The commonest side effects experienced with this drug are abdominal discomfort and diarrhoea but these are not usually of any great severity. Vomiting and transient urticaria have been more rarely reported.
3. The drug should be used with great care or avoided in patients with liver or cardiovascular disease.
4. The drug is not recommended for administration during pregnancy.

General notes
The drug should be stored at room temperature.

DICHLORPHENAMIDE (Daranide)

Presentation
Tablets—50 mg

Actions and uses
Dichlorphenamide is a carbonic anhydrase inhibitor with a similar mechanism of action to

Acetazolamide (q.v.). It is used for the treatment of glaucoma.

Dosage
Adults: Initially up to 200 mg 12-hourly with maintenance dosage in the range of 25–50 mg one to three times a day.

Nurse monitoring
The Nurse monitoring aspects of Acetazolamide (q.v.) apply to this drug.

General notes
The drug may be stored at room temperature.

DICLOFENAC (Voltarol)

Presentation
Tablets—25 mg, 50 mg
Tablets, slow release—100 mg
Suppositories—100 mg
Injection—75 mg in 3 ml

Actions and uses
See the section on non-steroidal anti-inflammatory analgesic drugs.

Dosage
The adult oral dose range is 25–100 mg three times a day or 100 mg once daily as slow release tablets. 100 mg may be administered at night by the rectal route and 75 mg by intramuscular injection once or twice daily.

Nurse monitoring
See the section on anti-inflammatory analgesic drugs, non-steroidal.

General notes
Diclofenac tablets may be stored at room temperature.

DICYCLOMINE (Merbentyl)

Presentation
Tablets—10 mg
Syrup—10 mg in 5 ml

Actions and uses
Dicyclomine is an anticholinergic drug. It has a specific antispasmodic action on the smooth muscle of the gastrointestinal tract. It is therefore used for the following conditions: irritable colon, spastic constipation, infant colic, spasm associated with colitis, diverticulitis, Crohn's disease, gastritis, peptic ulcer and cholecystitis.

Dosage
1. *Adults*: 10–20 mg three times daily taken before or after meals.
2. *Children*:
   a. Infants (less than 2 years): 5–10 mg 15 minutes before feeding. The total daily dose in this age group should not exceed 40 mg.
   b. Older children may receive dosages as necessary up to the equivalent of the adult dose.

Nurse monitoring
Dicyclomine has identical side effects to those described under Hyoscine-N-Butylbromide (Buscopan). In addition dizziness, nausea, vomiting, anorexia, headache, constipation, fatigue, sedation and skin rash may occur.

General notes
Dicyclomine preparations may be stored at room temperature. Syrup should however be protected from light by storing in amber glass bottles. For ease of administration, if required, the syrup may be diluted immediately before use with an equal quantity of water.

DIETHLCARBAMAZINE (Banocide)

Presentation
Tablets—50 mg

Actions and uses
This antihelminthic drug is used in the treatment of filarial infection due to *W. bancrofti, B. malayi, Onchocerciasis volvulus* and *loa loa* It may also be used for the prophylaxis of bancrofti in malarian filariasis and loaises.

Dosage
1. Treatment of disease for adults and children: An initial dose of 1 mg/kg body weight, gradually increased over 3 days to 6 mg/kg body weight daily in three divided doses is recommended. Duration of treatment should be three weeks.
2. For prophylaxis of bancrofti, malarian filariasis: 50 mg monthly.

3. For prophylaxis of loaiases: 4 mg/kg for three successive days each month.

Nurse monitoring
1. Allergic reactions caused by destruction of the organisms are common and take the form of generalised itching and conjunctival congestion. These may be reduced by increasing the dosage slowly as recommended above and by the concurrent administration of antihistamines or corticosteroids.
2. Anorexia, nausea, vomiting, dizziness and mild drowsiness may occur with this drug.

General notes
The drug may be stored at room temperature.

DIETHYLPROPION (Tenuate, Apisate)

Presentation
Tablets—25 mg and 75 mg (slow release)

Actions and uses
Anorexogenic drugs abolish hunger by a direct action on the central nervous system. They are thought to have a supplementary effect in that they increase the ability to perform mental and physical work without the need for increased food intake.

Dosage
1. *Adults*: Either
   a. 25 mg three times a day one hour before meals and 25 mg if necessary on retiring.
   or
   b. 75 mg slow release tablet taken mid-morning.
2. *Children* in the age range 6–12 years: 25 mg one hour before the mid-day and evening meal. Note: The 75 mg slow release tablet is not recommended for the treatment of children under the age of 12 years and the ordinary formulation of 25 mg tablet is not recommended for the treatment of children under 6 years.

Nurse monitoring
1. As this drug is related to the amphetamine group of drugs there is a definite risk of physical and psychological dependence and addiction developing. It is, therefore, recommended that patients receive this drug for short (6–8 week) courses only and that the drug should be immediately discontinued if patients fail to lose weight.
2. Again because of its relationship to the amphetamine group of drugs, this drug should not be given to patients who suffer from cardiovascular disease such as angina or hypertension.
3. The drug should never be given to patients who are undergoing treatment or have recently been given treatment with monoamine oxidase inhibitors (q.v.).
4. Side effects may be divided into three groups:
   a. Neurological: insomnia, nervousness, depression and anxiety.
   b. Gastrointestinal: nausea, vomiting and constipation.
   c. Cardiovascular: tachycardia, hypertension and headache.
5. Rare side effects include dry mouth and allergic skin rashes.
6. If an excess dose is taken psychosis may be produced. This rapidly resolves after discontinuation of the drug.

General notes
The drug may be stored at room temperature.

DIFLUCORTOLONE (Nerisone)

Presentation
Cream—0.1%
Ointment and oily cream—0.1%, 0.3%

Actions and uses
This potent corticosteroid (q.v.) is used topically in the treatment of inflammatory skin conditions such as psoriasis, eczema and dermatitis.

Dosage
Cream, oily cream and ointment are applied one to three times daily to affected areas.

Nurse monitoring
Although applied topically, significant amounts of this drug may be absorbed through the skin producing some or all of the side effects described in the section on corticosteroids.

General notes
1. The ointment, cream and oily cream should be stored under cool, dry conditions.
2. These products have a shelf life of five years from the date of manufacture.

DIFLUNISAL (Dolobid)

Presentation
Tablets—250 mg, 500 mg

Actions and uses
1. See the section on Aspirin.
2. Diflunisal is a long-acting Aspirin-like drug which is less irritant to the stomach and therefore may produce fewer gastrointestinal problems than Aspirin.

Dosage
1. *Adults*: The average adult dose is 250–500 mg twice daily. Occasionally higher doses are required.
2. *Children*: It is not recommended that children receive this form of Aspirin.

Nurse monitoring
1. See the section on Aspirin for general Nurse monitoring points on this drug.
2. It is important to note that there is an increased incidence of severe skin rashes with Diflunisal as compared to other salicylate drugs.

General notes
Diflunisal tablets may be stored at room temperature.

DIGITOXIN (Digitaline Nativelle)

Presentation
Tablets—0.1 mg
Injection—0.2 mg in 1 ml
Oral solution—0.1 mg in 5 drops

Actions and uses
A cardiac glycoside (see the section on Digoxin).

Dosage
Oral adult loading doses are 1–2 mg followed by maintenance doses of 0.05–0.2 mg daily.

Nurse monitoring
See the section on Digoxin.

General notes
Digitoxin preparations may be stored at room temperature.

DIGOXIN (Lanoxin)

Presentation
Tablets—0.0625 mg, 0.125 mg, 0.25 mg
Injection—0.5 mg in 2 ml
Elixir—0.05 mg in 1 ml

Actions and uses
1. 'Inotropic' effect: Digoxin increases the force of contraction of heart muscle, thus improving its pumping action. This makes it useful in the treatment of heart failure.
2. 'Chronotropic' effect: The rate at which impulses pass down the conducting pathways of the heart is slowed, allowing in turn more efficient pumping of blood through the heart. Thus the drug is useful in the treatment of atrial tachyarrhythmias, such as atrial fibrillation.

Dosage
1. 'Loading' dose: After administration the drug is distributed throughout a number of body tissues and therefore in order to obtain adequate plasma concentrations a 'loading' dose must be given. The amount given, and the route of administration depend on a number of factors.
   a. Amount given: This depends mainly on the age, weight and renal function of the patient, and also to a certain extent on how rapidly the drug's effect is required. Thus a patient under 60 with normal renal function who is in heart failure

because of a supraventricular tachycardia might be given 0.5 mg intravenous followed by 0.25 mg three times a day until adequate clinical effects were obtained, whereas an older patient with atrial fibrillation in mild heart failure might only be given 0.25 mg once or twice a day orally until a clinical response was obtained.

  b. Route of administration: This depends on the required rapidity of onset. As mentioned above, in cases of heart failure due to supraventricular tachycardia, intravenous administration may be preferred, whereas oral treatment would be the choice with less urgent cases. Intramuscular Digoxin may be given in emergency situations where absence of adequate monitoring facilities makes intravenous administration impossible.

2. Maintenance dose: This varies according to the age, weight and renal function of the patient. Two ways of approaching the problem of calculating the required dosage are as follows:
  a. The use of a 'nomogram', where dosage is calculated according to age, weight and renal function.
  b. By monitoring the clinical effects (i.e. pulse rate) and the appearance of side effects, and tailoring the dose to suit individual patient needs.

Plasma levels of Digoxin can be measured. These are particularly useful for testing patient compliance, and for detecting excessive dosage but the levels obtained do not reflect accurately the clinical effect of the drug. Suggested dosages (given as a guideline only):

1. Intravenous administration in adults: 0.5 mg diluted in 50 ml of saline and given over 30 minutes.
2. Oral loading dose: 0.25 mg three times a day.
3. Maintenance dosage: 0.25 mg once a day in the age groups 12–70 years old and 0.0625 mg once a day over the age of 70.
4. Children's dosage:
   Less than 1 year: loading dose 0.02 mg/kg three times a day (oral maintenance 0.01 mg/kg daily.
   1–5 years: loading 0.2 mg three times a day (oral) maintenance 0.01 mg/kg daily.
   6–12 years: loading 0.375 mg three times a day (oral) maintenance 0.25 mg per day.

Nurse monitoring
1. The nurse's role in patients on Digoxin therapy is a particularly important one for two reasons:
   a. Non-cardiac side effects (see below) are most likely to be observed by the nurse and therefore warning may be given and the dose changed before life threatening complications arise.
   b. The nurse has an active role to play in the day-to-day manipulation of drug dosage, as it is generally accepted that Digoxin should be withheld at least until medical staff are consulted, if the pulse rate is less than 55 per minute.
2. Non-cardiac side effects include anorexia, nausea, vomiting, diarrhoea, yellow vision, gynaecomastia.
3. Cardiac side effects include bradycardia, paroxysmal atrial tachycardia, ventricular arrhythmias of any kind.

General notes
1. The drug should be stored in a dry place at room temperature.
2. The drug should be protected from light.

DIHYDROCODEINE (DF 118)

Presentation
  Tablets—30 mg
  Elixir—10 mg in 5 ml
  Injection—50 mg in 1 ml

Actions and uses
Dihydrocodeine is a narcotic analgesic drug. Its general actions and uses are described in the section on narcotic analgesics. The oral form is used for the treatment of mild painful conditions which would not usually be considered appropriate for treatment with other more powerful drugs of the narcotic analgesic group.

Dosage
For *adults*:
1. Orally: 30 mg every 4 to 6 hours.
2. By intramuscular or deep subcutaneous injection: 50 mg 4 to 6 hourly as required.

Nurse monitoring
See the section on narcotic analgesic drugs.

General notes
1. It is important to note that although oral preparations are not subject to legal requirements of 'controlled drugs' Dihydrocodeine injection is a controlled drug and should be stored in a locked (controlled drug) cupboard.
2. The drug should be stored at room temperature.

DIHYDROTACHYSTEROL (Tachyrol, AT 10)

Presentation
Tablets—200 μm (Tachyrol)
Oral solution—250 μg/ml (AT 10)

Actions and uses
The actions and uses of Dihydrotachysterol are identical to those described for Vitamin D (q.v.).

Dosage
1. For the treatment of resistant rickets and hypoparathyroidism: 0.05–0.25 mg per day initially depending on the age of the patient and the severity of the disorder. The dosage should subsequently be adjusted according to individual needs.

Nurse monitoring
See the section on Vitamin D.

General notes
The drug may be stored at room temperature.

DIMENHYDRINATE (Dramamine)

Presentation
Tablets—50 mg
Injection—50 mg in 1 ml

Actions and uses
Dimenhydrinate is an antihistamine. The actions and uses of antihistamines in general are discussed in the section on antihistamines. Dimenhydrinate is used in clinical practice:
1. For the treatment of nausea and vomiting, particularly motion sickness.
2. For the treatment of vertigo and the symptoms of vertigo and nausea due to Meniere's disease.

Dosage
1. *Adults*:
   a. Orally 50–100 mg 4-hourly.
   b. By intravenous or intramuscular injection: 50–100 gm repeated as required to a total dose of 400 mg per day.
2. *Children*:
   1–6 years: 12.5–25 mg orally two to three times daily.
   7–12 years: 25–50 mg two to three times daily orally.

Nurse monitoring
See the section on antihistamines.

General notes
The drug may be stored at room temperature.

DIMETHINDENE (Fenostil Retard)

Presentation
Tablets—2.5 mg (slow release)

Actions and uses
Dimethindene is an antihistamine. The actions and uses of antihistamines in general are described in the section on antihistamines. In clinical practice Dimethindene is used:
1. To suppress generalised minor allergic responses to allergens such as foodstuffs and drugs.
2. To suppress local allergic reactions i.e. inflammatory skin responses to insect stings and bites, contact allergens, urticaria etc.

3. Orally for allergic inflammatory conditions e.g. hay fever and allergic rhinitis.
4. As an anti-pruritic agent.

Dosage
Adults: 2.5 mg twice daily.

Nurse monitoring
See the section on antihistamines.

General notes
The drug may be stored at room temperature.

DIMETHOTHIAZINE (Banistyl)

Presentation
Tablets—20 mg

Actions and uses
Dimethothiazine is an antihistamine. The actions and uses of antihistamines in general are described in the section on antihistamines. In clinical practice Dimethothiazine is used:
1. To suppress generalised minor allergic responses to allergens such as foodstuffs and drugs.
2. To suppress local allergic reactions i.e. inflammatory skin responses to insect stings and bites, contact allergens, urticaria etc.
3. As decongestant e.g. in the treatment of allergic rhinitis and hay fever.
4. As an anti-pruritic agent.

Dosage
1. *Adults*: 20 mg three times per day up to a maximum daily dose of 120 mg.
2. *Children*:
   6–12 years—10 mg twice daily.

Nurse monitoring
See the section on antihistamines.

General notes
The drug may be stored at room temperature.

DIOCTYL SODIUM SULPHOSUCCINATE (Dioctyl Medo)

Presentation
Tablets—20 mg, 100 mg
Syrup—12.5 mg in 5 ml

Actions and uses
The actions of laxatives are discussed in the section on laxatives. Dioctyl Sodium Sulphosuccinate falls into the third group, i.e. it is a wetting agent which softens hard, impacted stools. It is used in the treatment of constipation.

Dosage
1. *Adults*: Up to 600 mg per day in three divided doses.
2. *Children*:
   Infants up to 30 mg per day in three divided doses.
   Older children up to 60 mg per day in three divided doses.
3. The syrup may be given by the rectal route as an enema:
   Adults: 15–40 ml
   Children: 7.5–15 ml
   Infants: 5–10 ml

Nurse monitoring
There are no specific problems with this drug.

General notes
1. Preparations containing Dioctyl Sodium Sulphosuccinate may be stored at room temperature.
2. For an optimum effect doses should be taken with plenty of fluid.

DIPHENHYDRAMINE (Benadryl)

Presentation
Capsules—25 mg

Actions and uses
Diphenhydramine is an antihistamine. The actions and uses of antihistamines in general are described in the section on antihistamines. In clinical practice Diphenhydramine is most commonly used:
1. To suppress generalized minor allergic responses to allergens such as foodstuffs and drugs.
2. To suppress local allergic reactions i.e. inflammatory skin responses to insect stings and bites, contact allergens, urticaria etc.
3. Orally for allergic inflammatory conditions e.g. hay fever and allergic rhinitis.
4. As nasal decongestant e.g. in the treatment of allergic rhinitis and

hay fever. It is also added to a few proprietary cough preparations because of its decongestant action.
Dosage
Adults: 25 mg three times a day, and 50 mg at bedtime.
Nurse monitoring
See the section on antihistamines.
General notes
The drug may be stored at room temperature.

DIPHENOXYLATE (Lomotil)
Presentation
Tablets—2.5 mg
Liquid—2.5 mg in 5 ml
Diphenoxylate is combined with a small quantity of Atropine and occasionally also with Neomycin.
Actions and uses
This drug is chemically related to morphine-like compounds, all of which tend to produce constipation by a direct action on the motility of the gut. It is frequently combined with Atropine because Atropine also affects gut movement and the two drugs have, therefore, an additive effect. It is occasionally also combined with Neomycin because Neomycin was in the past used to treat episodes of diarrhoea thought to be due to bacterial infection.
Dosage
1. *Adults*: Initially 10 mg followed by 5 mg every 6 hours until control of symptoms is achieved.
2. *Children*:
   1–3 years: 2.5 mg twice daily
   4–8 years: 2.5 mg three times daily
   9–12 years: 2.5 mg four times daily.
   12–16 years: 5 mg three times daily
   All until control of symptoms is achieved.
Nurse monitoring
1. Perhaps the most important point for the nurse to note about this drug is that although it is used for a frequently trivial and self-limiting disorder, it has potentially serious side effects and may be fatal in overdosage. It should only, therefore, be used in the short-term and patients must be continually encouraged to use it only as directed.
2. Diphenoxylate may produce nausea, vomiting, sedation, dizziness, skin rash, restlessness and depression.
3. The inclusion of Atropine in the preparation may give rise to side effects including dry mouth, tachycardia and urinary retention the latter being particularly frequent in children.
4. If this drug is taken in overdose, particularly in young children, it has a marked depressive function on the respiratory system and the central nervous system which may lead to fatality. Overdoses, therefore, should be referred immediately to hospital.
5. The drug should not be given to children under the age of 1 year.
6. The drug should not be given to patients who also are in receipt of sedative drugs such as barbiturates and tranquillisers.
7. Patients should be advised that the combination of this drug and alcohol may cause excessive sedation.
8. The drug should not be given to patients receiving monoamine oxidase inhibiting drugs (q.v.).
9. The drug should not be given to patients with jaundice.
General notes
Preparations containing Diphenoxylate may be stored at room temperature.

DIPHENYLPYRALINE (Histryl)
Presentation
Capsules, slow release—2.5 mg, 5 mg
Actions and uses
Diphenylpyraline is an antihistamine. The actions and uses of antihistamines in general are described in the section on antihistamines. Diphyenylpyraline is used in clinical practice:
1. To suppress gneralised minor

allergic responses to allergens such as foodstuffs and drugs.
2. To suppress local allergic reactions i.e. inflammatory skin responses to insect stings and bites, contact allergens, urticaria etc.
3. As a nasal decongestant e.g. in the treatment of allergic rhinitis and hay fever.

Dosage
1. *Adults*: 5–10 mg of the slow release preparation twice daily.
2. *Children*:
   Over 7 years—2.5 mg of the slow release preparation twice daily.

Nurse monitoring
See the section on antihistamines.

General notes
The drug may be stored at room temperature.

DIPIPANONE (Diconal)

N.B. Diconal tablets contain Dipipanone 10 mg in combination with Cyclizine 30 mg.

Actions and uses
Dipipanone is a narcotic analgesic drug and its actions and uses are described in the section on narcotic analgesics. It is produced in combination with Cyclizine for the latter drug's anti-emetic effect.

Dosage
For adults: 1–3 tablets 6-hourly as required.

Nurse monitoring
See the section on narcotic analgesic drugs.

General notes
1. This drug is subject to the legal requirements of 'controlled drugs' and should be kept in a locked (controlled drug) cupboard.
2. The drug should be stored at room temperature.

DIPROPHYLLINE (Silbephylline)

Presentation
Tablets—200 mg
Syrup—100 mg in 5 ml
Injection—500 mg in 2 ml
Suppositories—400 mg

Actions and uses
This drug is chemically related to Aminophylline and its actions and uses (q.v.). It is used in the management of bronchospasm associated with asthma and other conditions such as chronic bronchitis. It is also occasionally used in the treatment of congestive heart failure.

Dosage
1. Orally:
   a. *Adults*: 200–400 mg three times daily with two suppositories at night if necessary.
   b. *Children*:
      Under 1 year—10–30 mg daily.
      1–2 years—40 mg daily.
      3–5 years—60 mg daily.
      6–12 years—100 mg daily.
      All the above children's doses should be taken four times a day.
2. Intravenously: 500 mg by slow intravenous injection over 1–2 minutes as required.

Nurse monitoring
1. The Nurse monitoring notes on Aminophylline apply to this drug (q.v.).

General notes
1. Preparations containing this drug may be stored at room temperature.
2. For ease of administration the syrup may be diluted with syrup BP and the injection by Water for Injection BP.

DIPYRIDAMOLE (Persantin)

Presentation
Tablets—25 mg, 100 mg
Injection—10 mg in 2 ml

Actions and uses
1. The drug reduces the blood pressure by dilating peripheral blood vessels and thus reduces the work done by the heart.
2. It dilates coronary vessels increasing blood flow and oxygen supply to the heart. The combination of these two actions

makes the drug potentially useful for the treatment of angina. It is not effective in relieving the pain of an acute attack but is more useful when administered on a regular basis for the prevention of attacks of angina, usually when control of symptoms has been found to be difficult or impossible with established anti-anginal drugs (i.e. β-blockers, nitrates, nifedipine, perhexiline).
3. It also affects blood clotting by reducing platelet aggregation.

Dosage
1. For the prophylaxis of angina: Oral: 50 mg three times a day, intravenous: 10–20 mg three times a day.
2. To decrease platelet aggregation: Oral: 100 mg three to four times a day increasing to 800 mg if necessary.

Nurse monitoring
1. After an intravenous dose a bitter taste in the mouth, facial flushing and hypotension may occur.
2. With oral therapy-hypotension manifest by dizziness and fainting may occur. Other side effects such as skin rash, gastric upset, and diarrhoea are rare.

General notes
Dipyridamole tablets and injection solution can be stored at room temperature.

DISOPYRAMIDE (Rythmodan)

Presentation
Capsules—100 mg, 150 mg
Tablets—250 mg, slow release
Injection—50 mg in 5 ml

Actions and uses
Disopyramide has a number of effects on the heart muscle and the conducting tissues of the heart, which make it useful in the treatment of the supraventricular and ventricular tachyarrhythmias. These effects are:
1. Prolongation of the refractory period of cardiac muscle
2. Decrease in excitability of cardiac muscle
3. Decrease in conduction velocity.

Dosage
1. Intravenous:
Initial dose: 2 mg/kg body weight given over 5 minutes (to a maximum of 150 mg irrespective of body weight).
Maintenance infusion.
0.4 mg/kg/hour (to a maximum of 800 mg in 24 hours).
2. Oral dose range for adults is 300–800 mg/day divided into four equal doses.
3. Alternatively, an oral dose of 250–375 mg twice daily may be given using slow release tablets.

Nurse monitoring
1. Disopyramide has anticholinergic side effects such as dry mouth, blurred vision, and urinary retention, the latter being especially important in elderly men particularly those with prostatism
2. Nausea, diarrhoea and dizziness may also occur
3. Occasionally heart failure may be precipitated
4. Serious rhythm disturbances may occur in patients with hypokalaemia or heart block
5. Too rapid intravenous injection may cause profuse sweating

General notes
Disopyramide capsules, tablets and injections may be stored at room temperature. When given by intravenous infusion the injection solution may be added to sodium chloride, dextrose, compound sodium chloride or Ringers injection solution.

DOBUTAMINE (Dobutrex)

Presentation
Injection—250 mg vials

Actions and uses
Dobutamine indirectly stimulates heart muscle and leads to an increase in its force of contraction, thus improving cardiac output. It is used intravenously by infusion to try to increase cardiac output in patients who are suffering from cardiogenic shock, the commonest cause of this being a massive heart

attack, with subsequent severe impairment of the heart's ability to pump blood and therefore maintain blood pressure.

Dosage
For adults 2.5–10 μg/kg/minute. Doses up to 40 μg/kg/minute have been used if lower dosages fail to produce a reasonable effect.

Nurse monitoring
See the section on Dopamine.

General notes
Dobutamine injection as dry powder in vials may be stored at room temperature. The injection solution is reconstituted by adding Water for Injection or 5% dextrose injection to the vial. Reconstituted solution may be stored in a refrigerator for up to 48 hours or at room temperature for 6 hours. This solution is further diluted by addition to solutions of sodium chloride, dextrose, dextrose/saline, laevulose or compound sodium lactate injection. Infusion solutions must be used within 24 hours of preparation; they may develop a slight pink discolouration which does not necessarily indicate an alteration in potency.

DOMPERIDONE (Motilium)

Presentation
Tablets—10 mg
Suspension—5 mg in 5 ml
Injection—10 mg in 2 ml

Actions and uses
Domperidone has similar actions and uses to those of Metoclopramide, though it does not produce the adverse effects on the CNS which are associated with Metoclopramide. Its major use is as an anti-emetic.

Dosage
1. *Adults*:
   10–20 mg every 4–8 hours by the oral, intramuscular or intravenous routes.
2. Children: 0.2–0.4 mg/kg body weight every 4–8 hours by the oral, intramuscular or intravenous routes.

Nurse monitoring
1. While it is generally considered that this drug produces few, if any, side effects, patients should be carefully assessed for the occurrence of adverse effects similar to those described for Metoclopramide.
2. Children are usually very sensitive to Metoclopramide-produced CNS effects and treatment in children should be restricted to the control of nausea and vomiting associated with anti-cancer therapy.

General notes
Preparations containing Domperidone are stored at room temperature.

DOPAMINE (Intropin)

Presentation
Injection—200 mg in 5 ml

Actions and uses
Dopamine is inactive orally but when given intravenously it directly stimulates the heart's action increasing its force of contraction. It also increases the blood flow through the kidneys, by dilating renal blood Vessels. Urine output may be increased. This effect may be reversed at higher dosage. It is used in the treatment of cardiogenic shock (see the section on Dobutamine, its actions and uses).

Dosages
Adult intravenous dosage is initially 2–5 μg/kg/minute increasing by 1–4 μ/kg/minute every 15–30 minutes until an adequate effect is achieved. Doses of up to 50 μg/kg/minute have been used but 9 μg/kg/minute is the average maintenance dose needed.

Nurse monitoring
This drug is rarely used outwith intensive or coronary care units. The major problem with administration is an increase in the heart rate which may progress to fatal cardiac tachyarrhythmia. Cardiac monitoring is therefore obligatory. Both Dopamine and Dobutamine are less

likely to produce this effect than Isoprenaline which is an alternative treatment for cardiogenic shock. High dosages of Dopamine may produce peripheral vasoconstriction, hypertension, cardiac conduction defects, and reduced renal blood flow.

General notes
Dopamine injection solution may be stored at room temperature. An infusion solution is prepared by adding the injection to solutions of sodium chloride, dextrose, laevulose, dextrose/saline and compound sodium lactate injection.

DOTHIEPIN (Prothiaden)

Presentation
Capsules—25 mg
Tablets—75 mg

Actions and uses
Dothiepin is a tricyclic antidepressant drug. Its actions and uses are described in the section dealing with these drugs.

Dosage
For the treatment of depression 75–150 mg may be given daily orally in three divided doses or alternatively the total daily dose may be taken in the evening on retiring.

Nurse monitoring
1. For general notes on Nurse monitoring see the section on tricyclic antidepressant drugs.
2. It is worth noting that Dothiepin produces a lesser incidence of the troublesome anticholinergic side effects described in the section on tricyclic antidepressant drugs, and may therefore be particularly suitable for use in elderly patients.

General notes
Dothiepin capsules and tablets may be stored at room temperature.

DOXAPRAM (Dopram)

Presentation
Injection—100 mg in 5 ml
Intravenous infusion—1 g in 500 ml dextrose 5%

Actions and uses
This drug has a direct stimulant action on centres in the brain associated with respiration. It is, therefore, used to stimulate respiration in:
1. Acute respiratory failure associated with overdosage of drugs which depress breathing such as barbiturates and opiates.
2. Depressed respiration produced by anaesthesia in the postoperative recovery period.

Dosage
Doxapram is administered by intravenous injection or infusion:
1. For the treatment of acute respiratory failure due to overdosage of drugs: 0.5–4 mg/minute by infusion.
2. To aid recovery from anaesthesia: hourly injections of 1–1.5 mg/kg are given.

Nurse monitoring
1. The drug is contraindicated for use in patients who suffer from severe hypertension, coronary artery disease, thyrotoxicosis, status asthmaticus and cerebrovascular accident. It should be used with great care in patients who are either epileptic or are on monoamine oxidase inhibiting drugs.
2. Side effects include raised blood pressure and a fast pulse rate.
3. In postoperative conditions restlessness, muscle twitching, sweating, confusion, nausea and vomiting may be produced.

General notes
1. Solutions for intravenous injection and infusion are stored at room temperature, and should never be refrigerated.
2. Doxapram is unstable when added to infusion fluids containing alkaline substances such as Aminophylline, Frusemide and barbiturates.

DOXEPIN (Sinequan)

Presentation
Capsules—10 mg, 25 mg, 50 mg, 75 mg

Actions and uses
Doxepin is a tricyclic antidepressant drug. Its actions and uses are described in the section on these drugs.
Dosage
10–100 mg three times daily.
Nurse monitoring
1. For general notes see the section on tricyclic antidepressant drugs.
2. Doxepin induces fewer of the troublesome anticholinergic side effects described in the section on tricyclic antidepressant drugs and may therefore be particularly useful for treating elderly patients.
General notes
Doxepin capsules may be stored at room temperature.

DOXORUBICIN (Adriamycin)

Presentation
Injection—10 mg vials, 50 mg vials
Actions and uses
Doxorubicin is an anthracycline antibiotic which is used in clinical practice for its cytotoxic effect. It inhibits the division of cells, particularly those of rapidly multiplying malignant tumours. It is often used in combination with other cytotoxic drugs to treat a wide range of neoplastic diseases including acute leukaemias, lymphomas, soft tissue and bone malignancies in childhood and solid tumours (in particular breast and lung carcinoma).
Dosage
The drug is given by intravenous injection over 2–3 minutes to the drip tubing of a running infusion. The dosage is usually calculated on a body surface area basis. When used alone 60–75 mg/m^2 is the recommended dose to be given at intervals of three weeks. When used in combination with other cytotoxic drugs, 30–40 mg/m^2 at intervals of three weeks is recommended. Occasionally a dose regime of 1.2–2.4 mg/kg body weight is used.
Nurse monitoring
1. The drug is extremely caustic and must be given into a fast running infusion to prevent severe local effects. It is therefore important to ensure than an infusion is working correctly prior to administration of the drug.
2. An important side effect peculiar to this type of antibiotic is its cardiotoxicity. Initially tachycardia and electrocardiogram changes are seen but this can progress to gross cardiomyopathy resulting in cardiac failure and death.
3. Bone marrow suppression produces anaemia, leucopenia and thrombocytopenia with a resultant increased rish of severe infection and haemorrhage.
4. Gastrointestinal side effects such as oral ulceration, nausea, vomiting and diarrhoea may occur.
5. The drug must be used at a reduced dose level in patients with impaired renal function.
6. The drug usually produces a red discolouration of the urine. It is important that the patient be warned of this side effect in advance and be reassured that the red discolouration is of no significance.
7. The nurse should be constantly aware that most cytotoxic drugs are irritant to the skin and mucous surfaces, and are in general very toxic. Great care should therefore be exercised when handling these drugs, and in particular spillage or contamination of personnel or the environment must be avoided. If cytotoxic drugs are handled regularly it is theoretically possible that repeated skin contact or inhalation may produce systemic toxic effects and in nurses who have developed hypersensitivity, severe local and general reactions.
General notes
1. Doxorubicin dry powder in vials may be stored at room temperature.

2. The solution is prepared by adding 5 ml of Water for Injection or sodium chloride 0.9% injection to the 10 mg vial. 25 ml of these solvents may be added to the 50 mg vial.
3. Solutions thus prepared are injected into the drip tubing of a running sodium chloride 0.9%, dextrose 5% or dextrose saline infusion.

DOXYCYCLINE (Vibramycin)

(See Note 3, p. 310)
Presentation
Capsules—100 mg
Syrup—50 mg in 5 ml
Actions and uses
See the section on tetracyclines.
Dosage
1. *Adults*: 100–200 mg once or twice daily.
2. *Children*: 4 mg/kg initially, then 2 mg/kg body weight in total per day given as one or two doses.

Nurse monitoring
The general Nurse monitoring notes for tetracyclines (q.v.) apply to Doxycycline with two important exceptions:
1. Doxycycline is less likely to cause deterioration of renal function in patients with renal impairment.
2. Food and milk are less likely to affect its absorption and therefore the timing of administration in relation to meals is less important with this drug.

General notes
1. The drug should be stored at room temperature.
2. Once prepared the syrup should be used within fourteen days.

DROSTANOLONE (Masteril)

Presentation
Injection—100 mg in 1 ml
Actions and uses
1. The actions and uses of androgenic hormones in general are described in the section dealing with these drugs.
2. Drostanolone is used in clinical practice mainly for the treatment of breast carcinoma.

Dosage
For the treatment of breast carcinoma: 300 mg weekly by intramuscular injection is recommended.

Nurse monitoring
See the section on androgens and anabolic steroids.

General notes
1. The drug may be stored at room temperature.
2. The drug should not be exposed to direct sunlight.

DYDROGESTERONE (Duphaston)

Presentation
Tablets—10 mg
Actions and uses
1. The actions and uses of progestational hormones in general are described in the section dealing with these drugs.
2. In clinical practice Duphaston is recommended for the treatment of:
   a. Endometriosis
   b. Threatened abortion
   c. Habitual abortion
   d. Irregular menstrual cycles
   e. Functional uterine bleeding
   f. Infertility
   g. Premenstrual tension

Dosage
1. For the treatment of endometriosis: 10 mg two to three times per day from day 5–25 of the cycle.
2. For the treatment of threatened abortion: 40 mg initially and then 10 mg 8-hourly until symptoms remit. Persistence of symptoms or return of symptoms during treatment are indications to double the dose. The effective dose must be maintained for a week after the symptoms have ceased and should be gradually decreased thereafter.
3. For the treatment of habitual abortion, infertility or irregular

cycles: 10 mg twice daily from day 11–25 of the cycle.
4. For the treatment of dysmenorrhoea: 10 mg twice daily from day 5–25 of the cycle.
5. For the treatment of functional bleeding:
   a. To arrest bleeding: 10 mg twice daily together with an oestrogen for 5–7 days.
   b. To prevent bleeding: 10 mg twice daily together with an oestrogen from day 11–25 of the cycle.
6. For the treatment of amenorrhoea: 10 mg twice daily in combination with an oestrogen from day 11–25 of the cycle.
7. For the treatment of premenstrual tension: 10 mg twice daily from day 12–26 of the cycle.

Nurse monitoring
1. The Nurse monitoring aspects of progestational hormones in general are described in the section dealing with these drugs.
2. No contraindications are known to the administration of this drug.
3. Side effects are rare and the only one of note is that breakthrough bleeding may occur in a few patients.

General notes
The drug may be stored at room temperature.

E

ECONAZOLE (Ecostatin, Pevaryl)
Presentation
Cream and lotion—1%
Pessaries—150 mg
Actions and uses
Econazole is effective in the treatment of fungal infection due to candida albicans and Its main use in clinical practice is for the treatment of vaginal and vulval candidiasis (thrush).
Dosage
1. Pessaries: one pessary should be inserted at bedtime for three consecutive nights.
2. Cream: The cream should be applied twice daily, in the morning and the evening, to the ano-genital area.

Nurse monitoring
1. It is important that patients should be advised that should menstruation commence the course of treatment may be continued.
2. The nurse may play an important role in emphasising to the patient that despite disappearance of symptoms full courses of treatment should be taken.
3. Occasional local irritation may be produced giving symptoms of burning, stinging or itching.

General notes
The drug may be stored at room temperature.

EDROPHONIUM CHLORIDE (Tensilon)
Presentation
Ampoules containing 10 mg Edrophonium Chloride in 1 ml
Actions and uses
Tensilon has the same mechanism of action as Neostigmine (q.v.). It has a very short mechanism of action and its major clinical use arises when clinicians are faced with a patient who has myasthenia gravis and who is already on an anticholinergic drug, but who has developed an increase in weakness. This may be due to under- or overdosage with the anticholinergic drug and administration of Edrophonium will produce a rapid, short-lived improvement in muscle power if inadequate dosage is the cause of weakness, but it will not have this effect if the patient has already received too much anticholinergic drug. It may also be used to confirm the diagnosis of myasthenia gravis as its administration to a patient with myasthenia gravis produces a rapid and short-lived improvement in muscle power.

Dosage
1. In adults with myasthenia gravis to differentiate the cause of an increase in weakness: 10 mg is given intravenously two hours after the last dose of their treatment. If therapy has been inadequate there is a rapid, transient increase in muscle strength. If the patient has been over-treated there is a transient increase in muscle weakness.
2. As a dianostic test for myasthenia gravis: 2 mg is given intravenously initially. If no reaction occurs with 30 seconds a further 8 mg is administered.

Nurse monitoring
This drug has a very short duration of action and therefore only high dosage or prolonged administration

may lead to problems. It has the potential to produce the same problems described under the Nurse monitoring section of Neostigmine (q.v.).
General notes
The ampoule solution should be protected from light.

EMEPRONIUM BROMIDE (Cetiprin)
Presentation
Tablets—100 mg
Actions and uses
This drug has an anticholinergic action, one effect of which is to relax bladder muscle thus increasing its capacity and reducing the desire to void urine. The drug is used in clinical practice for the management of urinary frequency and incontinence in the elderly or following bladder or prostatic surgery.
Dosage
200 mg three times a day or 200–400 mg at night for nocturnal frequency.
Nurse monitoring
1. The most important side effect of this drug is that it is irritant to the gastrointestinal tract. Patients should be advised not to suck or chew tablets as this might cause ulceration of the gum and mouth tablets should not be broken up prior to administration.
2. More rarely oesophageal stricture and ulceration may be produced.
3. It is absolutely essential that patients receiving this drug maintain an adequate fluid intake and the nurse may play an important role in making sure this is achieved.
4. The anticholinergic side effects of this drug include dry mouth and blurred vision.
5. The drug should not be used in patients who suffer from glaucoma.
6. The elderly are particularly at risk of developing the problems associated with administration of this drug and it should therefore be administered to elderly patients with great caution.

General notes
The drug may be stored at room temperature.

ERGOMETRINE MALEATE
Presentation
Tablets—250 μg and 500 μg
Injection—500 μg in 1 ml
Actions and uses
This drug produces powerful rhythmic contractions of the uterus by direct action on the uterine muscle. In clinical practice it is administered in the management of third stage labour to assist in the delivery of the placenta and the cessation of bleeding, thereby reducing the risk of post-partum haemorrhage.
Dosage
1. Orally: 500 μg to 1 mg up to a maximum of 3 mg.
2. By subcutaneous, intramuscular or intravenous injection: up to 1.5 mg.

Nurse monitoring
1. Nausea and vomiting may occasionally be produced.
2. This drug should be used with caution in patients who are suffering from toxaemia of pregnancy.

General notes
1. The tablets may be stored at room temperature.
2. Injection solution should be protected from light and preferably stored in a refrigerator.

ERGOTAMINE (Migril, Cafergot)
N.B. These preparations contain Ergotamine in combination with Caffeine.
Presentation
Tablets—1 mg and 2 mg
Inhaler—0.36 mg in each metered dose
Suppositories—2 mg
Actions and uses
Migraine classically causes severe throbbing, unilateral headache. It is

caused by alteration in the cerebral blood vessels and Ergotamine in clinical practice is found to be effective in the treatment of this condition as it reverses the changes in cerebral vasculature.

Dosage
1. Orally: 1 or 2 mg repeated every 30 minutes until relief is obtained to a maximum of 6 mg in one day and 12 mg in any one week.
2. Rectally: 2 mg at the onset of an attack, repeated half-hourly to a total of 6 mg per day or 12 mg per week.
3. Inhalation: One dose repeated after five minutes if required to a total of six doses per day or 15 doses per week.

Nurse monitoring
1. If it is to be effective in the acute attack it should be administered as soon as possible after the onset of either the premonitory symptoms if they occur, or the headache.
2. This drug causes generalised vasoconstriction which may produce in minor cases coldness of the skin and limbs and in extreme cases gangrene.
3. Other side effects include nausea, vomiting, diarrhoea, dizziness, ocular disturbance, muscular weakness, confusion, anxiety, drowsiness and convulsion.
4. The drug should be used with great care in patients who suffer from heart diseases as it may produce angina, alter the blood pressure and alter the rhythm of the heart.
5. The nurse may play an important role in reminding patients that they must never exceed the maximum advised doses.

General notes
The drug may be stored at room temperature.

ERYTHROMYCIN (Erythrocin, Ilotycin, Ilosone)

(See Note 3, p. 310)
Presentation
Tablet—250 mg, 500 mg
Capsules—250 mg
Syrup—100 mg in 5 ml
   125 mg in 5 ml
   250 mg in 5 ml
   500 mg in 5 ml
Injection—100 mg in 5 ml
   (intramuscular)
   300 mg and 1 g vials
   (intravenous)

Actions and uses
Erythromycin is an antibiotic with a bacteriostatic action. This means that it inhibits growth and multiplication of bacterial cells in the body but does not kill them. It is effective principally against staphylococci and streptococci. Unfortunately resistance to Erythromycin can develop if treatment persists longer than one week. It is a useful alternative to Penicillin for the treatment of staphylococcal and streptococcal infections, when the infections have been proven to be resistant to Penicillin or when the patient is allergic to Penicillin. It is also used in the treatment of rarer infections due to mycoplasma, rickettsia, chlamydia and in the treatment of Legionnaire's disease.

Dosage
1. *Adults*:
   a. Orally: 250–500 mg four times a day.
   b. Intramuscularly: 100 mg 4–8 hourly.
   c. Intravenously: 300 mg 6-hourly or 600 mg 8 hourly. These intravenous doses may be doubled in the case of severe infection.
2. *Children*:
   Less than 1 year: 12 mg/kg orally four times day.
   1–7 years: 125–250 mg orally four times a day.
   Over 7 years: adult doses may be given.
   Intramuscular injections should be avoided in children as they usually have insufficient muscle mass to tolerate the injection. Intravenous doses in children are identical to the above oral doses.

Nurse monitoring
1. Mild gastrointestinal upset with nausea and vomiting may occur.

This may be reduced by ensuring that the tablets are taken with meals.
2. The estolate form of Erythromycin (Ilosone) has been associated with liver injury which usually manifests as fever, pain and obstructive jaundice. This occurs only very rarely but it is recommended that the dosage of Erythromycin estolate be reduced in patients with previously diagnosed liver disease.
3. Erythromycin for intravenous administration and infusion must be in a final concentration of not more than 1% i.e. 10 mg per ml. It is usually diluted in 0.9% sodium chloride or 5% dextrose.

General notes
1. The drug may be stored at room temperature.
2. Intravenous Erythromycin is prepared by adding Water for Injection to the vial before addition to infusion fluid.
3. As noted above the maximum concentration of an intravenous injection should be 10 mg per ml.

ESTRAMUSTINE (Estracyt)

Presentation
Capsules—140 mg

Actions and uses
This drug is a combination of an oestrogenic substance (oestradiol) and a cytotoxic agent (mustine). It readily concentrates in prostatic tissue and is used for the treatment of cancer of the prostate, particularly when unresponsive to conventional oestrogenic treatment.

Dosage
The daily dose may vary from 140 mg to 1400 mg and it is usually divided to be taken with meals. An average dose is of the order of 560 mg.

Nurse monitoring
1. Relatively common side effects include nausea, vomiting and diarrhoea.
2. Thrombocytopenia with resultant increased risk of haemorrhage may occur with this drug.
3. Other side effects noted have been altered liver function, gynaecomastia and increased risk of myocardial infarction.
4. This drug should be avoided in patients with active peptic ulcer disease and those with severe liver or cardiac disease.
5. It should be used with great caution in patients who already have existing impairment of bone marrow function.
6. The nurse should be constantly aware that most cytotoxic drugs are irritant to the skin and mucous surfaces, and are in general very toxic. Great care should therefore be exercised when handling these drugs, and in particular spillage or contamination of personnel or the environment must be avoided. If cytotoxic drugs are handled regularly it is theoretically possible that repeated skin contact or inhalation may produce systemic toxic effects and in nurses who have developed hypersensitivity, severe local and general hypersensitivity reactions.

General notes
Capsules of Estramustine should be stored in a refrigerator.

ETHACRYNIC ACID (Edecrin)

Presentation
Tablets—50 mg
Injection—50 mg as dry powder

Actions and uses
Ethacrynic acid is a 'loop' diuretic and has a similar mode of action and spectrum of use to Frusemide (q.v.). Ethacrynic acid has a longer duration of action than Frusemide of 6–8 hours.

Dosage
1. *Adults*:
   a. The oral adult dose range is 50–150 mg per day. Dosages of up to 400 mg may occasionally be required for the treatment of refractory oedema. Where the total daily dose exceeds 100 mg, divided

dosage regimes should be used.
b. The usual intravenous dose is 50 mg or 0.5–1 mg/kg up to a maximum of 100 mg.
2. *Children*: Oral therapy only should be used. Dosages are as follows:
Up to 1 year: 2.5 mg/kg
1–7 years: 2.5 mg/kg
7 years plus: 50 mg taken as a single dose

Nurse monitoring
1. The Nurse monitoring notes for thiazide diuretics (q.v.) are applicable to Ethacrynic acid.
2. Ethacrynic acid is a very irritant drug and should never be given by the intramuscular or subcutaneous routes.
3. Ethacrynic acid is commonly associated with hearing dysfunction including persisting deafness. For this reason it is very rarely used as a first line 'loop' diuretic and if it is used, large single doses should never be given as they produce an increased incidence of this effect.

General notes
Ethacrynic acid tablets and powder for injection may be stored at room temperature. To make up solutions for injection 50 ml sodium chloride 0.9% or dextrose 5% injections are added to the vial containing powder (occasionally dextrose solutions may produce a cloudy appearance and such solutions must be discarded.) The injection is given slowly (over several minutes) either directly or via the drip tube of a running infusion. Unused solution must be discarded after 24 hours.

ETHAMBUTOL (Myambutol)

Presentation
Tablets—100 mg, 400 mg
N.B. Ethambutol is often used in combination with Isoniazid in the preparation 'Mynah'.

Actions and uses
Ethambutol is an antibacterial drug which is of use only for the treatment of tuberculosis caused by the organism *Mycobacterium tuberculosis*. Its action may be either bacteriostatic (inhibiting growth and replication of the organism) or bacteriocidal (killing the organism), depending on the concentration achieved in the tissues. If used on its own for the treatment of tuberculosis it will be, in a large number of cases, ineffective as the organism gradually develops resistance to it and therefore it is usually used in combination with other antituberculous drugs (q.v.).

Dosage
1. For initial treatment and for prophylaxis against tuberculosis: A single daily oral dose of 25 mg/kg is recommended.
2. For maintenance treatment a single oral dose of 15 mg/kg body weight is recommended.

Nurse monitoring
1. Patients undergoing treatment for tuberculosis receive their drugs for considerable periods of time. The nurse may play an important role in reminding patients that their drug therapy must be taken regularly for as long as recommended by medical staff, whether or not they themselves feel that they have recovered.
2. Ethambutol is generally well tolerated by most patients. Rare side effects include:
   a. An optic neuritis with visual disturbance including colour blindness to green and red
   b. Gastrointestinal upset
   c. Skin rash
   d. Jaundice
   e. Peripheral neuritis
   f. Raised serum urate level (which may give rise to joint pain due to gout).
3. It is recommended that the drug be used with great caution in patients with impaired renal function, gout or reduced visual acuity. In the latter group, regular testing of visual acuity should be performed if it is decided that it is necessary to commence such a patient on Ethambutol.

General notes
The drug may be stored at room temperature.

ETHINYLOESTRADIOL

Presentation
Tablets—1, 10, 50, 100 μg and 1 mg

Actions and uses
This drug is an oestrogenic substance. In clinical practice it is used for the treatment of:
1. Menopausal symptoms
2. The suppression of lactation
3. The treatment of malignant disease of prostate and breast
4. The treatment of primary amenorrhoea
5. It is used in conjunction with a progestational agent as an oral contraceptive.

Dosage
1. For the treatment of menopausal symptoms: 10–50 μg thrice daily is given initially and subsequent maintenance doses range from 10–20 μg per day.
2. For the suppression of lactation: 100 μg is given twice daily for three days, reducing to 50 μg twice daily for six days.
3. For the treatment of malignant disease of prostate and breast: Between 1 and 3 mg is given daily.
4. For the treatment of primary amenorrhoea: 10–50 μg is given thrice daily for 14 consecutive days every four weeks.

Nurse monitoring
See the section on oestrogenic hormones

General notes
The drug may be stored at room temperature.

ETHOSUXIMIDE (Zarontin, Emeside)

Presentation
Capsules—250 mg
Syrup—250 mg in 5 ml

Actions and uses
1. The actions and uses of anticonvulsant drugs in general are discussed in the section on these drugs.
2. Ethosuximide is particularly useful for the treatment of petit mal epilepsy.

Dosage
N.B. Individaul dosage requirements vary greatly. The following doses are given as a guide only.
1. *Adults*: The usual maintenance dose range is 1–1.5 g daily.
2. *Children*: An initial dose of 250 mg is recommended in children less than 6 years and 500 mg in children older than 6 years. The dose should thereafter be gradually increased until an optimum response is achieved.

Nurse monitoring
1. See Nurse monitoring aspects in the section on anticonvulsant drugs in general.
2. Gastrointestinal upset including nausea, vomiting and anorexia commonly occur with this drug.
3. Neurological effects are fairly common and include drowsiness, lethargy, euphoria, dizziness, headache and behavioural disorders such as restlessness, agitation, anxiety and aggression.
4. Skin rashes and disorders of the blood may rarely occur.

General notes
The drug may be stored at room temperature.

ETHOTOIN (Peganone)

Presentation
Tablets—500 mg

Actions and uses
The actions and uses of anticonvulsant drugs in general are discussed in the section on these drugs.

Dosage
N.B. Individual dosage requirements vary greatly. The following doses are given as a guide only.
1. *Adults*: An initial total dose of 1 g per day is given and is gradually increased until the disorder is controlled. The usual

maintenance dose range for adults is 2–3 g per day in total. The total daily dose is usally divided and given up to four or six times per day.
2. *Children*: An initial total daily dose of 500 mg is recommended and 1 g per day in total is usually found to be adequate for younger age groups. The total daily dose is usually divided and given four to six times daily.

Nurse monitoring
1. See the Nurse monitoring aspects in the section on anticonvulsant drugs in general.
2. Ethotoin is a member of the same group as Phenytoin and therefore the Nurse monitoring aspects of this drug (q.v.) are applicable to Ethotoin.

General notes
The drug may be stored at room temperature.

F

FENBUFEN (Lederfren)

Presentation
Capsules—300 mg
Tablets—300 mg

Actions and uses
See the section on non-steroidal anti-inflammatory analgesic drugs.

Dosage
The usual adult dose is 600 mg at night and 300 mg in the morning.

Nurse monitoring
See the section on anti-inflammatory analgesic drugs, non-steroidal.

General notes
Fenbufen capsules and tablets may be stored at room temperature.

FENFLURAMINE (Ponderax)

Presentation
Tablets—20 mg and 40 mg
Capsules—60 mg sustained release

Actions and uses
Anorexogenic drugs abolish hunger by a direct action on the central nervous system. They are thought to have a supplementary effect in that they increase the ability to perform mental and physical work without the need for increased food intake.

Dosage
1. *Adults*: Either
   a. 20–40 mg twice or three times daily half an hour before meals or
   b. 60–120 mg once daily of the slow release capsules taken before breakfast.
2. *Children*:
   Less than 6 years: This drug should not be given.
   6–10 years: One 20 mg tablet daily.
   10 years and over: 20 mg twice a day.

Nurse monitoring
1. Perhaps the most important point to note about Fenfluramine is that although it, like other anorexogenic drugs, is a member of the amphetamine group, it does not produce the neurological effects of drugs of this group and it, therefore, does not produce dependence or addiction and is unlikely to be abused in this way.
2. The drug is contraindicated for the treatment of patients who have recently received or are at present receiving treatment with monoamine oxidase inhibiting drugs (q.v.).
3. Patients should be warned that the mild sedative effect of this drug will be markedly increased if alcohol is taken.
4. The mild sedative effect on its own may occasionally impair driving skills and again patients should be warned of this potential effect.
5. The drug is not recommended for the treatment of patients who have a history of depressive illness.
6. Side effects which include sedation, dizziness, diarrhoea, nausea and headache may be minimised by initiating treatment with low doses and subsequently increasing doses gradually.

General notes
The drug may be stored at room temperature.

FENOPROFEN (Fenopron)

Presentation
Tablets—300 mg, 600 mg
Actions and uses
See the section on non-steroidal anti-inflammatory analgesic drugs.
Dosage
The usual adult dose is 300–600 mg three or four times day.
Nurse monitoring
See the section on anti-inflammatory analgesic drugs, non-steroidal.
General notes
Fenoprofen tables may be stored at room temperature.

FENOTEROL (Berotec)

Presentation
Inhaler—200 micrograms/dose of metered aerosol
Nebuliser solution–0.5%
Actions and uses
This drug has a highly selective action on receptors in bronchial muscle causing relaxation of muscle tone. It is used, therefore, for the treatment of reversible airways obstruction (bronchospasm) in asthma and other conditions such as bronchitis and emphysema.
Dosage
By inhalation:
1. One or two inhalations (metered doses) three times a day using the pressurised inhaler.
2. 0.1–0.5 ml of nebuliser solution may be inhaled up to four times a day for the control of acute, severe, symptoms.

It should be noted that this drug has a long duration of action.
Nurse monitoring
1. Rarely this drug may cause palpitation, tachycardia, headache and fine muscle tremor.
2. The drug should be used with great care in patients suffering from heart disease, hypertension or hyperthyroidism.
3. The drug should be used with great care if patients are receiving monoamine oxidase inhibitors or tricyclic antidepressants.

General notes
1. The pressurised aerosol should be stored at room temperature.
2. The container should never be punctured or incinerated at the end of use.

FERROUS FUMARATE

Presentation

Name	Also Contains
B.C. 500 with Iron	Vitamins B and C
Co-Ferol	Folic acid
Ferrocap	Vitamin B
Ferrocap-F 350	Folic Acid
Fersaday	
Fersamal	
Folex 350	Folic Acid
Galfer	
Gerifit	Vitamins B and C
Givitol	Vitamins B and C + Folic Acid
Pregaday	Folic Acid

Actions and uses
See the section on Irons (oral).
Dosage
300 mg of Ferrous Fumarate contains 100 mg of elemental iron.
1. For the treatment of iron deficiency anaemia:
    a. *Adults*: 300 mg of Ferrous Fumarate twice daily.
    b. *Children*:
    Less than 1 year: 100–150 mg of Ferrous Fumarate per day.
    1–7 years: 200–300 mg per day.
    Over 7 years: 300–450 mg per day.
    Children over 12 years should receive the adult dose.
2. For the prevention of iron deficiency anaemia during pregnancy: 300 mg of Ferrous Fumarate once per day.

Nurse monitoring
See the section of Irons (oral).
General notes
Most iron tablets may be stored safely at room temperatures.

FERROUS GLUCONATE
Presentation

Name	Also Contains
Ferfolic	Vitamins B and C + Folic Acid
Fergluvite	Vitamins B and C
Fergon	
Sidros	Vitamin C

Actions and uses
See the section on Irons (oral).

Dosage
900 mg of Ferrous Gluconate contains 100 mg of elemental iron.
1. For the treatment of iron deficiency anaemia:
   a. *Adults*: 900–1800 mg of Ferrous Gluconate per day.
   b. *Children*:
      Less than 1 year: 225–450 mg of Ferrous Gluconate per day.
      1–7 years: 450–700 mg of Ferrous Gluconate per day.
      7–12 years: 750–900 mg of Ferrous Gluconate per day.
      Over 12: Adult doses apply.
2. For the prevention of iron deficiency anaemia in pregnancy 900 mg of Ferrous Gluconate per day.

Nurse monitoring
See the section on Irons (oral).

General notes
Most iron tablets may be stored safely at room temperature.

FERROUS SUCCINATE
Presentation

Name	Also Contains
Ferromyn	
Ferromyn B	Vitamin B
Feeromyn S	Succinic acid
Ferromyn S Folic	Succinic acid + Folic acid

Actions and uses
See the section on Irons (oral).

Dosage
280 mg of Ferrous Succinate contains 100 mg elemental iron.
1. For the treatment of iron deficiency anaemia:
   a. *Adults*: 280–560 mg of Ferrous Succinate per day.
   b. *Children*:
      Less than 1 year: 70–140 mg of Ferrous Succinate per day.
      1–7 years: 140–210 mg of Ferrous Succinate per day.
      7–12 years: 210–280 mg of Ferrous Succinate per day.
      Over 12: Adult doses apply.
2. For the prevention of iron deficiency anaemia in pregnancy: 280 mg of Ferrous Succinate per day.

Nurse monitoring
See the section on Irons (oral).

General notes
Most iron tablets may be stored safely at room temperature.

FERROUS SULPHATE

Proprietary preparations containing Ferrous Sulphate are:

Name	Also Contains
Feac	Vitamins B and C
Fe-Cap	Glycine
Fe-Cap C	Glycine + Vitamin C
Fe-Cap Folic	Glycine + Folic Acid
Fefol	Folic Acid
Fefol Vit	Folic Acid + Vitamins B and C
Feospan	
Ferraplex B	Vitamins B & C + minerals
Ferrlecit 100	Vitamin C + Citrate
Ferrocontin	Glycine
Ferrocontin Folic	Glycine + Folic Acid
Ferrograd C	Vitamin C
Ferrograd Folic	Folic Acid
Ferro-Gradumet	
Fesovit	Vitamins B and C
Folicin	Folic Acid + Minerals
Folvron	Folic Acid
Gastrovite	Glycin + Vitamin C + Vitamin D + Calcium
Iberet 500	Vitamins B and C + liver extract (B12)
Irofol C	Folic Acid + Vitamin C

Kelferon	Glycine
Kelfolate	Glycine + Folic Acid
Plesmet	Glycine
Pregfol	Folic Acid
Pregnavite Forte	Vitamins C + D + B + Calcium
Pregnavite Forte F	Vitamins C + D + B + Calcium + Folic Acid
Slow Fe	
SlowFeFolic	Folic Acid

Actions and uses
The actions and uses of Ferrous Sulphate are identical to those described for iron (q.v.).

Dosage
200 mg of Ferrous Sulphate dried contains 60 mg of elemental iron; 300 mg of Ferrous Sulphate contains 60 mg of ferrous iron. The appropriate daily dosage is therefore as follows:
1. For the treatment of iron deficiency anaemia:
   a. *Adults*: Ferrous Sulphate 300 mg two of three times a day Ferrous sulphate dried: 200 mg two to three times a day
   b. *Children*:
      Less than 1 year: 100–150 mg of Ferrous Sulphate per day
      1–7 years: 200–300 mg per day
      Over 7 years: 300–450 mg per day
      Children over 12 years should receive the adult dose
2. For the prevention of iron deficiency anaemia during pregnancy: 300 mg two or three times per day of Ferrous Sulphate is advised.

Nurse monitoring
See the section on Irons (oral).

General notes
Most iron tablets may be stored safely at room temperature.

FLAVOXATE (Urispas)

Presentation
Tablets—100 mg

ons and uses
This drug has anticholinergic actions which in clinical pratice make it useful for the treatment of disorders associated with spasm of the smooth muscle of the lower urinary tract. It is used in the treatment of dysuria, urgency, nocturia and painful spasm of the bladder due to catheterisation or cystoscopy.

Dosage
100–200 mg three times a day in adults.

Nurse monitoring
1. Due to its anticholinergic action the drug produces dry mouth and blurred vision and should not be used in patients who suffer from glaucoma.
2. The drug is contraindicated in patients who have gastrointestinal obstruction.
3. Common side effects experienced by the patient include nausea, headache and fatigue.

General notes
The drug should be stored at room temperature.

FLUCLOROLONE (Topilar)

Presentation
Cream and ointment—0.025%

Actions and uses
This potent corticosteroid (q.v.) is used topically in the treatment of inflammatory skin conditions such as psoriasis, eczema and dermatitis.

Dosage
Cream and ointment are applied sparingly once or twice per day.

Nurse monitoring
Although used topically, sufficient may be absorbed through the skin for this drug to produce some or all of the side effects described in the section on corticosteroids.

General notes
1. Fluclorolone ointment and cream may be stored at room temperature but excessively warm storage areas should be avoided.
2. Dilution with other creams may alter the stability of the drug and are therefore contraindicated;

however, white soft paraffin may be used if necessary.

FLUCLOXACILLIN (Floxapen)

(See Note 3, p. 310)
Presentation
Capsules—250 mg, 500 mg
Syrup—125 mg in 5 ml
Injection—Vials containing 250 mg and 500 mg

Actions and uses
Flucloxacillin is a member of the Penicillin group of antibiotics and has the same actions and uses as those described for Benzylpenicillin (q.v.). It has a number of important advantages over Benzylpenicillin and these are as follows:
1. It is very well absorbed from the gut and therefore is indicated when oral treatment is desired.
2. It is often highly effective against organisms especially of the staphylococcal group which are likely to be resistant to Benzylpenicillin.

Dosage
1. *Adults*:
   a. Orally: 250–500 mg four times a day
   b. Intramuscular or intravenous: 250–500 mg four times a day.
   c. Intrapleural and intra-articular: 250–500 mg per day.
2. *Children*:
   Less than 2 years: one-quarter of the adult dose.
   Over 2 years: one-half of the adult dose

Nurse monitoring
See the section on Benzylpenicillin.

General notes
1. Preparations containing Flucloxacillin may be stored at room temperature
2. Once reconstituted injection solutions must be used immediately
3. Once reconstituted the syrup should be used within seven days
4. Injections are prepared as follows:
   a. For intramuscular injection: The vials should be diluted with 1.5–2 ml of Water for Injection
   b. For intravenous injection: 1 g should be dissolved in 20 ml of Water for Injection and given either directly over 3–4 minutes or added to 0.9% sodium chloride, 5% dextrose or dextrose/saline mixtures and infused over 4–6 hours
   c. For intra-articular or intrapleural injection: The vials should be diluted with 5–10 ml of Water for Injection.

FLUCYTOSINE (Alcobon)

Presentation
Tablets—500 mg
Intravenous infusion—2.5 g in 250 ml

Actions and uses
This drug is effective in the treatment of certain systemic fungal infections. It acts by inhibiting the production of a crucial component necessary for fungal growth and development. It is indicated for the treatment of systemic infections with *Crytococcus neoformans*, *Candida albicans* and other candida species, *Torulopsis glabrata*, *hansenula, chromomycosis* and other rare fungal diseases.

Dosage
The total daily dose in adults and children is 200 mg/kg body weight divided into four doses. It should be administered via the giving set provided which contains a special filter. It may be administered directly into a vein, through a central venous catheter or by intraperitoneal infusion. The duration of each section of the infusion should be of the order of 20–40 minutes. It should be noted that recommendations are produced by the manufacturers giving recommendations of total daily dosage related to creatinine clearance (an indication of renal function). It should be noted that

the total daily dose by either oral or intravenous route is identical.

Nurse monitoring
1. The drug should never be given to patients with severe renal failure unless blood levels of the drug can be monitored.
2. Disease of the bone marrow is a relative contraindication to the use of this drug.
3. Nausea, vomiting, diarrhoea, skin rash, thrombocytopenia and bone marrow suppression may occur.
4. Tests of liver function may be altered by administration of this drug.

General notes
1. Infusions are supplied ready for use by direct request to the manufacturers.
2. Storage conditions for both tablets and infusion are critical. The tablets should be stored in a well-closed container, protected against moisture and light. The infusion should be stored between 15 and 20°C. Deviation outside this range in either direction will lead to degeneration and render the infusion useless.

FLUDROCORTISONE (Florinef)

Presentation
Tablets—0.1 mg, 1 mg

Actions and uses
Fludrocortisone is a corticosteroid drug which has primarily mineralocorticoid actions. It is therefore not used for the indications described under corticosteroid rugs (q.v.). Its only use in clinical practice is in the treatment of disorders associated with deficiency of adrenal gland function such as Addison's disease.

Dosage
For replacement of mineralocorticoid function in Addison's disease 0.1 mg daily or on alternative days is given. Adequacy of dosage is monitored by checking the urea and electrolytes and blood pressure of the patient under treatment.

Nurse monitoring
1. Fludrocortisone has mainly mineralocorticoid actions. A deficiency of replacement treatment will be manifest by weakness, nausea, vomiting, hypotension and in extreme cases shock and excessive dosage will be manifest by hypertension and hyperkalaemia. Both an excess and deficiency of Fludrocortisone are highly dangerous situations and constitute a medical emergency requiring immediate further assessment in hospital.
2. It is worth noting that very few patients require more than 0.1 mg per day for replacement treatment in diseases such as Addison's disease. If these patients are accidentally given 1 mg per day they may becomes severely ill and die. The only indication for using 1 mg tablets is in very rare circumstances where suppression of adrenal gland over-activity is required.

General notes
Fludrocortisone tablets may be stored at room temperature.

FLUNITRAZEPAM (Rohypnol)

Presentation
Tablets—1 mg

Actions and uses
Flunitrazepam is a benzodiazepine and the section on these drugs should be consulted for a brief general account. It has a marked sedative effect and is taken as a hypnotic, to induce sleep. Of particular interest is the short action of this drug in the body which tends to produce a normal length sleep of up to 8 hours without the hang-over effect which occasionally extends into the following day with other hypnotics.

Dosage
Adults: 0.5 mg to 1 mg taken on retiring. Elderly patients should receive the lower dosage.

Nurse monitoring
See the section on benzodiazepines.

General notes
Tablets containing flunitrazepam may be stored at room temperature.

FLUOCINOLONE (Synandone, Synalar)
Presentation
Ointment and cream—0.01%, 0.025%, 0.2%
Gel—0.025%
Lotion—0.025%
Actions and uses
This potent corticosteroid (q.v.) is used topically fo-, for the treatment of inflammatory skin conditions such as psoriasis, eczema and dermatitis.
Dosage
Cream or ointment is applied sparingly to the affected area four times daily.
Nurse monitoring
Although applied topically, significant absorption through the skin may occur and produce some or all of the side effects described in the section on corticosteroids.
General notes
1. Preparations containing Fluocinolone should be stored in a cool, dry place.
2. The stability of the drug may be markedly altered by dilution with other ointments, creams or lotions.

FLUOCINONIDE (Metosyn)
Presentation
Cream and ointment—0.05%
Actions and uses
This potent corticosteroid (q.v.) is used topically for the treatment of inflammatory skin conditions such as psoriasis, eczema, dermatitis.
Dosage
Cream or ointment is applied sparingly to the affected area one to four times daily.
Nurse monitoring
Although Fluocinonide is applied topically, sufficient absorption may occur through the skin to produce some or all of the effects described in the section on corticosteroids.
General notes
1. The cream may be stored at room temperature but warm areas, such as around a radiator should be avoided.
2. If absolutely necessary the ointment may be diluted with white soft paraffin but other creams and ointments should not be mixed with Fluocinonide.

FLUOCORTOLONE (Ultradil)
Presentation
Ointment and cream—a mixture of the pivalate and hexanoate esters containing 0.1% and 0.25% of each.
Actions and uses
This moderately potent corticosteroid (q.v.) is used topically for the treatment of inflammatory skin conditions such as psoriasis, eczema and dermatitis.
Dosage
Ointment or cream is applied sparingly to the affected area one to three times daily.
Nurse monitoring
Although applied topically, significant amounts of this drug may be absorbed through the skin to produce some or all of the side effects described in the section on corticosteroids.
General notes
1. Fluocortolone ointment and cream should be stored in a cool, dry place.
2. These preparations may be used for up to five years from the date of manufacture.

FLUOXYMESTERONE (Ultandren)
Presentation
Tablets—5 mg
Actions and uses
1. For a description of the actions and uses of this drug see the section on adrogenic and anabolic steroids.
2. Fluoxymesterone in clinical practice has two main uses:
   a. For the treatment of hypogonadism in males
   b. For the treatment of breast cancer in females.

Dosage
This depends on the condition under treatment and individual response.
Nurse monitoring
See the section on androgens and anabolic steroids.
General notes
The drug may be stored at room temperature.

FLUPENTHIOXOL (Depixol, Fluanxol)
Presentation
Tablets—0.5 mg and 1 mg (as dihydrochloride)
Injection — 20 mg in 1 ml
40 mg in 2 ml
200 mg in 10 ml (all as decanoate)
Actions and uses
Flupenthixol is a neuroleptic and antidepressant drug used for its tranquillising or calming effect in the management of patients with severe behavioural disorders including depression. It shares many of the actions and uses described for phenothiazine major tranquillisers in the section on phenothiazines.
Dosage
Adults:
1. 1–2 mg by the oral route once daily or up to 6 mg daily in 2 divided doses.
2. As a long acting intramuscular depot injection it is administered every 2–4 weeks in doses of 20–40 mg or more.

Nurse monitoring
See the section on Phenothiazines.
General notes
Flupenthixol tablets and injection should be stored at room temperature.

FLUPHENAZINE (Modecate, Moditen)
Presentation
Tablets—1 mg, 2.5 mg, 5 mg (as hydrochloride)
Elixir—0.5 mg in 1 ml (hydrochloride)
Injection—25 mg in 1 ml: 0.5 ml, 1 ml, 2 ml and 10 ml oil injection as the decanoate or enanthate
Actions and uses
Fluphenazine is a member of the phenothiazine group of drugs and its actions and uses are described in the section on these drugs. It may be taken orally or more frequently it is administered by deep intramuscular injection. The latter method of administration ensures a prolonged effect lasting several days to some weeks. The use of long-acting intramuscular preparations of Fluphenazine allows many schizophrenic patients to be treated at home with their drug being administered at regular clinic visits.
Dosage
1. *Adults*:
   a. Orally: 1–4 mg daily as a single daily dose
   b. By deep intramuscular injection: 25 mg is administered in a single dose at intervals varying between 10 days and 4 weeks according to clinical effect.
2. *Children*:
   a. Orally for behavioural disorders: 0.25–1 mg per day is given.

Nurse monitoring
1. The Nurse monitoring points on Fluphenazine are identical to those described for phenothiazines (q.v.).
2. The muscle twitching and tremors described in the section on Fluphenazine which occur as side effects of phenothiazines are particularly likely to occur with this drug and usually occur with this drug and usually require treatment with anti-Parkinsonian preparations.

General notes
1. Preparations containing Fluphenazine may be stored at room temperature.
2. Oral liquid and solution for injection must be protected from direct sunlight.

FLUPREDNYLIDENE (Decoderm)
Presentation
Cream—0.1%
Actions and uses
This corticosteroid drug (q.v.) is

normally only used as a topical application in the treatment of inflammatory skin disorders such as psoriasis, eczema and dermatitis.

Dosage
The cream is applied sparingly to the affected area one to three times per day.

Nurse monitoring
Although applied topically to the skin, sufficient may be absorbed for all the effects of corticosteroids (q.v.) described to occur.

General notes
The cream may be stored at room temperature.

FLURANDRENOLONE (Haelan)

Presentation
Cream and ointment—0.0125%, 0.05%

Actions and uses
A moderately potent corticosteroid (q.v.) which is applied topically for the treatment of inflammatory skin conditions e.g. psoriasis, eczema, dermatitis etc.

Dosage
Apply sparingly two or three times daily to the affected area.

Nurse monitoring
Although applied topically, significant amounts of this drug may be absorbed to produce some or all of the side effects described in the section on corticosteroids.

General notes
1. Flurandrenolone cream and ointment should be stored at room temperature.
2. If necessary these preparations may be diluted with aqueous cream B.P. (in the case of cream) or for ointment, white soft paraffin B.P.

FLURAZEPAM (Dalmane)

Presentation
Capsules—15 mg, 30 mg

Actions and uses
Flurazepam is a benzodiazepine drug (q.v.). Its marked sedative action makes it useful for use at night as an hypnotic.

Dosage
15–30 mg taken on retiring

Nurse monitoring
See the section on benzodiazepines.

General notes
Preparations containing Flurazepam may be stored at room temperature.

FLURBIPROFEN (Froben)

Presentation
Tablets—50 mg, 100 mg

Actions and uses
See the section on non-steroidal anti-inflammatory analgesic drugs.

Dosage
The usual adult dose is 150–200 mg daily in three or four divided doses.

Nurse monitoring
See the section on anti-inflammatory analgesic drugs, non-steroidal.

General notes
Flurbiprofen tablets may be stored at room temperature.

FOLIC ACID

Presentation
Folic acid is available in a number of preparations either alone or in combination with iron and other vitamins.

Actions and uses
Folic acid is indicated for the treatment of megaloblastic anaemia (anaemia associated with large immature red cells in the blood). This type of anaemia may be produced by:
1. Nutritional deficiency
2. Pregnancy
3. Malabsorption.

Dosage
1. In the treatment of megaloblastic anaemia: Initially 10–20 mg a day for 14 days. Subsequently 5–10 mg per day.
2. For the prophylaxis of megaloblastic anaemia in pregnancy: 200–500 μg daily.

Nurse monitoring

No problems are encountered with the administration of this drug. An important point to note which primarily concerns medical staff is that when a megaloblastic anaemia is identified, folic acid should never be instituted prior to the elucidation of its cause as administration of folic acid to patients with megaloblastic anaemia due to vitamin B^{12} deficiency (q.v.) may be highly dangerous and cause severe and irreversible neurological symptoms.

FRUSEMIDE (Lasix)

Presentation
Tablets—20 mg, 40 mg, 500 mg
Injections — 20 mg in 2 ml
　　　　　　 50 mg in 5 ml
　　　　　　 250 mg in 25 ml
Paediatric liquid—1 mg in 1 ml

Actions and uses

All diuretics act on the kidney to increase excretion of water and electrolytes from the body. The functional unit of the kidney is called a nephron and is composed of a glomerulus and a tubule. The tubule has four sections, each of which has different functions. They are known as the proximal tubule, the loop of Henle, the distal tubule and the collecting tubule. Frusemide is the best known and most commonly used of the diuretics known as 'loop' diuretics. This particular group act on the loop of Henle and inhibit electrolyte and therefore water reabsorption. Diuretics which act on the loop of Henle tend to have a rapid onset of action and a much more marked diuresis than diuretics acting at other parts of the tubule. The indications for use of Frusemide therefore are in situations where a rapid loss of body salt and water is necessary such as acute left heart failure with pulmonary oedema, or where milder diuretics have proved ineffective. It is worth noting that Frusemide is not as effective in the management of hypertension as other thiazide type diuretics (q.v.).

Dosage

1. *Adults*:
   a. Intravenous injection in emergency situations. The usual initial dose is between 40 and 250 mg depending on the severity of the problem and response to previous doses.
   b. Intramuscular Frusemide may be given in emergency situations or where oral treatment is contraindicated, in equivalent doses to the intravenous dose.
   c. Oral dosage: Daily dosage is usually given once per day in the morning. Initial dosage is usually 40 mg, the dose being increased until an appropriate clinical response has been achieved. It is worth noting that doses of up to 2 g orally or 1 g intravenously may be given in patients with chronic renal failure.
2. Children's doses are as follows:
   1 year or less: 1–2 mg/kg
   1–5 years: 10–20 mg
   6–12 years: 20–40 mg
   Intramuscular or intravenous doses should be half of the recommended oral dose.

Nurse monitoring

1. The Nurse monitoring notes for thiazide diuretics (q.v.) are applicable to Frusemide.
2. When high doses of Frusemide are given transient deafness may occur.
3. Acute renal failure may be precipitated if Frusemide and other 'loop' diuretics are used in combination with cephalosporin antibiotics

General notes

Frusemide tablets, liquid and injection may be stored at room temperature. The injection solution is sensitive to light and is therefore packed in amber coloured ampoules. Other drugs must never be mixed with Frusemide injection in the same syringe and the drug should not be added to dextrose solutions before infusion. The recommended solutions for infusion are sodium chloride 0.9% injection or compound sodium lactate (Ringers) injection: the rate of infusion must not exceed 4 mg/minute.

FUSIDIC ACID/SODIUM FUSIDATE (Fucidin)

(See Note 3, p. 310)

Presentation
Capsules—250 mg
Tablets—250 mg (enteric coated)
Suspension—250 mg in 5 ml
Injection—500 mg vials with 50 ml diluent
Ointment—2%
Gel—2%
Medicated gauze dressing—2%

Actions and uses
Fucidin is an antibiotic which has been found to be particularly effective against staphylococcal infections. It has the advantage that it may be given to patients who are sensitive to Penicillin and in addition it is particularly good at penetrating most tissues including importantly bone. It has the disadvantage that when used alone bacteria rapidly become resistant to it and it is therefore often used in combination with other antibiotics such as Erythromycin (q.v.) or Novobiocin (q.v.). It is used in all types of staphylococcal infection including skin infection, wound infection, pneumonia, septicaemia, osteomyelitis and endocarditis.

Dosage
1. Oral:
   a. *Adults*: 500 mg–1 g three times a day.
   b. *Children*:
      Less than 1 year: 50 mg/kg body weight in total daily in three divided doses
      1–5 years: 250 mg three times per day
      5–12 years: 500 mg three times per day
2. Intravenous injection:
   a. *Adults*: 2 g in total per day in three or four divided doses.
   b. *Children*: 20 mg/kg per day in total usually given in three divided doses.
3. The ointment, gel or medicated gauze dressing should be applied to topical infections three or four times daily if uncovered and less frequently if covered.

Nurse monitoring
1. The drug itself is associated with very few side effects other than some reports of jaundice. It is usually recommended that patients with liver dysfunction or those receiving high doses of the drug should have periodic liver function tests performed.
2. The major Nurse monitoring aspects of this drug lie in the problems that may arise with the administration of Fucidin in its various forms:
   a. Fucidin for injection should never be given intramuscularly or subcutaneously as severe local tissue reaction and injury may occur.
   b. Fucidin may be infused in sodium chloride and it has also been given safely in plasma and 5% dextrose. Higher concentrations of dextrose lead to an opalescence being formed by the infusion of the drug and it is recommended that such infusions be discontinued.
   c. Fucide should not be infused with amino acid infusions or in whole blood.

General notes
1. The drug may be stored at room temperature.
2. Suspension should be protected from direct light.
3. After reconstitution the injection should be discarded if unused after 24 hours.
4. Powder for injections should be reconstituted with the diluent provided and it is customary to then dilute it in 500 ml of either normal saline or 5% dextrose and infuse over 2–4 hours or longer. Other problems with Fucidin for infusion are discussed above.

G

GENTAMICIN (Genticin, Cidomycin)

(See Note 3, p. 310)

Presentation
Injection—20 mg in 2 ml
80 mg in 2 ml
120 mg in 1.5 ml
1 mg and 5 mg in 1 ml (intrathecal)
Powder—1 mg (sterile) for preparation of intrathecal injections
Ointment—3 mg in 1 g (0.3%)
Cream—3 mg in 1 g (0.3%)
Eye/ear drops—0.3% in 10 ml dropper

Actions and uses
1. The actions and uses of aminoglycoside antibiotics in general are discussed in the section on these drugs.
2. Superficial infections of the eye, ear and skin may be effectively treated by topical applications.

Dosage
1. For systemic infection:
   a. *Adults*: The usual adult dose is 80 mg given 8-hourly by intramuscular or intravenous injection.
   b. Children receive a dose calculated on the basis of 2 mg/kg body weight 8-hourly. Blood levels of gentamicin may now be measured in most major centres and it is customary to adjust the dose according to the results of these investigations. By doing this the incidence of serious side effects has been reduced.
2. Dosage of topical applications are as follows:
   a. Gentamicin cream and Gentamicin ointment should be applied to the skin three to four times daily.
   b. Gentamicin eye and ear drops:
      i. 1–3 drops should be instilled into the affected eye 3–4 times daily or more frequently if required.
      ii. 2–4 ear drops should be instilled 3–4 times per day and at night.

Nurse monitoring
See the section on aminoglycoside antibiotics.

General notes
1. Preparations containing Gentamicin may be stored at room temperature.
2. The drug should never be mixed with other antibiotics prior to administration.

GLIBENCLAMIDE (Euglucon, Daonil)

Presentation
Tablets—5 mg, 2.5 mg

Actions and uses
See the section on hypoglycaemic drugs, oral (1).

Dosage
For adults: An initial dose of 2.5–5 mg is advised with gradual increments to a total of 20 mg as a single morning dose.

Nurse monitoring
See the section on hypoglycaemic drugs, oral (1).

General notes
Tablets may be stored at room temperature.

GLIBORNURIDE (Glutril)

Presentation
Tablets—25 mg
Actions and uses
See the section on hypoglycaemic drugs, oral (1).
Dosage
An initial dose of 12.5 mg is advised with gradual increments to a total dose of 50 mg daily. Doses are taken once daily or divided into a morning and evening dose.
Nurse monitoring
See the section on oral hypoglycaemic drugs (1).
General notes
Tablets may be stored at room temperature.

GLICLAZIDE (Diamicron)

Presentation
Tablets—80 mg
Actions and uses
See the section on hypoglycaemic drugs, oral (1).
Dosage
40–80 mg initially, increasing up to 320 mg daily.
Nurse monitoring
See the section on hypoglycaemic drugs, oral (1).
General notes
Tablets may be stored at room temperature.

GLIPIZIDE (Glibenese, Minodiab)

Presentation
Tablets—5 mg
Actions and uses
See the section on hypoglycaemic drugs, oral (1).
Dosage
An initial dose of 2.5–5 mg is advised with gradual increments to a total of 30 mg daily. Daily doses above 10 mg are given in 2–3 divided doses.
Nurse monitoring
See the section on hypoglycaemic drugs, oral (1).
General notes
Tablets may be stored at room temperature.

GLIQUIDONE (Glurenorm)

Presentation
Tablets—30 mg
Actions and uses
See the section on oral hypoglycaemic drugs (1).
Dosage
45–60 mg daily (maximum 180 mg) taken before meals.
Nurse monitoring
See the section on oral hypoglycaemic drugs (1).
General notes
Tablets may be stored at room temperature.

GLYCERYL TRINITRATE (Nitrocine, Nitrocontin, Nitrolingual, Percutol, Suscard, Sustac, Transiderm-Nitro, Tridil)

Presentation
Sublingual tablets—500 μg and 600 μg
Slow release tablets—2.6 mg and 6.4 mg
Sublingual aerosol spray—400 μg per metered dose
Buccal tablets—1 mg, 2 mg, 3 mg and 5 mg
Ointment—2%
Skin patches—5 mg and 10 mg
Injection — 5 mg in 10 ml
10 mg in 10 ml
50 mg in 10 ml
50 mg in 50 ml
Actions and uses
Glyceryl trinitrate reduces the work of the heart by a complex process. It would appear that its major action is the result of venous dilatation and reduction in the return of blood to the right side of the heart. This leads to a subsequent reduction in the amount of blood the heart pumps and therefore a reduction in the work that it performs. It is used to treat acute attacks of angina

pectoris and also prophylactically particularly before exercise which would normally produce angina. The reduction in the venous return to the heart which glyceryl trinitrate produces gives the drug a further use in treatment of severe congestive cardiac failure (often secondary to acute myocardial infarction) and for this purpose intravenous infusions are administered.

A bewildering range of different preparations are available. For acute attacks of angina a sublingual tablet is placed under the tongue and sucked vigorously in this position. Alternatively a metered dose is sprayed into the mouth.

For prophylaxis, the drug may be sucked or chewed, stuck to the gum, swallowed whole, sprayed into the mouth, smeared on the skin or stuck to the skin.

Dosage
1. Acute attacks of angina: One sublingual tablet (500 µg or 600 µg) administered as described above, or one metered dose (400 µg) sprayed into the mouth.
2. Prophylaxis of angina:
   a. Sublingual route: One tablet held under the tongue immediately before exercise.
   b. Buccal route: One tablet (1, 2, 3 or 5 mg) stuck to the gum.
   c. Topical route: One dose of ointment (measured on a special ruler) smeared onto the skin or one skin patch applied to skin.
3. Intravenous route (for the treatment of heart failure): the dose range varies according to the individual response and is in the range 10–200 µg/minute infused in 5% dextrose or 0.9% sodium chloride.

Nurse monitoring
The nurse may contribute greatly towards the management of patients on this drug as follows.
1. She should ensure that the patient knows exactly how a particular form of the drug is administered, particularly when confusion exists due to the variety of alternatives available.
2. Patients may dislike using preparations containing glyceryl trinitrate because of the side effects of flushing, headaches, syncope and hypotension which are all due to an extension of the pharmacological activity of the drug. Often, however, these effects diminish with continued use of the drug. If they occur after sublingual tablets are sucked during an acute attack of angina, patients should be instructed to terminate the action of the drug by spitting out or swallowing the tablet once the angina is relieved.
3. Should an attack of angina be unresponsive to one or two doses of glyceryl trinitrate and should its duration exceed 15 minutes, a myocardial infarction should be suspected and medical assessment and appropriate treatment must be organised.
4. Tablets deteriorate with age, and may become ineffective. Loss of a bitter taste in the mouth may give an indication that this has occurred. This is especially important to note in patients who only rarely require to use the drug.

GLYCOPYRROLATE (Robinul)

Presentation
Tablets—2 mg
Powder—for reconstitution with saline solution

Actions and uses
1. It has an anticholinergic effect identical to that described for Poldine Sulphate (q.v.) and is used in the treatment of peptic ulceration.
2. This drug may be given as an application to the skin to reduce excess sweating.

Dosage
1. Peptic ulceration: The adult dose is 1–4 mg two to three times per day.

2. For hyperhydrosis a 0.05% solution in distilled water is used.

Nurse monitoring
The Nurse monitoring notes on this anticholinergic drug are identical to those for Hyoscine-N-Butylbromine (Buscopan) (q.v.).

General notes
Preparations containing glycopyrrolate may be stored at room temperature.

GLYMIDINE (Gondafon)

Presentation
Tablets—500 mg

Actions and uses
See hypoglycaemic drugs, oral (1).

Dosage
500 mg—1.5 g daily taken in the morning.

Nurse monitoring
See hypoglycaemic drugs, oral (1).

General notes
Tablets may be stored at room temperature.

GRISEOFULVIN (Fulcin, Grisovin)

Presentation
Tablets—125 and 500 mg
Suspension—125 mg in 5 ml

Actions and uses
Griseofulvin is an effective antifungal agent which in clinical practice is used most commonly for the treatment of fungal infections of skin, scalp and nails.

Dosage
1. *Adults*: 500 mg per day which may be given once daily or divided into four doses. Severe infections may be treated by doubling the dose.
2. *Children*: A total daily dose of 10 mg/kg may be administered as a single dose or in four divided doses.

Nurse monitoring
1. Headache and gastrointestinal upset may occur especially during the early stages of treatment. The nurse may make a positive contribution by encouraging the patient to persist with treatment despite these effects.
2. Urticaria, erythematous rashes and photosensitivity reactions may occur.
3. Patients suffering from severe liver disease should not receive this drug.
4. Patients suffering from the rare condition of porphyria should not receive this drug.
5. The dosage of Warfarin required for anticoagulation may have to be altered if Griseofulvin is given.

General notes
The drug may be stored at room temperature.

GUANETHIDINE (Ismelin)

Presentation
Tablets—10 mg, 25 mg
Injection—10 mg in 1 ml

Actions and uses
A simplified description of the action of Guanethidine is as follows: Arterioles are small arteries present throughout the body. The degree to which these arterioles are constricted is one of the major determinants of blood pressure and depends on stimuli which pass to the arterioles from the brain via the sympathetic nervous system. Stimuli are transmitted between nerves in this system by the release of noradrenaline. Any drug which reduces the amount of noradrenaline present, or blocks its release, will reduce the number of stimuli passing along the system and lead to vasodilation and the lowering of blood pressure. Guanethidine is one of these drugs and is known as an 'adrenergic neurone blocker.' The drug is usually given orally but may be given intramuscularly if required in an emergency situation.

Dosage
1. The intramuscular dosage for emergency use is 10–20 mg repeated every 3–4 hours if

necessary. Intramuscular doses for children are the same as oral doses outlined below.
2. Oral maintenance treatment:
   a. Adult doses vary widely. Normally 20–40 mg per day is sufficient, but up to 100 mg may be given for severe degrees of hypertension. Initial dosages do not usually exceed 10 mg. As Guanethidine has a long duration of action and may be given as a single daily dose.
   b. Children's doses:
      Up to 1 year old: 0.2 mg/kg orally.
      Between 1–6 years: 2.5 mg orally.
      Above 7 years: 5 mg or as a single daily dose.
      These are initial children's doses and, as in the case of adults, they may be increased gradually up to 20 times the dose stated.

Nurse monitoring

Guanethidine and the other adrenergic neurone blockers have a number of serious side effects.
1. Bradycardia may commonly be produced.
2. Postural hypotension occurs frequently. The nurse may be the first to notice this, when patients may complain of dizziness or fainting when rising from a chair, or more commonly getting out of bed.
3. Diarrhoea, nasal congestion, weakness, paraesthesia, myalgia and impotence may all occur.
4. Adrenergic neurone blocking drugs interact with tricyclic antidepressants such as Imipramine or Amitryptyline and control of blood pressure may be lost.
5. The antihypertensive action of Guanethidine is increased by alcohol and patients should be advised to restrict their alcohol intake when on these drugs.

General notes

Guanethidine tablets and solution for injection may be stored at room temperature.

H

HALCINONIDE (Halciderm)

Presentation
Cream—0.1%

Actions and uses
This is a very potent corticosteroid (q.v.) which is used most frequently as a topical preparation for the treatment of inflammatory skin conditions such as eczema, dermatitis and psoriasis.

Dosage
The cream is applied sparingly to the affected area two or occasionally three times per day.

Nurse monitoring
1. Although Halcinonide is applied to the skin only, it is important to remember that prolonged excessive use can result in significant absorption and all the effects described under the Nurse monitoring section of corticosteroids (q.v.) can occur.

General notes
1. Halcinonide creams may be stored at room temperature.
2. The creams should not normally be diluted as chemical stability may be affected.

HALOPERIDOL (Fortunan, Haldol, Serenace)

Presentation
Tablets—0.5 mg, 1.5 mg, 5 mg, 10 mg, 20 mg
Oral liquid—10 mg & 50 mg in 5 ml
Injection—5 mg/ml, 1 & 2 ml ampoules 100 mg in 1 ml (as decanoate) depot injection

Actions and uses
Haloperidol is a neuroleptic drug which is used for its tranquillising or calming effect in severely agitated patients with a range of behavioural disorders including schizophrenia, mania and other psychoses. In this respect Haloperidol possesses many of the properties of the phenothiazine tranquillisers which are discussed in the section on phenothiazines.

Dosage
1. *Adults*: The dosage varies widely according to the nature and severity of the disorder under treatment. Initially 1–15 mg daily in single or divided doses with gradual increments up to 200 mg until control is achieved. Thereafter maintenance doses are tailored to individual patients.
2. Emergency control of severely disturbed patients may be treated by an intramuscular or intravenous injection 5–30 mg repeated at 6-hourly intervals.
3. Haloperidol decanoate is a depot injection for long-term control administered as 100–300 mg by deep intramuscular injection each month.

Nurse monitoring
1. Adverse effects which are associated with the phenothiazine tranquillisers are also commonly encountered with Haloperidol. In particular a degree of unwanted sedation, extrapyramidal (Parkinsonian) symptoms and tardive dyskinesia occur. See the section on phenothiazines.
2. Photosensitivity reactions occasionally occur and patients should be warned to avoid excessive exposure to strong sunlight.

3. The endocrine side effects of the phenothiazines are also associated with Haloperidol as is the depressant action on the bone marrow affecting the production of white blood cells. Since this latter effect makes the patients more susceptible to infection, patients developing even simple symptoms such as sore throat should have their white blood cell count checked.

General notes

All preparations containing Haloperidol should be stored at room temperature. The drug is very sensitive to light and accordingly oral solution or solutions for injections should be suitably protected during storage. Note that Haloperidol decanoate injection, if stored for long periods in the cold, may precipitate (turn cloudy), though the injection should clear on re-storage at room temperature.

HEPARIN (Pularin, Calciparine, Minihep)

Note. Heparin is available as both the sodium and calcium salt

Presentation

Injection (intravenous)—5 ml vials contain 1000, 5000 and 25 000 units in 1 ml

Injection (subcutaneous)—5000 units in 0.2 ml

Actions and uses

Heparin is an anticoagulant drug which acts by inhibiting one stage of the formation of clot from its constituent factors. It is given by intravenous injection in the treatment of arterial and venous thrombosis and by subcutaneous injection for the prophylaxis of thrombo-embolic complications following surgery and myocardial infarction.

Dosage

1. For the treatment of arterial and venous thrombosis: Heparin may be administered by continuous or intermittent intravenous infusion:
   a. Continuous intravenous infusion: It is normal to administer 1000 units/hour and regularly check the thrombin time which is the test of choice for anticoagulant effect in patients on Heparin. Depending on the results of this test the dose may be adjusted up or down until appropriate anticoagulation is obtained.
   b. Intermittent intravenous infusion: 5000–10 000 units is administered intravenously by bolus injection four to six hourly and individual requirements are then adjusted according to the results of the thrombin time.
2. For the prevention of thromboembolic complications following surgery or myocardial infarction: The drug is administered subcutaneously in a dose of 5000 units 8–12 hourly. Clotting studies are not usually estimated when Heparin is given by this route as it does not achieve a full anticoagulant effect but still proves useful in the prevention of thromboembolism.

Nurse monitoring

1. As with all anticoagulant therapy the two major risks to the patient are:
   a. Overcoagulation with resultant bleeding
   b. Undercoagulation with failure to treat or prevent problems of thrombosis or embolism.

The nurse may play a very important role in the successful administration of Heparin by ensuring that intravenous infusions proceed at the appropriate rate and intermittent intravenous treatment or subcutaneous treatment is administered at appropriate times and in the appropriate dosage.

2. It is important to note that subcutaneous injections may be very painful.
3. Occasional urticaria, fever and thrombocytopenia may be produced by Heparin.
4. The drug should never be administered by bolus injection by the intramuscular route.

5. Heparin is contraindicated for administration to patients with blood clotting disorders such as haemophilia and patients who have a history of active peptic ulceration or severe, uncontrolled hypertension.
6. When symptoms of overcoagulation occur the effect of Heparin may be rapidly reversed by the administration of protamine sulphate.

HEPTABARBITONE (Medomin)

Presentation
Tablets—200 mg

Actions and uses
Heptabarbitone is a barbiturate drug (q.v.) which is used to induce sleep.

Dosage
100–200 mg on retiring.

Nurse monitoring
See the section on barbiturate drugs.

General notes
Heptabarbitone tablets may be stored at room temperature.

HORMONES (1)

OESTROGENS AND DRUGS WITH MAINLY OESTROGENIC ACTIONS

Introduction
This group of drugs includes: Stilboestrol, Dinoestrol, Ethinyloestradiol, Mestranol, Oestradiol valereate, Oestrogens conjugated (equine), Oestriol, Quinestrol, Piperazine oestrone sulphate, Quinestradiol.

Presentation
See individual drugs.

Actions and uses
1. The contribution of oestrogens to oral contraceptive therapy is discussed in the section on contraceptives—oral.
2. Oestrogens are used widely for a number of disorders including:
    a. Obstetric problems:
        i. Habitual and threatened abortion
        ii. Suppression of lactation
        iii. Puerperal depression
    b. Gynaecological problems:
        i. Menstrual irregularities
        ii. Functional uterine bleeding
        iii. Endometriosis
        iv. Menopausal symptoms
        v. Premenstrual tension
        vi. Endometrial carcinoma
        vii. Atrophic or senile vaginitis
    c. Treatment of cancer:
        i. Mammary carcinoma
        ii. Endometrial carcinoma
        iii. Prostatic carcinoma
    d. Prevention of bone resorption: Oestrogens are used for the prevention and treatment of osteoporosis in postmenopausal women.

Dosage
See specific drugs.

Nurse monitoring
1. The nurse monitoring aspects of the oestrogen component of contraceptive therapy are discussed in the section on contraceptives.
2. The use of oestrogens in other clinical situations is associated with the following problems:
    a. In females, increased uterine growth, withdrawal bleeding and amenorrhoea may occur
    b. Breast tenderness, gynaecomastia and loss of sexual characteristics in males
    c. Nausea, vomiting, depression, headache and dizziness may commonly occur
    d. Salt and water retention leading to hypertension and weight gain may occur
    e. Treatment with oestrogens occasionally produces jaundice due to liver damage
    f. Rare side effects include hypercalcaemia, skin rashes e.g. urticaria and erythema multiforme.
3. Oestrogens may stimulate the growth of malignant tumours and are contraindicated in patients with a history of neoplastic disease of the breast or genital tract.
4. Oestrogens should not be administered to patients with a

history of liver disease or previous thrombo-embolic disorders.
5. The administration of oestrogens to diabetic patients may alter insulin or oral hypoglycaemic requirements.
6. The administration of oestrogens to epileptics may lead to an increase in fit frequency and the need to alter their anticonvulsant regime.

General notes
See specific drugs.

HORMONES (2)

PROGESTOGENS AND DRUGS WITH PROGESTATIONAL ACTION

Introduction
This group of drugs includes: Allyloestranol, Medroxyprogesterone, Hydroxyprogesterone, Progesterone, Dydrogesterone.

Presentation
See individual drugs.

Actions and uses
1. The contribution of progesterone to oral contraceptive therapy is discussed in the section on contraceptives.
2. Progesterones are used widely for a number of disorders including:
   a. Obstetric problems:
      i. Habitual and threatened abortion
      ii. Suppression of lactation
      iii. Puerperal depression
   b. Gynaecological problems:
      i. Menstrual irregularities
      ii. Functional uterine bleeding
      iii. Endometriosis
      iv. Menopausal symptoms
      v. Premenstrual tension
      vi. Endometrial carcinoma
      vii. Atrophic or senile vaginitis
   c. Treatment of cancer:
      i. Mammary carcinoma
      ii. Endometrial carcinoma
      iii. Prostatic carcinoma.

Nurse monitoring
1. The administration of progestogens can lead commonly to symptoms of gastrointestinal upset, headache, depression, urticaria, pruritis vulvae and change in menstrual function.
2. Acne, weight gain and hypertension due to salt and water retention, gynaecomastia, vaginal candidiasis and vaginal discharge may occur when patients receive this drug.
3. Less frequently jaundice and liver damage have been produced.
4. Progestogen drugs should be used with caution in patients with heart and kidney disease due to their salt and water retaining effects.
5. Progestogens should not be given to pregnant women as they cause masculinisation of the female fetus.
6. The administration of progestogens to asthmatics and epileptics may lead to an exacerbation of their symptoms.

HORMONES (3)

DRUGS WITH MIXED OESTROGENIC AND PROGESTOGENIC ACTIONS

Introduction
Norethisterone is the commonest drug in use with mixed oestrogenic and progestogenic actions.

Presentation
See individual drugs.

Actions and uses
The actions and uses of this group of drugs are identical to those described for oestrogens (q.v.).

Nurse monitoring
The Nurse monitoring aspects of this drug are identical to those described for oestrogens (q.v.) and progestogens (q.v.).

HORMONES (4)

DRUGS WITH ANDROGENIC AND ANABOLIC ACTIONS

Introduction
This group of drugs includes: Fluoxymesterone, Testosterone

preparations, Mesterolone, Methyltestosterone.
Presentation
See individual drugs.
Actions and uses
Drugs with androgens and anabolic actions have a limited number of uses. They include:
1. The treatment of male patients with deficiency states involving these hormones.
2. The treatment of mammary carcinoma in females.
3. These drugs are occasionally used to treat rare haematological disorders including aplastic anaemia and haemolytic anaemia.

Dosage
See individual drugs.
Nurse monitoring
1. All patients receiving these drugs may experience an increase in weight, an increase in muscle bulk and salt and water retention with resultant hypertension and oedema.
2. When these drugs are given to female patients menstrual function is suppressed and virilisation may occur characterised by deepening of the voice, hirsutism (excess body hair), atrophy of the breasts. Increased libido is a further feature.
3. Prolonged treatment with these drugs has been noted to cause an increased incidence of tumours of the liver.
4. These drugs should never be given to patients with carcinoma of the prostrate as they appear to stimulate the tumour growth.
5. These drugs should be used with great caution in patients with cardiac failure, renal failure or liver impairment as they may lead to a worsening of the patient's condition.
6. They should be used with great caution in patients suffering from epilepsy as an increased frequency of seizures may be precipitated.
7. They should be used with caution in patients with migraine as symptoms may be aggravated.

HORMONES (5)

DRUGS OF THE ANDROGEN GROUP WHICH HAVE MAINLY ANABOLIC ACTIVITY

Introduction
This group of drugs includes: Drostanolone, Nandrolone, Oxymethalone, Stanazolol, Norethandrolone.
Presentation
See individual drugs.
Actions and uses
1. These drugs stimulate skeletal growth by affecting protein metabolism. They may rarely be used in clinical situations for this effect.
2. This group of drugs is also occasionally used for the treatment of rare disorders involving bone marrow function including aplastic anaemia and haemolytic anaemia.
3. These drugs inhibit bone resorption in the elderly male and are used therefore in the treatment of senile osteoporosis in males.

Dosage
See individual drugs.
Nurse monitoring
The Nurse monitoring notes for these drugs are identical to those described for androgen and anabolic steroids (q.v.).
General notes
See individual drugs.

HYALURONIDASE (Hyalase)

Presentation
Ampoules containing 1500 international units of Hyaluronidase
Actions and uses
This substance breaks down hyaluronic acid which is a substance concerned with maintaining structure in cells. It is used in clinical practice as an aid to the dispersal of infusions administered subcutaneously or intramuscularly. It may also be used to reduce local inflammation and oedema.

Dosage
Adults: In general 1500 international units are sufficient for the administration of 500–1000 ml of most fluids.

Nurse monitoring
1. This drug should never be administered to the site of bites or stings or at sites where infection or malignancy are present.
2. The drug should never be given intravenously.
3. Side effects are due to sensitisation and may be severe enough to produce anaphylactic shock.

General notes
The drug should be stored in a cool, dry place.

HYDRALAZINE (Apresoline)

Presentation
Tablets—25 mg, 50 mg
Injection—20 mg powder in 2 ml ampoule

Actions and uses
Hydralazine has a direct action on the small arteries (arterioles) causing them to dilate. The effect of this is to reduce the blood pressure. Administration of the drug often leads to a degree of fluid retention and tachycardia and is often therefore given along with thiazide diuretics and/or beta-blocking drugs.

Dosage
1. It may be given by slow intravenous injection or intravenous infusion for hypertensive emergencies. The usual dose is 20–40 mg.
2. The adult oral maintenance dose is 25–50 mg two to three times daily. The maximum dose advisable is 200 mg per day.

Nurse monitoring
1. The nurse should be aware that the presence of tachycardia in a patient on Hydralazine may be due to the drug therapy.
2. Fluid retention and heart failure may develop if patients who are on Hydralazine are not on a diuretic.
3. Headache and flushing may be caused by the vasodilator action of the drug. As these side effects are often poorly tolerated there may be a reduction in compliance with treatment and patients should always be asked therefore whether they are suffering from these effects.
4. A serious side effect usually seen only with high dosage, is a development of a syndrome similar to systemic lupus erythematosus which is associated with widespread danger to the arterial system reflected in skin rashes, renal and hepatic dysfunction etc. The development of the features of this syndrome are an indication for immediate withdrawal of drug therapy.

General notes
Hydralazine tablets and powder for injection may be stored at room temperature. Solutions for injection are prepared by adding 1 ml of Water for Injection to each ampoule which is then further diluted with sodium chloride 0.9% (normal saline) injection. It is given by slow intravenous injection or added to an infusion of sodium chloride 0.9% or compound sodium lactate (Ringers) injection. Any unused solution must be immediately discarded.

HYDROCHLOROTHIAZIDE (Hydrosaluric)

Presentation
Tablets—25 mg, 50 mg

Actions and uses
See the section on thiazide and related diuretics.

Dosage
The daily adult dose range is 25–50 mg twice daily. Hydrochlorothiazide is effective for 6–12 hours after an oral dose.

Nurse monitoring
See the section on thiazide and related diuretics.

General notes
Hydrochlorothiazide tablets may be stored at room temperature.

HYDROCORTISONE (Hydrocortone, Efcortesol, Efcortelan, Solu-cortef)

Numerous other preparations containing Hydrocortisone (often combined with other substances) are available.

Presentation
Tablets—10 mg, 20 mg
Injection—intravenous or
  intramuscular — 100 mg in 1 ml and 2 ml
    — 500 mg in 5 ml
  intra-articular—25 mg in 1 ml
Ointment and cream—0.5%, 1% and 2.5%
Eye drops—1%
Eye ointment—2.5%

Actions and uses
See the section on corticosteroids.

Dosage
Dosages vary considerably with the nature and severity of the illness being treated and it is not therefore appropriate to quote specific instances.

Nurse monitoring
See the section on corticosteroids.

General notes
1. Preparations containing Hydrocortisone may be stored at room temperature.
2. Intravenous use: Sodium succinate or sodium phosphate salts only should be used. Hydrocortisone acetate is for intra-articular injection only.
3. Intravenous injections are given slowly over a period of one minute to several minutes.
4. Intravenous infusions are prepared by adding the required dose to a volume of 5% dextrose or 0.9% sodium chloride injection. The volume of diluent varies from 100 ml to 1 litre.

HYDROFLUMETHIAZIDE (Hydrenox)

Presentation
Tablets—50 mg

Actions and uses
See the section on thiazide and related diuretics.

Dosage
The adult dose range is 25–100 mg daily in divided doses. The duration of action of hydroflumethiazide is about 4–6 hours.

Nurse monitoring
See the section on thiazide and related diuretics.

General notes
Hydroflumethiazide tablets may be stored at room temperature.

HYDROXYCHLOROQUINE (Plaquenil)

Presentation
Tablets—200 mg

Actions and uses
This anti-malarial drug has been found to be useful in the treatment of the following conditions:
1. Malaria
2. Giardiasis
3. Rheumatoid disease
4. Lupus erythematosus

Dosage
1. Malaria:
   a. Prophylactically 400 mg once per week during the period of exposure and for 4–8 weeks afterwards.
   b. Treatment of an acute attack of malaria: Initial dose of 800 mg followed by 400 mg after 6–8 hours and then 400 mg on two successive days.
2. Giardiasis: 200 mg three times daily for five days.
3. Rheumatoid disease and lupus erythematosus: 400–500 mg per day are given initially usually at mealtimes and if a response is obtained the dose is reduced after several weeks to a maintenance dosage of 200–400 mg per day.

Note: All the above doses are for adults only.

Nurse monitoring
The Nurse monitoring notes on Chloroquine (q.v.) are entirely similar to those for Hydroxychloroquine.

General notes
Hydroxychloroquine tablets may be stored at room temperature.

VITAMIN B12—HYDROXOCOBALAMIN (Neo-Cytamen, Cobalin-H)

Presentation
Injection — 250 µg in 1 ml
1000 µg in 1 ml

Actions and uses
Hydroxocobalamin (Vitamin B12) us indicated for the treatment of megaloblastic anaemia where this has been shown to be due to a deficiency of Vitamin B12 by the appropriate laboratory test. Deficiency of Vitamin B12 occurs either where there is a deficiency in the gut of a substance (intrinsic factor) normally produced by the stomach which is essential for the absorption of Vitamin B12, this condition being known as pernicious anaemia, or it may be due to other forms of malabsorption. More rarely Vitamin B12 deficiency may be seen in people who have a strict vegetarian diet.

Dosage
1. For pernicious anaemia: Initially 250–1000 µg i.m. on alternative days for 1–2 weeks, and then 1000 µg every 2–3 months.
2. For the prophylaxis of megaloblastic anaemia due to gastrectomy or malabsorption syndromes or strict vegetarianism: 250–1000 µg monthly.

Nurse monitoring
1. Sensitisation to Vitamin B12 is extremely rare. It may present as an itching skin rash and very exceptionally as anaphylactic shock.
2. Hydroxocobalamin is preferable as the form of Vitamin B12 for replacement therapy as it has the advantage over Cyanocobalamin that it does not contain Cyanide. This is especially important when Vitamin B12 is being given to patients with either tobacco amblyopia or optic atrophy and optic neuritis due to Leber's optic atrophy when Cyanide containing compounds are specifically contraindicated.
3. Hydroxocobalamin has an additional advantage over Cyanocobalamin in that it is longer acting and therefore the interval between injections can be at least monthly.

General notes
Ampoules should be protected from light.

HYDROXYPROGESTERONE HEXANOATE (Proluton Depot)

Presentation
Injection—250 mg/ml

Actions and uses
1. See the section describing the actions and uses of progestational hormones in general.
2. Prolution Depot in clinical practice is used for the treatment of threatened abortion and habitual abortion.

Dosage
1. For the treatment of habitual abortion: 250–500 mg at weekly intervals during the first half of pregnancy.
2. For the treatment of threatened abortion: 500 mg of Proluton Depot intramuscularly daily until bleeding has stopped. Subsequently 250–500 mg intramuscularly every three days for three doses and then weekly throughout the first half of pregnancy.

Nurse monitoring
1. See the section describing the Nurse monitoring aspects of progestational hormones in general.
2. Rarely local reactions may occur at the site of injection.

General notes
The drug may be stored at room temperature.

HYDROXYZINE (Atarax)

Presentation
Tablets—10 mg and 25 mg
Syrup—10 mg in 5 ml

Actions and uses
Hydroxyzine is a depressant affecting the CNS. It has a calming effect in anxious patients, an anti-emetic activity and via its

antihistamine action, an antipruritic action. In clinical practice the drug is used mainly for its ability to suppress itch in various dermatological conditions, particularly in patients who have an associated anxiety.

Dosages
1. *Adults*: 25–100 mg taken three or four times daily.
2. *Children*:
   a. Under 6 years: 30–50 mg daily in divided doses
   b. Over 6 years: 50–100 mg daily in divided doses

Nurse monitoring
1. Hydroxyzine is a CNS depressant drug and marked sedation may follow its use, particularly if other sedative drugs are taken.
2. In the above context patients should be warned of the dangers of taking alcohol, even in moderate amounts, concurrently with hydroxyzine.
3. Some patients may complain of dryness of the mouth with this drug.
4. Rarely tremor or abnormal muscle activity is produced. This symptom is indicative of excessive dosage and if it occurs, should be brought to the attention of the doctor.

General notes
Tablets and syrup containing hydroxyzine should be stored at room temperature.

HYOSCINE-N-BUTYLBROMIDE (Buscopan)

Presentation
Tablets—10 mg
Injection—20 mg in 1 ml

Actions and uses
Hyoscine-N-Butylbromide is an anticholinergic drug. It has a specific antispasmodic action on the smooth muscle of the gut, renal and biliary tracts. It is therefore used to relieve pain associated with acute spasm, i.e. renal colic, biliary colic and spasm produced by diagnostic procedures such as gastric or duodenal endoscopy.

Dosage
1. *Adults*:
   a. Oral: 20 mg four times a day.
   b. By injection: 20 mg intramuscularly or intravenously repeated at half-hourly intervals as required.
2. *Children*:
   Oral: 10 mg three times daily is the ideal dose range for the 6–12 year age group.

Nurse monitoring
1. Patients may frequently suffer the common anticholinergic side effects of dryness of the mouth, visual disturbance and tachycardia.
2. More serious side effects which may be encountered are:
   a. Intra-ocular pressure may be raised, thus the drug is contraindicated in patients with glaucoma and may on occasions precipitate glaucoma in patients who had not previously had this problem recognised.
   b. Patients may have difficulty in initiating micturition and occasionally urinary retention may result.
   c. The drug should not be used in patients with heart disease or intestinal obstruction.

General notes
Hyoscine-N-Butylbromide tablets and injection may be stored at room temperature. The injection solution however should be protected from light. Should it be necessary to dilute the injection solution, dextrose 5% injection may also be mixed with commonly used radiological contrast media e.g. diodone, sodium diatrizoate, before intravenous pyelography when spasm and pain in the urinary tract may be produced.

HYPOGLYCAEMIC DRUGS, ORAL (1)

THE SULPHONYLUREAS

Presentation
See individual drugs.

Actions and uses
Sulphonylurea drugs stimulate the islet cells of the pancreas to

produce more insulin. They are, therefore, useful in the management of patients who have been found to have diabetes mellitus which is not adequately controlled by diet only but which is not sufficiently severe to require insulin. It should be pointed out that as they stimulate production of insulin by the pancreas, at least some degree of insulin production by the pancreas must already be present.

Dosage

The dosage required for each of the drugs in this group should tailored to individual patient requirements and should be monitored by regular estimation of plasma glucose and urine glucose. For specific doses see individual drugs.

Nurse monitoring

1. Sulphonylurea drugs should be avoided if possible in patients who are overweight as their stimulation of insulin production may lead to further gain in weight.
2. With the longer acting members of this group of drugs such as Chlorpropamide, hypoglycaemia may be produced especially in the early hours of the morning and in elderly patients. The nurse should be alerted to the possibility of this by noting the occurrence of any faintness, dizziness or confusion in elderly patients at the appropriate time.
3. Common side effects include gastrointestinal upset manifest by nausea, vomiting and epigastric pain, neurological side effects including dizziness, weakness, paraesthesiae and headache.
4. Less common side effects include hypersensitivity reactions such as fever, skin rash and jaundice and blood dyscrasias such as leucopenia, thrombocytopenia, aplastic anaemia and agranulocytosis.
5. A proportion of patients receiving sulphonylureas will experience facial flushing, tachycardia, sweating, breathlessness, headache, vomiting and dizziness if they take alcohol. Patients should be warned of the potential development of these effects and if they occur the only alternatives are to change to another drug or to avoid alcohol.
6. A number of important problems may arise when diabetic patients on sulphonylurea drugs receive other drugs. These are as follows:
   a. Beta blockers: These may be dangerous because patients on beta blocking drugs may not experience the early symptoms which normally warn them that they are about to become hypoglycaemic, and they might then proceed to sudden hypoglycaemic coma.
   b. Corticosteroids: These may affect glucose metabolism in the body in such a way that increased requirements for insulin or oral hypoglycaemics are necessary.
   c. Diuretics: These have two effects:
      i. They may raise blood glucose levels and result in the need for change in dosage.
      ii. They may potentiate hyperosmolar diabetic states.
   d. Alcohol: Alcohol has two actions:
      i. It may produce symptoms with sulphonylurea drugs described in the section above.
      ii. Alcohol itself may produce hypoglycaemia of a transient nature.
   e. Monoamine oxidase inhibitors: These drugs enhance and/or prolong the hypoglycaemic response to oral hypoglycaemic drugs and a reduction in dosage may be necessary.
   f. Phenylbutazone: This durg interferes with the liver metabolism of oral hypoglycaemic drugs and a change in dosage may be necessary.

g. Salicylates: These may displace oral hypoglycaemic drugs from the proteins to which they bind in blood and a change in dosage may be necessary.
h. Sulphonamides: These may affect both the metabolism and protein binding of the sulphonylureas, making a change in dosage necessary.
7. When dealing with diabetic patients, the nurse may be faced with the problem of a patient presenting with coma or altered level of consciousness. This is further discussed in the Nurse monitoring section (6) on insulins (q.v.).

General notes
Sulphonylurea drugs may be stored at room temperature.

HYPOGLYCAEMIC DRUGS, ORAL (2)

THE BIGUANIDES

Note: Since the withdrawal of Phenformin due to its potential to produce serious and life-threatening side effects, Metformin is currently the only drug of this type available.

Presentation
See individual drugs.

Actions and uses
Biguanide drugs do not stimulate insulin secretion. Their precise mechanism of action is not clearly understood but they appear to increase the utilisation of glucose in the tissues.

Dosage
See individual drugs.

Nurse monitoring
1. Biguanide drugs would appear to be the treatment of choice in obese diabetic who do not require insulin.
2. Metformin (though to a lesser extent than Phenformin) may cause a serious alteration in the blood biochemistry known as lactic acidosis. For this reason Phenformin has now been withdrawn from clinical use. It remains, however, that there is still a risk of this effect occurring with Metformin. The clinical features of lactic acidosis are of general malaise, impaired consciousness and other symptoms suggestive of diabetic ketoacidosis, but ketones are not detectable on the breath or in the urine, and this gives the clue to the diagnosis.
3. Gastrointestinal upsets are relatively common and symptoms include nausea, vomiting and diarrhoea.
4. A metallic taste may be produced by these drugs.
5. Less common side effects include muscle weakness, lassitude and skin rash.
6. The coincident administration of other drugs may affect patients on Biguanide therapy in varying ways:
   a. Beta blockers: These may be dangerous because patients on beta blocking drugs may not experience the early symptoms which normally warn them that they are about to become hypoglycaemic and they might then proceed to sudden hypoglycaemic coma.
   b. Corticosteroids: These may affect glucose metabolism in the body in such a way that increased requirements for insulin or oral hypoglycaemics are necessary.
   c. Diuretics: These have two effects:
      i. They may raise blood glucose levels and result in a need for change in dosage
      ii. They may potentiate hyperosmolar diabetic states.
   d. Alcohol: Alcohol has three effects:
      i. It may produce symptoms with biguanide drugs as described under section (5) of the Nurse monitoring notes on sulphonylurea drugs (q.v.)
      ii. Alcohol itself may produce

hypoglycaemia of a transient nature
   iii. Patients who take alcohol are at an increased risk of developing the metabolic complication of lactic acidosis (see above).
  e. Monoamine oxidase inhibitors: These drugs enhance and/or prolong the hypoglycaemic response to oral hypoglycaemic drugs and a reduction in dosage may be necessary.
  f. Phenylbutazone: This drug interferes with the liver metabolism of oral hypoglycaemic drugs and a change in dosage may be necessary.
  g. Salicylates: These may displace oral hypoglycaemic drugs from the proteins to which they bind in blood and a change in dosage may be necessary.
  h. Sulphonamides: These may affect both metabolism and protein binding of the biguanides, making a change in dosage necessary.
7. When dealing with diabetic patients, the nurse may be faced with the problems of a patient presenting with coma or altered level of consciousness. This is further discussed in the Nurse monitoring section (6) on insulins (q.v.).

General notes
Biguanide hypoglycaemic drugs may be stored at room temperature.

IBUPROFEN (Brufen)

Presentation
Tablets—200 mg, 400 mg, 600 mg
Suspension—100 mg in 5 ml

Actions and uses
See the section on anti-inflammatory analgesic drugs, non-steroidal.

Dosage
1. *Adults*:
   a. Initial dosage is 1200 mg per day in three or four divided doses
   b. Maintenance dosage is 600–1200 mg per day in divided dosage.
2. *Children*: A dosage of 20 mg/kg has been used but the total daily dose should not exceed 500 mg in those weighing less than 30 kg.

Nurse monitoring
See the section on anti-inflammatory analgesic drugs, non-steroidal.

General notes
Ibuprofen tablets and suspension may be stored at room temperature.

IDOXURIDINE (Herpid, Dendrid)

Presentation
Paint—5% in Dimethylsulphoxide (DMSO)
Eye drops—0.1%
Eye ointment—0.5%

Actions and uses
This compound is effective against viral infections. Unfortunately, it is only available for topical use and in clinical practice it may be used to treat the following diseases:
1. Cutaneous herpes zoster (shingles)
2. Ocular herpes zoster
3. Skin infections due to herpes simplex
4. Acute dendritic ulcer.

Dosage
1. If the paint is used it should be applied carefully and sparingly to the skin lesion and the immediate surrounding erythematous area four times per day for 4–5 days.
2. Eye drops should be administered at the rate of one drop each hour during the day and one drop two-hourly throughout the night.
3. Eye ointment should be applied sparingly four-hourly.
4. Idoxuridine 0.1% (using eye drop solution) is applied to oral or peri-oral lesions (the 5% paint is not suitable in this case). Adults and children should hold approximately 2 ml in the mouth in contact with the lesion for 2–3 minutes at least 3 times a day. Alternatively the solution may be applied 4–5 times daily.

Nurse monitoring
1. The Dimethylsulphoxide component of the paint preparation will damage normal skin and care should be taken to apply the paint only to the infected area.
2. The paint may produce stinging and an unpleasant taste if applied to the mouth.
3. Irritation, pain, itching and inflammation may follow the use of ophthalmic preparations.
4. It is worth noting that topical corticosteroid preparations should never be used where viral infection is suspected.

General notes
1. The paint preparation may be stored at room temperature.
2. Ophthalmic preparations should be refrigerated.

IMIPRAMINE (Tofranil)
Presentation
Tablets—10 mg, 25 mg
Syrup—25 mg in 5 ml
Injection—25 mg in 2 ml
Actions and uses
Imipramine is a tricyclic antidepressant drug. Its actions and uses are described in the section dealing with these drugs.
Dosage
1. For the treatment of depression:
   a. Oral doses range from 75–200 mg daily in total usually given in three or four divided doses. Lower doses i.e. up to 30 mg daily may be sufficient, in older patients who often have difficulty in tolerating the standard doses described.
   b. In patients who require injection i.e. those who are uncooperative or have severe depression which requires rapid control, intramuscular injections of 25 mg up to six times daily may be administered.
2. For the treatment of enuresis in children dose ranges are as follows:
   5–12 years: 25 mg taken as a single dose at bed time.
   Over 12 years: 50 mg taken as a single dose at bed time.
Nurse monitoring
See the section on tricyclic antidepressant drugs.
General notes
1. Preparations containing Imipramine should be stored at room temperature.
2. Solution for injection and syrup should be protected from light.

INDAPAMIDE (Natrilix)
Presentation
Tablets—2.5 mg
Actions and uses
1. When given in a dosage of 2.5 mg per day, the drug has a weak diuretic but much more pronounced hypotensive action. It is therefore useful in the treatment of hypertension.
2. Higher doses have a more pronounced diuretic action and therefore it may be used as such.
Dosage
For adults the usual dose is 2.5 mg taken once daily in the morning.
Nurse monitoring
1. When given in the above dosage for hypertension side effects may be seen in the form of nausea, vomiting and headache. Hypotension and its clinical features may also be produced.
2. If higher doses are used the diuretic effect becomes more pronounced and all the adverse effects associated with thiazide diuretics (q.v.) may occur.
General notes
Indapamide tablets may be stored at room temperature.

INDOMETHACIN (Indocid)
Presentation
Capsules—25 mg, 50 mg, 75 mg (sustained release)
Suspension—25 mg in 5 ml
Suppositories—100 mg
Actions and uses
See the section on non-steroidal anti-inflammatory analgesic drugs.
Dosage
1. *Adults*:
   a. The usual adult dose range is 25 mg twice or three times daily up to 200 mg per day in divided doses.
   b. A sustained release capsule on a once or occasionally twice daily dosage regime can be used.
   c. One suppository (100 mg)

inserted at night is often useful in relieving the troublesome morning stiffness in joints affected by rheumatoid arthritis.

Nurse monitoring
1. See the section on anti-inflammatory analgesic drugs, non-steroidal.
2. A specific problem with Indomethacin is the production of headache and dizziness in a proportion of patients. These symptoms may be sufficiently severe to warrant a change to an alternative non-steroidal anti-inflammatory drug.

General notes
Indomethacin capsules, suspension and suppositories may be stored at room temperature.

INOSITOL NICOTINATE (Hexopal)

Presentation
Tablets—500 mg
Suspension—1 g in 5 ml

Actions and uses
The actions and uses of this drug are identical to those described for Nicofuranose (q.v.)

Dosage
Adults: 500 mg–1 g three times per day.

Nurse Monitoring
See the section on Nicofuranose.

General notes
The drug should be stored at room temperature.

INSULIN

Insulin is available in the United Kingdom in several forms. The various preparations available may differ according to a number of important factors:
1. *Source of insulin*: Insulins in use today are derived from the pancreas of cattle or pigs when they are known as bovine and porcine insulin respectively. More recently the so-called human insulins have been developed in the laboratory to provide an insulin which chemically resembles the human type. It has been found that patients may react differently to equivalent doses of bovine, porcine and human insulin. Therefore if a patient is changed from one insulin to another from a different source, requirements may vary.
2. *Formulation of insulin*: Soluble insulin i.e. a simple solution of insulin, has a characteristically rapid onset and brief duration of action. In order to achieve prolonged control, various preparations have been produced which release insulin at varying rates and thus prolong its action.
3. *Concentration*: Since 1983, all diabetics in the United Kingdom have started insulin therapy with a standard 100 unit per ml strength. All existing diabetics have been transferred from the old 20, 40, and 80 unit per ml to this new strength which is widely known as U100. U100 insulin has been developed so that the treatment of all diabetics may be standardised and in future errors are less likely to arise over confusion with insulin strengths.
Two new insulin syringes, 0.5 ml and 1 ml syringes, have been introduced for use with U100 insulin. The 0.5 ml syringe is graduated at one unit intervals and numbered 0, 10, 20 . . . 50. The 1 ml syringe, which is only slightly longer than the 0.5 ml syringe, has been graduated at 2 unit intervals (one unit intervals would be too close for legibility), numbered 0, 10, 20 . . . 100.
It is important to note that all prescriptions for U100 insulin will indicate the number of units to be injected and the term 'marks' will disappear.
4. *Purity*: Several years ago important changes in the manufacturing process enabled insulins of a high purity to be

produced. Thus the previous problems with low purity insulin, poor diabetic control, reactions at injection sites and insulin resistance, are no longer important problems since all insulins now produced, i.e. in U100 form, are of the highly purified type.
5. *Preservative*: Different preparations of insulin contain different preservatives. As patients may be allergic to one or other preservative this factor may be important in the choice of insulin used. Note that the nature and concentration of preservative present in any insulin preparation is indicated on the insulin package.

Actions and uses
Insulin is used for the treatment of patients suffering from diabetes mellitus, a disease caused by failure of the insulin producing endocrine cells of the pancreas.

Dosage
The total daily dosage required by individual patients varies greatly.

Nurse monitoring
1. In insulin-dependant diabetic patients the nurse, both in the hospital and community, may play an extremely important role in educating the patient in the calculation of dosage of insulin required, the method of administration, the avoidance of side effects, and in general, health measures necessary to avoid complications of diabetes.
2. Several important points arise concerning the mixing of various available preparations of insulin.
   a. Soluble insulin or neutral soluble insulin may be mixed with other insulins, with the exception of Protamine Zinc insulin, without affecting the duration of action of either preparation.
   b. The order of mixing should ensure that the soluble or soluble neutral insulin is drawn up first into the syringe before drawing up the long-acting preparation. In this way soluble insulins are never contaminated.
   c. The mixing of insulins from different sources (bovine, porcine and human) is irrational and should be avoided.
   d. When insulins containing different preservatives are mixed, the risk of a local or general reaction is increased.
   e. Insulins mixed in a syringe should be immediately injected. If they are not immediately used they should be discarded.
3. Local reactions consisting of itchy red lumps at injection sites may occur during the early phase of treatment. They tend to remit spontaneously within about one month of starting treatment in newly diagnosed diabetics. Local reactions are extremely rare with the use of insulins of high purity, and if they do occur allergy to a component of the preparation, e.g. preservative, may be the cause.
4. To prevent local fat atrophy patients should be encouraged to vary the site of administration of daily injections of insulin. High purity insulins rarely cause this local reaction.
5. Following the introduction of U100 insulin and the new syringes, it was decided to restrict the supply of syringes to 'glass only' on NHS prescriptions. Despite this, many patients prefer to obtain, at their own expense, plastic disposable insulin syringes. These patients may be instructed to use plastic syringes repeatedly for a limited period e.g. one week and even up to 2 weeks. If this is done patients should be instructed to store their insulin syringe with needle attached in a refrigerator when the possibility of bacterial contamination is minimised. In addition, they should be instructed not to wash the syringe/needle but rather leave any residual insulin in the barrel

since preservatives present in the insulin will tend to minimise bacterial contamination.
6. When dealing with diabetic patients, the nurse may be faced with the problems of a patient presenting with coma or altered level of consciousness, which may be due to hyperglycaemia or hypoglycaemia; and differentiation may be difficult. A history of recent weight loss, malaise, thirst and polyuria, or recent intercurrent infection, along with signs of dry lax skin, a dry tongue and ketotic (deep and rapid) breathing would suggest the former, while a history of previous good health, recent alcohol consumption, a missed meal, rapidity of onset of coma, and signs of tachycardia, sweating and pallor would suggest the latter. If in doubt, and while awaiting emergency medical assessment, the administration of oral or intravenous glucose will correct hypoglycaemia and will not significantly worsen hyperglycaemia, whereas insulin administered in such doubtful cases is contraindicated, as death might result if hypoglycaemia exists.

General notes

Insulin should be stored in a cool place. In hospital a refrigerator should be used as everyday ward temperatures tend to be too high.

IPRATROPIUM BROMIDE (Atrovent)

Presentation
Metered aerosol—0.02 mg per dose.
Nebuliser solution—0.25 mg in 1 ml

Actions and uses
Ipratropium bromide is a drug with anticholinergic actions. When inhaled via an aerosol it exerts a direct effect on the airways causing dilation and relief from the symptoms of wheeze and breathlessness due to airways obstruction in diseases such as a emphysema and chronic bronchitis.

Dosage
1. *Adults*: One or two inhalations (0.02–0.04 mg) three or four times daily. If necessary up to four inhalations may be given four times daily to obtain maximum benefit.
2. *Children*:
Under 6 years: One inhalation three times daily.
6–12 years: One or two inhalations three times daily.
3. In severe breathlessness solution may be administered via a nebuliser: The usual dose is 0.4–2 ml administered up to 3 times a day in children or 4 times a day in adults.

Nurse monitoring
1. This drug has minor anticholinergic side effects and may produce a dry mouth.
2. Systemic toxic effects rarely occur.

General notes
1. Ipratropium bromide inhaler may be stored at room temperature.
2. As with all pressured aerosols the container should never be punctured or incinerated after use.

IPRINDOLE (Prondol)

Presentation
Tablets—15 mg, 30 mg.

Actions and uses
Iprindole is a tricyclic antidepressant drug. Its actions and uses are described in the section dealing with these drugs.

Dosage
15–30 mg three times daily is the normal oral dosage for the treatment of depression in adults. If necessary a maximum daily dose of up to 180 mg may be used.

Nurse monitoring
See the section on tricyclic antidepressant drugs.

General notes
Iprindole tablets may be stored at room temperature.

Available U100 insulins i.e. containing 100 units in 1 ml

Insulin type	Beef	Pork	Human	Onset of action	Duration of action
Soluble	No brand name—Wellcome Quicksol—Boots Neusulin—Wellcome Hypurin NS—Weddel No brand name—Evans	Velosulin—Nordisk Actrapid MC—Novo	Humulin S—Eli Lilly Human Celosulin—Nordisk Human Actrapid—Novo	½–1 h ½–1 h	6–8 h 6–8 h
Neutral Soluble					
Protamine Zinc	Hypurin PZ—Weddel				
Isophane	Monophane—Boots Neuphane—Wellcome Hypurin I—Weddel No brand name—Evans	Insulatard—Nordisk	Humulin I—Eli Lilly Human Insulatard—Nordisk	4–6 h 2–3 h	30 h 24 h
Insulin Zinc Suspension Amorphous (Semilente)		Semitard MC—Novo	—	1 h	14–16 h
Mixed (Lente)	Tempulin—Boots Neulente—Wellcome Hypurin L—Weddel No brand name—Evans Lentard MC—Novo (30% Pork (amorphous) 70% Beef (crystalline)	Monotard MG—Novo	Human Monotard—Novo	2–3 h	24 h+
Crystalline (Ultralente)	Ultratard MC—Novo	—		4–6 h	30 h+
Biphasic Insulins	Rapitard MC—Novo (25% Pork (neutral soluble) 75% Beef (crystalline) Mixtard 30/70—Nordisk (30% Neutral Sol./70% Isophane) Initard 50/50—Nordisk (50% Neutral Sol./50% Isophane)		Human Mixtard 30/70—Nordisk (30% Neutral Sol./70% Isophane) Human Initard 50/50—Nordisk (50% Neutral Sol./50% Isophane)	½–1 h	20–24 h

N.B. Other forms of human insulin are currently under development.

IPRONIAZID (Marsilid)

Presentation
Tablets—25 mg, 50 mg

Actions and uses
Iproniazid is a monoamine oxidase inhibiting drug. Its actions and uses are described in the section on these drugs.

Dosage
25–150 mg daily as a single dose.

Nurse monitoring
See the section on monoamine oxidase inhibiting drugs.

General notes
Iproniazid tablets may be stored at room temperature.

IRON (Parenteral)
Iron Sorbitol injection BP (Jectorer)
Iron Dextran injection BP (Imferon)

Presentation
See individual drugs.

Actions and uses
The indications for parenteral iron are identical to those described for oral iron. Parenteral therapy is usually resorted to only when patients are in a state of gross iron deficiency and are intolerant of oral preparations.

Dosage
The total replacement dose required is determined by reference to tables produced by the manufacturers of the parenteral preparations of iron, which allow the total dosage to be computed on the basis of the patient's body weight and haemoglobin level. The total dose may then be administered as a series of daily intramuscular of intravenous injections of 1.5 mg/kg body weight or by one or two large dose intravenous infusions in normal saline of 5% dextrose given over 6–8 hours.

Nurse monitoring
1. Parenteral iron is very toxic and should only be used when the oral route has been tried and found to be totally unsuccessful.
2. The administration of parenteral iron may lead to hypersensitivity reactions including fever, urticaria, skin rash, muscle pain, lymphadenopathy and occasionally anaphylactic shock which is potentially fatal.
3. Test doses should always be given and facilities for emergency resuscitation and the administration of intravenous adrenaline, antihistamines and corticosteroids should be available.

General notes
Iron for injection may be stored at room temperature.

IRONS (Oral)

Presentation
A wide range of preparations contain iron, either on its own or in combination with Folic Acid or in combination with Vitamins. Iron is available for administration either as the fumarate, succinate, gluconate or sulphate.

Actions and uses
Iron may be administered usefully in two situations:
1. Where patients, due to inadequate diet or disease of the gut, have been shown by laboratory testing to be deficient in iron.
2. Where patients are known to be at risk of developing iron deficiency anaemia such as in pregnancy.

Dosage
The dosage of any iron preparation may be expressed in terms of elemental iron it supplies i.e.:
1. For the treatment of iron deficiency anaemias:
100–200 mg of elemental iron daily is required in adults for 3–6 months.
2. For the prevention of iron deficiency anaemias during pregnancy: 100 mg of elemental iron (Fe) per day is recommended.

The four major salts of iron available i.e. Ferrous Sulphate, Ferrous Fumarate, Ferrous Gluconate and

Ferrous Succinate are discussed individually in the text and the tablet dosage equivalent to the elemental iron requirements is given.

Nurse monitoring
1. Iron is irritant to the gastrointestinal tract. It may produce nausea, vomiting, constipation or diarrhoea. These symptoms may be so troublesome that patients may not take their treatment. The nurse may play an important role in identifying whether patients are complying with their therapy in emphasising to them the importance of continuing with therapy. She may advise them to seek alternative preparations of iron from their doctor should the particular preparation they are taking be causing severe side effects. Patients may find their symptoms are reduced if they take iron with food.
2. The gastrointestinal side effects described above vary and therefore where side effects are troublesome different types of iron salts may be administered until one with lesser effects is obtained.
3. Iron always produces a black stool. This may alarm patients and the nurse may play an important role in patient management by warning them of the possible occurrence of black stools and reassuring them of its innocence.
4. In excessive dosage iron is an extremely dangerous compound, especially in children. The nurse may contribute to the management of this problem by emphasising to patients the importance of keeping iron preparations out of the reach of children and also by warning patients to take their children immediately to hospital for treatment should they accidentally swallow any number of iron tablets.

General notes
Most iron tablets may be stored safely at room temperature.

IRON DEXTRAN INJECTION BP (Imferon)

Presentation
50 mg Fe/ml in 2 ml, 5 ml and 20 ml ampoules for intramuscular, intravenous injection or intravenous infusion.

Actions and uses
See the section on iron (parenteral).

Dosage
See the section on iron (parenteral).

Nurse monitoring
See the section on iron (parenteral).

General notes
Iron for injection may be stored at room temperature.

IRON SORBITOL INJECTION BP (Jectofer)

Presentation
100 mg of elemental iron (Fe) in 2 ml ampoules for intramuscular injection.

Actions and uses
See the section on iron (parenteral).

Dosage
See the section on iron (parenteral).

Nurse monitoring
See the section on iron (parenteral).

General notes
Iron for injection may be stored at room temperature.

ISOCARBOXAZID (Marplan)

Presentation
Tablets—10 mg

Actions and uses
Isocarboxazid is a monoamine oxidase inhibiting drug. Its actions and uses are described in the section on these drugs.

Dosage
10–30 mg daily.

Nurse monitoring
See the section on monoamine oxidase inhibitors.

General notes
Isocarboxazid tablets may be stored at room temperature.

ISONIAZID

Presentation
Tablets—50 mg, 100 mg
Injection—50 mg in 2 ml
N.B. Isoniazid is generally used in combinations containing other drugs. These are as follows:
1. Isoniazid and sodium aminosalicylate (Inapasade)
2. Isoniazid and ethambutol (Mynah)
3. Isoniazid and Rifampicin (Rifinah, Rimactazid).

Actions and uses
Isoniazid is an antibacterial drug which is of use only for the treatment of tuberculosis caused by the organism mycobacterium tuberculosis. Its action may be either bacteriostatic (inhibiting growth and replication of the organism) or bacteriocidal (killing the organism), depending on the concentration achieved in the tissues. If used on its own for the treatment of tuberculosis it will be, in a large number of cases, ineffective as the organism gradually develops resistance to it and therefore it is usually used in combination with other antituberculous drugs (q.v.).

Dosage
For oral or intramuscular administration:
1. *Adults*: 300–600 mg daily in total given in three divided doses.
2. *Children*: 16 mg/kg body weight daily in two divided doses.

Nurse monitoring
1. Patients undergoing treatment for tuberculosis receive their drugs for considerable periods of time. The nurse may play an important role in reminding patients that their drug therapy must be taken regularly for as long as recommended by medical staff, whether or not they themselves feel that they have recovered.
2. Gastrointestinal upset including nausea and vomiting commonly occur in patients receiving this drug.
3. Isoniazid is associated with a high incidence of neurological side effects, the most common of which is peripheral neuropathy (altered sensation and motor function of the limbs). Peripheral neuropathy may be treated by giving Pyridoxine 50–100 mg orally per day in addition to the Isoniazid. Other neurological side effects include mental disturbance, convulsion, inco-ordination, encephalopathy and alcohol intolerance. If the patient is not receiving too high a dose of the drug then the occurrence of these side effects is an indication for change of treatment to alternative drugs.
4. Isoniazid interferes with the metabolism of a substance known as Pyridoxine. This may cause peripheral neuropathy and more rarely anaemia or a deficiency syndrome known as pellagra which is characterised by diarrhoea, dementia and dermatitis of the light exposed areas of the skin.
5. Other side effects include disorders of the blood such as haemolytic anaemia aplastic anaemia or agranulocytosis, skin rashes and metabolic disturbances such as hyperglycaemia and acidosis.
6. The drug should be used with caution in patients with liver disease, epilepsy or those with reduced renal function.
7. The drug should be given with caution to patients receiving Phenytoin as it increases the effects of Phenytoin and may precipitate Phenytoin toxicity (q.v.).

General notes
The drug may be stored at room temperature.

ISOPRENALINE (Saventrine, Suscardia)

Presentation
Tablets—30 mg sustained release
Injection—2 mg in 2 ml
Isoprenaline is included in several

proprietary aerosol preparations for inhalation therapy.

Actions and uses
Isoprenaline is a powerful stimulant of the beta-adrenergic receptors which form a part of the sympathetic branch of the autonomic nervous system. It is sufficient to note that the stimulation of these beta-receptors will result in dilation of the bronchioles (small airways) in the lungs, and increase in heart rate and cardiac output. Isoprenaline therefore has a number of possible actions.

1. If given by inhalation it may reverse the constriction of bronchioles in bronchial asthma. Because of its effects on heart rate and because there are other drugs now available which have the same effect on the lungs but do not have the effect on heart rhythm the drug is rarely used for this purpose nowadays.
2. It may be used orally or intravenously to stimulate the heart rate in patients with bradycardia due to disease of the tissues which conduct electrical impulses through the heart.
3. The effect of stimulation of both heart rate and cardiac output makes it a potentially useful drug when given intravenously for the state of cardiogenic shock.

Dosage
1. The dose administered via aerosol depends on the proprietary preparation used.
2. When used in the treatment of bradycardia the dose range is 90–270 mg in three divided doses orally. It may be given by intravenous infusion at a rate of 0.5–40 µg/minute. The intravenous dosage is usually titrated by observing the effect on blood pressure and pulse.

Nurse monitoring
1. As mentioned above, Isoprenaline has the potentially serious side effects of tachycardia when given by aerosol. Other preparations such as Salbutamol (Ventolin) which do not have this effect are more suitable. However, should the nurse encounter patients on this drug, she should be aware that it may cause tachycardia, and in extreme cases, cardiac arrest due to ventricular fibrillation may occur.
2. When given orally or intravenously for bradycardia there is still a risk of the production of a serious tachycardia or other cardiac dysrhythmia should an excessive dose be given. Patients on oral treatment should have their pulse checked regularly and intravenous treatment should never be given unless facilities are available for ECG monitoring or unless the drug is given as an emergency treatment to sustain the patient while transfer to hospital for further treatment is effected.
3. Side effects other than tachycardia are palpitations, tremor, precordial pain, sweating, facial flushing and headache.

General notes
Isoprenaline tablets may be stored at room temperature. The solution for injection should be stored in a refrigerator and protected from light. When given by intravenous infusion the injection solution should be added to 5% dextrose.

ISOSORBIDE DINITRATE (Cedocard, Isordil, Sorbitrate, Vascardin)

Presentation
Tablets—5 mg (sublingual), 10 mg and 20 mg (sustained release)

Actions and uses
This drug reduces heart work in a similar manner to Glyceryl Trinitrate (q.v.). It is used prophylactically to prevent angina pectoris. Its advantages over Glyceryl Trinitrate is that it has a longer duration of action.

Dosage
The usual adult dose for prevention

of angina is 10 mg three or four times a day or 20 mg twice daily of the sustained release preparation. It may be taken in an acute attack in a similar way to Glyceryl Trinitrate (i.e. held under the tongue).
Nurse monitoring
See the section on Glyceryl Trinitrate.
General notes
Isosorbide Dinitrate tablets may be stored at room temperature.

ISOSORBIDE MONONITRATE (Elantan, Isomo, Monit, Mono-Cedocard)
Presentation
Tablets—20 mg and 40 mg
Actions and uses
This drug reduces heart work in a similar manner to Glyceryl Trinitrate. It has the actions and uses described for Glyceryl Trinitrate (though it has a much longer duration of action) and Isosorbide Dinitrate but unlike these drugs it is not appreciably destroyed by the liver and hence has a more predictable action. Isosorbide mononitrate is used mainly for the prophylaxis of angina pectoris.
Dosage
Usually 20–40 mg is taken three times a day.
Nurse monitoring
See the section on Glyceryl Trinitrate.
General notes
Isosorbide Mononitrate tablets may be stored at room temperature.

ISOXSUPRINE (Duvadilan, Defencin)
Presentation
Tablets—20 mg
Capsules—40 mg slow release
Injection — 10 mg in 2 ml
  50 mg in 10 ml
Actions and uses
This drug acts at two sites of the sympathetic nervous system to produce vasodilation. It is therefore used in the treatment of:
1. Raynaud's phenomenon
2. Intermittent claudication
3. Night cramps
4. Chilblains
5. Frost bite
6. It has also been proposed that the drug may be useful in the treatment of cerebrovascular insufficiency
7. Its effect on one component of the sympathetic nervous system leads to a reduction of uterine motility and the drug has been used for the treatment of premature labour.

Dosage
1. For the treatment of peripheral vascular disease.:
   a. Orally: 10–20 mg three or four times a day. Slow release capsules should be administered in a dose of 40 mg twice per day.
   b. Intramuscularly: 5–10 mg two or three times a day.
   c. Intravenously: 100 mg is dissolved in 500 ml of 0.9% sodium chloride or 5% dextrose and infused over a period of up to one hour.
   d. 10 mg may be given intra-arterially up to four times daily.
2. For the treatment of premature labour: 100 mg of the drug in 500 ml of dextrose 5% or sodium chloride 0.9% injection is infused at a rate of 1–1.5 ml/minute according to patient response up to a maximum of 2.5 ml/minute. Subsequent treatment consists of intramuscular injections of 10 mg every three hours for 24 hours, then 4–8 hourly for a further 48 hours and then 20–40 mg by mouth four times per day.

Nurse monitoring
The Nurse monitoring aspects of this drug are identical to those described for Cyclandelate (q.v.).
General notes
1. The tablets and capsules may be stored at room temperature.
2. The injection solution should be refrigerated.

ISPAGHULA (Fybogel, Isogel)

Presentation
Sachets—3.5 g
Granules

Actions and uses
See the section discussing the actions of laxatives. Ispaghula falls into the second group, i.e. it is a bulking agent. The Ispaghula husk, like bran, is a natural dietary fibre supplement and it is used in those disorders of the bowel thought to be associated with reduced dietary fibre i.e.:

1. Diverticular disease
2. Spastic or irritable colon
3. Constipation.

Dosage
One sachet (3.5 g) or two 5 ml spoonfuls of granules taken twice daily after meals, stirred into a glass of cold water.

Nurse monitoring
There are no specific problems associated with this drug.

General notes
Sachets and granules containing Ispaghula husk may be stored at room temperature.

K

KANAMYCIN (Kantrex)

(See Note 3, p. 310)

Presentation
Capsules—250 mg
Injection—1 g in 3 ml

Actions and uses
Kanamycin is an aminoglycoside antibiotic and its actions and uses are described in the section dealing with these drugs. It is in addition recommended for the following conditions:
1. It may be used for the treatment of respiratory tract infections including tuberculosis.
2. It may be used for the treatment of genito-urinary tract infections (including gonorrhoea).
3. It may be used in the treatment of meningitis, septicaemia, bacteraemia and peritonitis.
4. It may be used in the treatment of bone and joint infections.
5. It may be used in the treatment of skin and soft tissue infections.
6. It may be used for post-surgical infection.
7. It may also be given orally in order to attempt gut sterilisation.

Dosage
1. Intramuscular route:
   a. *Adults*: 1 g in total is administered daily in divided doses every 6 or 12 hours. The daily dose should never exceed 1.5 g.
   b. For *children* under 50 kg: 15 mg/kg body weight in total daily is given in two divided doses.
   c. For *premature infants* weighing less that 2.5 kg: The recommended dose is 7.5–10 mg/kg body weight per day given in two divided doses.
2. The drug may be given intravenously but this is not recommended unless it is felt that the intramuscular route is inappropriate. Dosage should be 15 mg/kg body weight in total per day given in two divided doses. The injection is diluted with sterile normal saline or 5% dextrose in water to a concentration of 2.5 mg/ml and administered slowly.
3. For the treatment of gonorrhoea a single dose of 2 g is an effective regime.
4. When used in the treatment of tuberculosis: 1–2 g should be given two or three times a week. Treatment should be given for three to four months.
5. If administered by the intraperitoneal route, the recommended dose for adults is 0.5 g as a single injection.
6. If given by aerosol 250 mg two to four times a day is recommended.
7. The drug may also be given into abscess cavities, pleural spaces, peritoneal and ventricular cavities. It has also been given intrathecally but this latter route is inappropriate as adequate concentrations may be obtained by intramuscular administration.
8. To attempt gut sterilisation: 1–2 g daily given in four divided doses is recommended for adults.

Nurse monitoring
The Nurse monitoring notes on aminoglycoside antibiotics (q.v.) are applicable to Kanamycin with the

exception that Kanamycin may be given by infusion rather than intravenous bolus injection.
General notes
Preparations containing Kanamycin may be stored at room temperature.

KAOLIN
Presentation
Kaolin is included in many anti-diarrhoeal mixtures.
Actions and uses
Kaolin is a highly absorbent powder which absorbs toxic and other substances from the alimentary tract and increases the bulk of the faeces. This has an effect of reducing the frequency and severity of diarrhoea. It is administered in a suspension.
Dosage
1. *Adults*: 5–25 g as required.
2. *Children*: 1–5 g as required.

Nurse monitoring
1. Kaolin is not absorbed and therefore has no systemic effects.
2. The only point worthy of note is that as it produces bulk within the gut it is contraindicated in patients with intestinal obstruction.

General notes
Preparations containing Kaolin may be stored at room temperature. The powder however does not dissolve in water and such mixtures must be thoroughly shaken before each dose is withdrawn.

KETAZOLAM (Anxon)
Presentation
Capsules—15 mg and 30 mg
Actions and uses
Ketazolam is a benzodiazepine drug which has long duration of action. It is used in the management of anxiety neurosis.
Dosage
Adults: 15–60 mg usually taken as a single dose with doses in the lower range preferred for elderly patients.

Nurse monitoring
See the section on benzodiazepines.
General notes
Capsules containing ketazolam may be stored at room temperature.

KETOCONAZOLE (Nizoral)
Presentation
Tablets—200 mg
Actions and uses
Ketoconazole is an anti-fungal drug. It has a major advantage over other anti-fungal agents in that effective blood levels may be obtained after oral administration. It is used in the treatment of the following disorders:
1. Treatment of fungal infections of skin and hair by dermatophytes and/or yeasts i.e. dermatomycosis, pityriasis versicolor, chronic mucocutaneous candidosis
2. Treatment of yeast infections of the mouth (*Candida albicans*)
3. For gut sterilisation
4. For treatment of systemic mycoses i.e. systemic candidosis, paracoccidioidomycosis, histoplasmosis, coccidioidomycosis etc.
5. Recurrent vaginal candidosis
6. It may be used prophylactically in 'at risk' groups i.e. those with reduced immunity due to cytotoxic therapy for malignant disease.

Dosage
1. For the uses described under 1, 2, 3, 4 and 6 above
   a. Adults: Initittally 200 mg once daily is given. The dose may be doubled if a satisfactory response is not achieved. The treatment is continued for at least one week after symptoms have cleared and the usual duration of treatment varies widely according to the condition under treatment i.e. 10 days for oral thrush, 6 months for systemic infections with

paracoccidioidomycosis, coccidioidomycosis and histoplasmosis
  b. Children: the single daily dose is calculated on the basis of 3 mg per kg
 2. For the treatment of recurrent vaginal candidosis—200 mg twice daily for 5 days.

Nurse monitoring
 1. The commonest problems associated with administration of this drug are gastro-intestinal upset, predominantly nausea
 2. Skin rash and pruritus is also fairly common
 3. Any drug which reduces the acid content of the stomach such as antacids, cimetidine, ranitidine and anticholinergic drugs will impair absorption of ketoconazole and therefore at least two hours should be allowed between administration of ketoconazole and any of these agents.
 4. Ketoconazole tablets should be taken with meals when gastric acidity is high
 5. The drug should be avoided in pregnancy.

General notes
Tablets may be stored at room temperature.

KETOPROFEN (Alrheumat, Orudis)

Presentation
Capsules—50 mg

Actions and uses
See the section on non-steroidal anti-inflammatory analgesic drugs.

Dosage
The usual adult dose is 50–100 mg twice daily although 50 mg three or four times daily is used occasionally in a few cases some patients achieve adequate control with a single (bed-time) dose of 100–200 mg

Nurse monitoring
See the section on anti-inflammatory analgesic drugs, non-steroidal.

General notes
Ketoprofen capsules may be stored at room temperature.

KETOTIFEN (Zaditen)

Presentation
Capsules—1 mg

Actions and uses
Ketotifen binds to cells present in the airways which under certain conditions would normally release chemicals which would cause an increase in muscle tone in the airways thereby causing bronchospasm manifest as dyspnoea and wheezing. It is, therefore, useful for the prophylactic treatment of conditions associated with bronchospasm.

Dosage
The usual adult dosage is 1–2 mg twice daily with food.

Nurse monitoring
 1. It is important to note that this drug is of prophylactic use only and will not be of any benefit in the treatment of an established attack of bronchospasm.
 2. The nurse may play an important role in encouraging patients to persevere with the therapy in the early stages when symptomatic benefit may not be obtained. It has been found in practice that symptomatic benefit is only established after several weeks of treatment.
 3. The nurse may also play an important role in encouraging patients to persist with this therapy despite disturbing symptoms in the early treatment period of drowsiness, dizziness and dry mouth, as she may confidently re-assure them that these symptoms will become far less troublesome as treatment continues.

General notes
Ketotifen capsules may be stored at room temperature.

L

LABETALOL (Trandate)

Presentation
Tablets—100 mg, 200 mg, 400 mg
Injection—100 mg in 20 ml

Actions and uses
Labetalol is a beta-adrenoreceptor blocker and therefore has all the actions of beta-adrenoreceptor blocking drugs (q.v.). However, it also blocks alpha receptor sites in peripheral blood vessels such as arterioles and produces dilation of these vessels. This additional effect adds to its capacity to reduce blood pressure and Labetolol's main use is in the treatment of hypertension.

Dosage
1. In hypertensive emergencies it may be given by slow intravenous injection (50 mg given over a period of at least one minute), or by intravenous infusion of a solution containing 200 mg in 200 ml given at a rate of 2 mg per minute. The maximum intravenous dosage is 300 mg.
2. The usual adult oral maintenance dose is 300–600 mg per day in three divided doses. Up to 2.4 g daily may be given in divided doses to establish control of hypertension.

Nurse monitoring
1. Labetalol has all the side effects of beta-adrenoreceptor blocking drugs (q.v.).
2. Its additional alpha blocking action makes it especially likely to produce postural hypotension. Patients must be warned of this and instructed on how to avoid its effects by changing posture slowly.
3. When patients receive intravenous doses of this drug they should be in a supine position to avoid hypotension.
4. Labetolol has a number of side effects not seen with other beta-blocking drugs and these include difficulty with micturition, epigastric pain, blurred vision, a lichenoid skin rash and tingling sensations in the scalp.

General notes
Labetalol tablets and injection may be stored at room temperature. The injection solution is however sensitive to light.

LACTULOSE (Duphalac)

Presentation
Syrup—3.35 g in 5 ml

Actions and uses
Lactulose is a sugar compound which is neither digested in nor absorbed from human gut. When taken it passes into the large bowel where it affects both the bowel bacteria and the amount of water present in the stool. It has two main uses:
1. As a laxative it falls into group 3 in terms of its mode of action (see the section on laxatives).
2. It is used for the treatment of patients with severe liver cell disease and hepatic encephalopathy. Its use in this condition is to reduce the amount of protein absorbed from the gut.

Dosage
1. For constipation:
   a. *Adults*: 15 ml syrup twice per day.

b. *Children*:
      Babies: 2.5 ml.
      Children under 5 years: 5 ml.
      5–10 years: 10 ml.
2. For the treatment of hepatic encephalopathy: doses of 30–50 ml three times daily are given initially and subsequently adjusted to produce two or three soft stools each day.

Nurse monitoring
1. This drug is largely without side effects, except in two very rare conditions:
   a. Galactosaemia where patients are intolerant of the sugar galactose which is contained in the commercial syrup preparation of this drug.
   b. There is a small group of patients who are actually intolerant to lactulose.

General notes
1. The syrup may be stored at room temperature.
2. It should not be stored in a refrigerator and never be allowed to freeze.
3. For ease of administration it may be diluted with water or with fruit juices etc.

LATAMOXEF (Moxalactam)

(See Note 3, p. 310)

Presentation
Injection—500 mg, 1 g and 2 g vials

Actions and uses
This drug is similar in almost all respects to drugs of the cephalosporin group of antibiotics and its actions and uses are described in the section dealing with this group. Latamoxef, for practical purposes, should be considered to be equivalent to a 3rd Generation cephalosporin.

Dosage
1. *Adults*: The total daily dose varies from 500 mg to 12 g daily, depending upon the nature and severity of infection, in 2–3 divided doses.
2. *Children*: Neonates: 25 mg/kg body weight every 8–12 hours
   Older children: 50 mg/kg body weight every 12 hours.
   Doses are administered by intramuscular or intravenous injection or be intravenous infusion.

Nurse monitoring
See the section on cephalosporins.

General notes
1. The drug should be stored at room temperature.
2. Intravenous infusions are prepared in sodium chloride 0.9%, dextrose 5% and dextrose/saline to produce a final concentration of about 5%.
3. If intramuscular injections prove painful, the injection may be prepared using lignocaine 0.5% injection.
4. Reconstituted solution in vials may be stored for up to 4 days in a refrigerator.

LAXATIVES

Presentation
See individual drugs.

Actions and uses
Laxatives act principally by one of three mechanisms:
1. They may irritate the bowel wall and produce increased bowel movement.
2. They may increase the amount of bulk with the stool and promote a more natural colonic action and more regular defaecation.
3. They may act as a 'wetting agent'. These substances either attract water into the stool or retain water already present in the stool causing an increase in volume and softening of consistency.

Dosage
See individual drugs.

Nurse monitoring
1. The taking of laxatives is a national pastime. However, the nurse may play an important role in detecting serious disease by noting change in bowel habit manifest by a need for an increase in frequency or dosage of regular laxatives or a failure of their action.
2. Individual side effects for the

various drugs are described under each drug in turn.
General notes
See individual drugs.

LEVODOPA (Larodopa)
Presentation
Tablets—500 mg
Actions and uses
In Parkinson's disease it has been shown that certain areas of the brain are depleted of a substance known as dopamine. It has further been shown that treatment with substances which increase concentrations of dopamine in these areas leads to an improvement in symptoms. Levodopa is a precursor of dopamine and is converted in the body to dopamine. It is used, therefore, for the treatment of Parkinson's disease.
Dosage
N.B. This drug is not recommended for administration to children. For adults: an initial dose of 125 mg twice daily immediately after food is recommended. The dose is doubled after a week and thereafter increased at weekly intervals by 375 mg per day, the total daily dose being given in four or five doses.
Nurse monitoring
1. It is important to note that there are now preparations available ('Madopar' and 'Sinemet', q.v.) which combine Levodopa with another compound which reduces the rate of metabolism of Levodopa in the body and therefore allows low doses to be administered and leads to a reduction in the incidence of side effects.
2. Side effects, usually dose-related, occur at some time in most patients. During the initiation of therapy nausea, vomiting, anorexia, weakness and hypotension (commonly postural) may occur. It is important for the nurse to note that nausea and vomiting may be reduced by the administration of the drug immediately after food. Occasionally, however, an anti-emetic drug may be necessary. At any stage in the treatment the following other side effects may occur.
   a. Psychiatric disturbance including elation, depression, anxiety, agitation, aggression, hallucination and delusion.
   b. Involuntary movements commonly in the form of oral dyskinesia (rhythmic writhing movements of the mouth and tongue) or similar writhing movements of the limbs. These effects are usually dose related and may disappear after a reduction in the dose. They are particularly likely to occur in the elderly.
   c. Abnormalities in liver function tests and other biochemical blood values may occur.
   d. Patients on Levodopa may notice a darkening in colour with a reddish tinge of the urine and further darkening if the urine is left to stand. They should be reassured that this is quite normal and does not imply any renal damage.

General notes
The drug may be stored at room temperature.

LEVORPHANOL TARTRATE (Dromoran)
Presentation
Tablets—1.5 mg
Injection—2 mg in 1 ml
Actions and uses
For an account of the actions and uses of this drug, see the general description in the section on narcotic analgesic drugs. It is important to note that Levorphenol tartrate has a more prolonged action than Morphine.
Dosage
For adults:
1. Orally: 1.5–3 mg once or twice daily
2. By intramuscular, subcutaneous or intravenous injection: 2–4 mg once or twice daily.

Nurse monitoring
See the section on narcotic analgesic drugs.
General notes
1. This drug is subject to the legal requirements of 'controlled drugs' and should be stored in a locked (controlled drug) cupboard.
2. The drug may be stored at room temperature.

LIGNOCAINE

1. Local anaesthetic—Lignostab, Lidothesin
2. Antidysrhythmic—Xylocard

1. LOCAL ANAESTHETIC
Presentation
Injection—0.5%, 1%, 1.5%, 2% for infiltration anaesthesia and spinal regional nerve block.
Tropical solution—4%
Antiseptic gel—2%
Oral gel—2%
Eye drops—4%
Local anaesthetic spray—10%
Ointment—5%
Preparations are also available with adrenaline added (see below).

Actions and uses
Lignocaine is a local anaesthetic with very wide uses and may be applied topically on the cornea, conjunctiva, and mucous surfaces of the mouth, rectum and urethra. It may be injected subcutaneously round specific sites e.g. before suturing, or into the region of a main nerve branch to block an area of pain receptors prior to dental procedures. It may also be injected around the spinal nerves as they leave the spinal cord to produce regional anaesthesia for obstetric and surgical procedures.

Dosage
Individual doses for infiltration and spinal or regional nerve block vary with the type of procedure—0.5% to 1.5% are generally used for infiltration and 1% to 2% for nerve block and spinal block. Preparations are available with added adrenaline, which by its vasoconstrictor effect reduces the rate at which Lignocaine leaves the site of injection, and therefore prolongs its effect.

Nurse monitoring
1. By far the most important aspect of Nurse monitoring in patients prescribed this drug takes place before the drug is given. Should Lignocaine with adrenaline be administered instead of plain Lignocaine, especially to the peripheries, severe tissue ischaemia leading perhaps to gangrene and loss of part of a limb may occur. Conversely, administration of plain Lignocaine instead of Lignocaine and adrenaline may considerably reduce the duration of analgesia, and lead to severe patient discomfort. Thus, the nurse and doctor must check thoroughly in advance that the type and strength of the solution is appropriate.
2. Pain or stinging may occur at the site of application before the onset of local anaesthetic effect.
3. Skin rashes due to local allergy may occur.
4. Excessive dosage may lead to side effects.

General notes
Lignocaine solution may be stored at room temperature.

2. ANTIDYSRHYTHMIC
Presentation
2%—Intravenous
20%—For infusion

Actions and uses
Lignocaine suppresses the conduction of electrical impulses through heart muscle and may be given intravenously to treat serious ventricular dysrhythmias.

Dosage
1. Bolus dosage at onset of treatment: 1 mg/kg given over 5 minutes. This may be repeated once or twice if necessary at 5–10 minute intervals.
2. Maintenance regime: Initially 2 mg per minute, increasing to 3 mg per minute and a maximum of 4 mg per minute if necessary. This regime is usually continued for 48 hours and prior to

discontinuation loading doses of oral antidysrhythmic are given.

Nurse monitoring
1. Lignocaine is often given in emergency situations i.e. at a cardiac arrest and it is imperative in a situation where mistakes can easily be made that the nurse remembers that the 20% solution is never appropriate for bolus injection.
2. Calcium chloride or gluconate cannot be injected into a solution containing Lignocaine or the calcium salt will precipitate in a solid form.
3. Too rapid or excessive intravenous dosage may be associated with the following effects: nervousness, dizziness, blurred vision, tremore and convulsions; nausea; hypotension and bradycardia; respiratory depression (with very high doses).
4. Patients with impaired liver function are more likely to develop adverse effects.

General notes
Lignocaine preparation may be stored at room temperature. Lignocaine 20% solution for cardiac use must be added to Dextrose 5% or laevulose 5% (1 g added to 500 ml if infusion fluid) to give a final concentration of 0.2%.

LINCOMYCIN (Lincocin)

(See Note 3, p. 310)

Presentation
Capsules—500 mg
Syrup—250 mg in 5 ml
Injection—300 mg in 1 ml

Actions and uses
Lincomycin is an antibiotic with a bacteriostatic action, in that it inhibits further growth and multiplication of cells in the body. It has been found to be particularly effective against the Gram-negative bacillus bacteroides. It has been found to be particularly useful for the treatment of:

1. Staphylococcal or streptococcal infections in patients who are sensitive to Penicillin.
2. Staphylococcal or streptococcal infections where the organism is known to be resistant to Penicillin.
3. Staphylococcal infections of the bone.

In general Lincomycin is reserved for use only in the above circumstances.

Dosage
1. *Adults*:
   a. Orally: 500 mg three or four times per day.
   b. Intramuscularly: 600 mg once or twice daily.
   c. Intravenously: 600 mg—8–12 hourly by i.v. infusion diluted in 500 ml of 0.9% sodium chloride or 5% dextrose.
2. *Children*:
   a. Orally:
      Less than 6 months: 1.25–2.5 ml of syrup three times per day.
      6 months–2 years: 2.5–5 ml of syrup three times per day.
      3–9 years: 2.5–5 ml of syrup four times per day.
      10–12 years: 5–10 ml of syrup four times per day.
      Over 12 years: adult doses are given.
   b. By intramuscular injection: 10 mg/kg is given once or twice per day.
   c. By intravenous injection: a total of 10–20 mg/kg body weight per day is given by infusion after appropriate dilution in two or three divided doses.

Nurse monitoring
1. In order to obtain optimal absorption, it is recommended that nothing be given orally except water for a period of one or two hours before and after oral administration.
2. Intramuscular injections should be made deeply into the gluteal muscles.
3. For intravenous injection: 600 mg should be diluted in 250 ml or

more of 5% glucose or normal saline and given over a period of not less than one hour. Children's doses should be diluted appropriately.
4. The only major side effects associated with Lincomycin are gastrointestinal. If any patient on Lincomycin develops diarrhoea the drug should be immediately stopped as a proportion of these patients may develop the serious condition—pseudomembranous enterocolitis.
5. The drug should not be given to the newborn or to patients with pre-existing kidney, liver, endocrine or metabolic disease.

General notes
1. Capsules and syrup may be stored at room temperature.
2. Injections should be refrigerated.

LITHIUM CARBONATE (Camcolit, Phasal, Priadel)

Presentation
Tablets — 250 mg, 400 mg
300 mg, 400 mg (both as slow release tablets)

Actions and uses
Lithium carbonate by an unknown mechanism, has been found to be useful for the treatment of depression in two particular instances:
1. It has been found to control both the manic and depressive phases of manic depressive psychosis.
2. It has been found that continuing treatment with Lithium reduces the recurrence of depressive and manic phases in patients who have already been found to have endogenous depression.

Dosage
For the treatment of depression in adults the precise dosage is that which maintains the plasma lithium level in the range 0.6–1.4 mmol/l. Treatment is usually taken once per day and it is important that all patients receiving the drug have their dosage carefully monitored to keep them within the above range.

Nurse monitoring
1. Side effects which are usually mainly seen if an excess dose is being taken include anorexia, nausea, vomiting, diarrhoea, thirst, polyuria, fatigue, malaise, dizziness, confusion, hypotension and cardiac dysrhythmias.
2. The drug should not be used in patients with renal failure or cardiac disease.
3. The drug may affect thyroid function rendering the patient clinically hypothyroid. The nurse may aid the detection of this side effect by noticing the formation of a goitre (thyroid swelling). Most patients on this drug are regularly monitored by clinical and biochemical testing for the development of this effect.
4. Elderly patients require lower doses of this drug if side effects are to be avoided.

General notes
Preparations containing Lithium carbonate may be stored at room temperature.

LOMUSTINE (CCNU)

Presentation
Capsules—10 mg, 40 mg

Actions and uses
Lomustine is a cytotoxic drug which inhibits cell growth and division by combining with and rendering useless important substances necessary for cell growth and also by inhibiting the enzymes responsible for the incorporation of these substances into the cell. It may be used alone, with radiotherapy, or in combination with other cytotoxic drugs in the treatment of the following conditions:
1. Brain tumours
2. Bronchogenic carcinoma
3. Malignant melanoma
4. Hodgkin's disease
5. It has been occasionally given for non-Hodgkin's lymphoma, myeloma, tumours of the gut,

kidney, testes, ovary, cervix, uterus and breast.

Dosage
The drug is taken orally. The dose for adults and children is up to 120–130 mg per m² as a single dose repeated every 6–8 weeks.

Nurse monitoring
1. Bone marrow suppression is an important side effect and the resultant leucopenia and thrombocytopenia leaves the patient at risk from severe infection and haemorrhage.
2. Other side effects include anorexia, nausea, vomiting, alopecia, stomatitis and altered liver function.
3. White blood cell counts, platelet counts and liver function tests are normally monitored during treatment.
4. The nurse should be constantly aware that most cytotoxic drugs are irritant to the skin and mucous surfaces, and are in general very toxic. Great care should therefore be exercised when handling these drugs, and in particular spillage or contamination of personnel or the environment must be avoided. If cytotoxic drugs are handled regularly it is theoretically possible that repeated skin contact or inhalation may produce systemic toxic effects and in nurses who have developed hypersensitivity, severe local and general hypersensitivity reactions.

General notes
Lomustine capsules may be stored at room temperature. It is important to note that they should be stored in the original container and protected from light and moisture.

LOPERAMIDE (Imodium)

Presentation
Capsules—2 mg
Syrup—1 mg in 5 ml

Actions and uses
Loperamide has a direct action on the nerves which control muscular movement of the intestinal wall. Its overall effect is to slow the passage of substances through the intestine and its use is therefore in the treatment of diarrhoea.

Dosage
1. *Adults*: 4 mg initially followed by 2 mg after each loose stool. The maximum daily dosage should not exceed 16 mg.
2. *Children*:
   4–8 years: 1 mg four times per day
   9–12 years: 2 mg four times per day

It is recommended that all the above doses be given until the diarrhoea is controlled.

Nurse monitoring
1. The drug is very poorly absorbed from the gut and therefore produces little in the way of side effects.
2. Continued use after diarrhoea has been controlled may produce constipation.
3. It should always be remembered that persistent diarrhoea may be indicative of a serious underlying condition and, therefore, the patients should be encouraged to consult their doctors should chronic use of this drug be discovered.

General notes
1. Loperamide preparations may be stored at room temperature.
2. For ease of administration the syrup may be diluted with water.
3. The commercial syrup is sugar-free and is, therefore, suitable for patients who are disaccharide intolerant.

LOPRAZOLAM (Dormonoct)

Presentation
Tablets—1 mg

Actions and uses
Loprazolam is a benzodiazepine and the section on these drugs should be consulted for a brief general account. It has a marked sedative effect and is taken as a hypnotic to induce sleep. Of particular interest is the short action of this drug in the

body which tends to produce a normal length sleep of up to 8 hours without the hang-over effect which occasionally extends into the following day with other hypnotics.

Dosage
Adults: 1 mg to 2 mg taken on retiring. Elderly patients should receive the lower dosage.

Nurse monitoring
See the section on benzodiazepines.

General notes
Tablets containing Loprazolam may be stored at room temperature.

LORAZEPAM (Ativan)

Presentation
Tablets—1 mg, 2, 5 mg
Injection—4 mg in 1 ml

Actions and uses
Lorazepam is a benzodiazepine drug (q.v.). It has a short duration of action compared to other drugs of this group. It has two major uses:
1. For the control of anxiety.
2. Because of its short duration of action it is sometimes used as an alternative to Diazepam for sedation prior to minor operative or dental procedures.

Dosage
1. For the treatment of anxiety adults receive 1–4 mg daily in divided doses.
2. For sedation prior to minor surgical or dental procedures: 2–4 mg is given as a single dose one or two hours before the procedure beings.
3. By intravenous and intramuscular injection: a dose of 0.03–0.05 mg/kg body weight may be given or a single dose of 4 mg (2 mg for children) has been given to control status epilepticus.

Nurse monitoring
See the section on benzodiazepines.

General notes
Tablets containing Lorazepam may be stored at room temperature.

LORMETAZEPAM (Loramet, Noctamid)

Presentation
Tablets—0.5 mg and 1 mg
Capsules—1 mg

Actions and uses
Lormetazepam is a benzodiazepine-like compound which has a marked sedative effect and is taken at night as an hypnotic. Of particular interest is the very short action of this drug in the body which tends to reduce the hang-over effect which occasionally extends into the following day with other hypnotics. It may have a particular role therefore in producing sleep in elderly patients who are very sensitive to the prolonged sedative effect of similar hypnotics.

Dosage
Adults: 0.5–1 mg taken on retiring. Elderly patients should receive the lower dosage.

Nurse monitoring
See the section on benzodiazepines.

General notes
Tablets containing Lormetazepam may be stored at room temperature.

M

MADOPAR

Presentation
Madopar 62.5 capsules containing 50 mg of Levodopa and 14.25 mg of Benserazide Hydrochloride. Madopar 125 capsules containing 100 mg of Levodopa and 28.5 mg Benserazide Hydrochloride. Madopar 250 capsules containing 200 mg of Levodopa and 57 mg of Benserazide Hydrochloride

Actions and uses
This drug contains Levodopa and Benserazide Hydrochloride. (See the section on Levodopa for a description of its actions and uses.) The advantage of combining Levodopa with Benserazide is that the latter drug inhibits conversion of Levodopa to Dopamine in tissues of the body other than brain, thus allowing more Levodopa to reach the brain resulting in an increased clinical effect. It is thought that this drug produces a more rapid response at initiation of therapy, has a simpler dosage regime and is associated with fewer gastrointestinal side effects.

Dosage
1. Patients not previously treated with Levodopa: Initially one capsule of Madopar 125 should be given twice daily and this dose may be increased by one capsule a day every third or fourth day until a full therapeutic effect is obtained or side effects supervene. The effective dose usually lies within the range of 4–8 capsules of Madopar 125 daily in divided doses and most patients require no more than six capsules of Madopar 125 daily. Optimal improvement is usually seen in one to three weeks.
2. Patients previously treated with Levodopa: Levodopa should be discontinued 24 hours prior to the first dose of Madopar and the patient may then be initiated on a total of one less Madopar 125 capsule daily than the total number of 500 mg Levodopa tablets or capsules previously taken. After a week the initial dose may be increased in the manner described for patients not on previous therapy, (see (1) above).
3. Madopar 62.5 capsules are used to gradually tailor individual dosage requirements and are of particular value in the elderly who may readily respond to small dosage increments.

Nurse monitoring
The Nurse monitoring aspects of Levodopa (q.v.) apply to this drug with two major exceptions:
1. The rate of onset of clinical improvement is faster with this drug.
2. There are fewer gastrointestinal side effects with this drug compared to Levodopa.

General notes
1. The drug should be stored at room temperature.
2. The drug should be protected from moisture.

MAGNESIUM HYDROXIDE (Cream/Milk of Magnesia)

Presentation
Magnesium hydroxide is used alone or more often combined with other

antacids in a range of oral liquid and solid dosage forms.

Actions and uses
This drug is an antacid and is often useful for the symptomatic relief of dyspeptic pain.

Dosage
This varies with the type of preparation used.

Nurse monitoring
1. Magnesium hydroxide on its own frequently causes diarrhoea and therefore it is often used in combination with aluminium salts which have the opposite side effect.
2. In patients with chronic renal failure, increased levels of magnesium in the blood may be produce, leading to signs of magnesium toxicity such as hypotension, flushing and a sensation of heat and thirst, progressing to nausea, vomiting, lethargy and finally coma with weakness and paralysis of all muscles.
3. The absorption and therefore the clinical effect of other drugs such as salicylates, digoxin and antibiotics may be impaired.
4. The dosage of oral anticoagulants may need to be altered if magnesium hydroxide is administered.

General notes
Preparations containing magnesium hydroxide may be stored at room temperature. To exert a maximum antacid effect tablets should be thoroughly chewed before swallowing.

MAPROTILINE (Ludiomil)

Presentation
Tablets—10 mg, 25 mg, 50 mg, 75 mg, 150 mg

Actions and uses
Maprotiline is an anti-depressant drug which is derived from and is closely related chemically to tricyclic antidepressants. Its actions and uses are similar to those described for tricyclic antidepressants (q.v.)

Dosage
For the treatment of depression in adults: 25–150 mg per day is given either in three divided doses or as a single evening dose taken on retiring.

Nurse monitoring
1. The Nurse monitoring notes on tricyclic antidepressants (q.v.) are applicable to this drug.
2. It is worth noting that there is a particularly high incidence of skin rashes with this drug.

General notes
Maprotiline tablets may be stored at room temperature.

MAZINDOL (Teronac)

Presentation
Tablets—2 mg

Actions and uses
This anorexogenic drug which is used in the treatment of obesity is not related to the amphetamine group but is in fact a derivative of the tricyclic antidepressant group of drugs (q.v.). The problems encountered with dependence and addiction in patients receiving amphetamine derivatives, therefore, do not occur when this drug is used.

Dosage
For adults only: 2 mg after breakfast

Nurse monitoring
1. The Nurse monitoring notes on tricyclic antidepressant drugs (q.v.) are applicable to this drug.
2. In addition to the above notes, it is worth remembering that constipation, dry mouth, insomnia, nervousness, headache, dizziness and skin rashes are common in patients receiving this drug.

General notes
The drug may be stored at room temperature.

MEBENDAZOLE (Vermox)

Presentation
Tablets—100 mg
Suspension—100 mg in 5 ml

Actions and uses
This drug is effective in the treatment of helminthic infections both in the United Kingdom and the tropics. It is used for the treatment of hookworm, roundworm (Ascaris), threadworm and whipworm.

Dosage
For adults and children aged 2 years and above:
1. Threadworm: A single dose of one tablet or one 5 ml spoonful.
2. Whipworm, roundworm and hookworm: One tablet or one 5 ml spoonful twice daily (morning and evening) for three consecutive days.

Nurse monitoring
1. It is important to note that no special procedures such as purging, use of laxatives, and/or dietary changes are required when using this drug.
2. The drug is not at present recommended for use in children under 2 years.
3. The drug should not be given to pregnant women.
4. Particularly for the treatment of threadworm, it is advisable that all members of a family whether obviously infected or not should be treated at the same time to ensure eradication.
5. Side effects are mild and consist of transient abdominal pain and occasional diarrhoea.

General notes
The drug may be stored at room temperature.

MEBEVERINE (Colofac)

Presentation
Tablets—135 mg

Actions and uses
Mebeverine relieves colonic spasm by a direct action on the smooth muscle of the colon. It is used to relieve abdominal pain, cramps, flatulence, and diarrhoea associated with irritable bowel syndrome and the gastrointestinal spasm associated with diverticular disease, gastritis, duodenitis, oesophagitis, cholecystitis, inflammatory bowel disease, peptic ulceration and hiatus hernia.

Dosage
The adult dose is 135 mg three times daily taken 20 minutes before meals. Lower maintenance doses may be used once a therapeutic effect has been achieved.

Nurse monitoring
No specific problems or side effects are associated with the administration of this drug.

General notes
Mebeverine tablets may be stored at room temperature.

MEBHYDROLIN (Fabahistin)

Presentation
Tablets—50 mg
Suspension—50 mg in 5 ml

Actions and uses
Mebhydrolin is an antihistamine. The actions and uses of antihistamines in general are discussed in the section dealing with these drugs. In clinical practice Mebhydrolin is used:
1. To suppress generalised minor allergic responses to allergens such as foodstuffs and drugs.
2. To suppress local allergic reactions i.e. inflammatory skin responses to insect stings and bites, contact allergens, urticaria etc.
3. Orally for allergic ocular inflammatory conditions e.g. due to hay fever and allergic rhinitis.
4. As a nasal decongestant e.g. in the treatment of allergic rhinitis and hay fever.

Dosage
1. *Adults*: 50–100 mg three times daily.
2. *Children*: 50–100 mg daily in total given in divided doses.

Nurse monitoring
See the section on antihistamines.

General notes
The drug may be stored at room temperature.

MEDAZEPAM (Nobrium)

Presentation
Capsules—5 mg, 10 mg

Actions and uses
Medazepam is a benzodiazepine drug (q.v.). Its principal use is in the treatment of anxiety.

Dosage
1. *Adults*: Initial doses of 5 mg two to three times daily increased to a maximum total dosage of 40 mg per day.
2. *Children*: Dosages are calculated on the basis of 1–1.5 mg/kg body weight in total per day, usually administered in two or three divided doses.

Nurse monitoring
See the section on benzodiazepines.

General notes
Medazepam capsules may be stored at room temperature.

MEDIGOXIN (Lanitop)

Presentation
Tablets—0.1 mg
Injection—0.2 mg in 2 ml

Actions and uses
This drug has identical effects to Digoxin (q.v.).

Dosage
1. Loading dose:
   a. Oral loading doses are usually 0.2 mg twice daily in the adult.
   b. The intravenous loading dose is 0.4 mg once daily for three to five days.
2. Maintenance dosage is usually 0.1 mg two or three times daily orally in the adult. Alternatively a single daily intravenous injection of 0.2–0.3 mg may be given.
3. Children's dosages are based on a calculation of 0.01 mg/kg every six hours until a therapeutic effect is achieved. Maintenance doses of 0.01 mg/kg daily orally are usually adequate thereafter.

It is worth noting that Medigoxin has a particularly rapid onset of action after oral administration.

Nurse monitoring
See the section on Digoxin.

General notes
Medigoxin tablets and injection may be stored at room temperature.

MEDROXYPROGESTERONE ACETATE (Provera, Depot-Provera)

Presentation
Tablets—5 mg, 100 mg, 200 mg
Injection—50 mg/ml

Actions and uses
1. The actions and uses of progestational hormones in general are discussed in the section on these drugs.
2. In clinical practice this drug is indicated for the treatment of threatened and recurrent abortion, functional uterine bleeding, secondary amenorrhoea, endometrial carcinoma, endometriosis, and short-term contraception.

Dosage
1. For the treatment of threatened abortion: 10–30 mg daily or higher if necessary to be continued 'until fetal viability is evident'.
2. For the treatment of habitual abortion: 10 mg daily during the first trimester, 20 mg daily during second trimester, 40 mg daily during third trimester. Continue therapy to the end of the 8th month.
3. For the treatment of secondary amenorrhoea: 2.5–10 mg per day for 5–10 days of the cycle.
4. For the treatment of functional uterine bleeding: 2.5–10 mg daily for 5–10 days commencing on the assumed or calculated 16th–21st day of the cycle.
5. For the treatment of endometriosis: 50 mg intramuscularly once weekly or 100 mg every two weeks.
6. For the treatment of endometrial carcinoma: 200–400 mg daily orally.
7. For contraception: 150 mg intramuscularly repeated every three months.

Nurse monitoring
1. When used as recommended

above few problems are encountered with this drug although it remains technically capable of producing the problems described under the Nurse monitoring section of progestational hormones (q.v.).

General notes
The drug may be stored at room temperature.

MEFENAMIC ACID (Ponstan)

Presentation
Tablets—500 mg
Capsules—250 mg
Paediatric suspension—50 mg in 5 ml

Actions and uses
See the section on anti-inflammatory analgesic drugs, non-steroidal.

Dosage
1. *Adults*: The recommended daily dosage is 250 mg to 500 mg three times per day.
2. *Children*: The recommended total daily doses are as follows:
Infants over 6 months: 25 mg/kg body weight
1 year plus: 150 mg
2–4 years: 300 mg
5–8 years: 450 mg
9–12 years: 600 mg

Nurse monitoring
1. See the section on anti-inflammatory analgesic drugs, non-steroidal.
2. It is worth noting that a particularly troublesome problem with Mefenamic acid is the production of diarrhoea which may on occasions be sufficiently severe to require cessation of treatment.

General notes
Tablets, capsules and paediatric suspension may be stored at room temperature. For ease of administration the paediatric suspension can be diluted with Syrup B.P. but such dilutions must be used up within a fortnight.

MEFRUSIDE (Baycaron)

Presentation
Tablets—25 mg

Actions and uses
See the section on thiazide and related diuretics.

Dosage
The adult dose is 25–100 mg which is usually taken once daily or occasionally on alternate days.

Nurse monitoring
See the section on thiazide and related diuretics.

General notes
Mefruside tablets may be stored at room temperature.

MEGESTROL ACETATE (Megace)

Presentation
Tablets—40 mg

Actions and uses
Megestrol Acetate is a progestational hormone and it therefore has the actions of those drugs which are described under Hormones (2). In clinical practice it is used to block the growth of oestrogen-dependent neoplasms, such as endometrial and breast carcinoma.

Dosage
Breast cancer: 160 mg daily
Endometrial cancer: 40–320 mg daily

Nurse monitoring
1. Megestrol Acetate can theoretically produce all effects described for Hormones (2), and the nurse monitoring section for Hormones (2) apply to this drug.
2. In practice the drug is generally well tolerated, producing a degree of weight gain, occasional urticaria and nausea.

General notes
Tablets may be stored at room temperature.

MELPHALAN (Alkeran)

Presentation
Tablets—2 mg, 5 mg
Injection—100 mg

Actions and uses
Melphalan is a member of the nitrogen mustard group. It prevents cell growth and division by inactivating important constituents of the cell necessary for these activities. Its uses are as follows:
1. It has proved to be of most value in the management of multiple myeloma.
2. It has also been used for the treatment of carcinoma of breast, soft tissue sarcoma, malignant melanoma and seminoma of the testes.

Dosage
1. In multiple myelomatosis a dose schedule of 0.15 mg/kg daily for four days in combination with Prednisolone is given. It is repeated at intervals of 6 weeks.
2. For treatment of other tumours regimes are variable:
   a. A single daily dose ranging from 2–35 mg may be given until a total dose of 150–200 mg has been received.
   b. By intravenous injection single doses of 1 mg/kg have been given.
   c. An isolated perfusion technique is used in the treatment of malignant melanoma. By this technique a much higher dose, i.e. up to 100 mg is circulated and confined to a particular part of the body affected by the tumour.

Nurse monitoring
1. Severe bone marrow suppression may occur even at low dose ranges. If these side effects arise patients may suffer severe and sometimes fatal infection or haemorrhage.
2. Nausea, vomiting and alopecia also occur but are more frequent with higher dosage.
3. The nurse should be constantly aware that cytotoxic drugs are highly dangerous and therefore must be handled with great care. Spillage and contamination of the skin of the patient or nurse may lead to a degree of absorption of the drug which, if chronically repeated, may cause damage and the skin may also be sensitised to the drug making it, in some cases, impossible for the nurse to continue working with the drug.

General notes
1. Melphalan is highly irritant and precautions should be taken to avoid contact with skin and eyes.
2. Melphalan tablets may be stored at room temperature.
3. The injection should be stored in a cool place and for this purpose refrigeration may be preferred.
4. The injection must be protected from light.
5. To prepare Melphalan injection 1 ml of special solvent is first added to the vial and the mixture shaken before a further 9 ml of diluent is added. Solutions for injection must be used within 15–30 minutes of preparation and unused injection immediately discarded.

MEPIVACAINE (Carbocaine)
Presentation
Injection—1%, 2%, 3% and 4%
Actions and uses
This local anaesthetic drug is used in dental practice and for minor surgical procedures to produce nerve block anaesthesia.
Dosage
The dosage may vary according to the procedure being undertaken and individual response.
Nurse monitoring
The Nurse monitoring aspects of Lignocaine (local anaesthetic) (q.v.) apply to this drug.
General notes
The drug may be stored at room temperature.

MEPROBAMATE (Equanil, Milonorm)
N.B. Commonly prescribed in the combination product, Equagesic
Presentation
Tablets—200 mg, 400 mg

Actions and uses

Meprobamate has sedative and tranquillising properties and is used in the management of anxiety neuroses, though it has been largely replaced by the newer and more effective benzodiazepines. In addition, the drug produces useful muscle relaxation by an inhibitory action on spinal cord reflexes and it is still widely prescribed in combination with simple analgesics to treat painful muscle injuries associated with muscle spasm.

Dosage

1. Anxiety states:
   Adults: 200 mg to 800 mg three times daily
   Children: a total daily dose of 50–100 mg per year of age in three divided doses.
2. Muscle injury:
   Adults: 300 mg 2–4 times daily.

Nurse monitoring

1. Elderly patients are particularly sensitive to this drug which may produce excessive sedation, confusion and inco-ordination. In general these patients should receive dosages in the lower range.
2. In common with many drugs which act in the CNS, meprobamate may produce dependency in some patients if taken for prolonged periods.
3. CNS depression, and thus the degree of sedation, is more marked in patients who take other sedative drugs and in this context patients should be warned of the danger of taking alcohol in even moderate amounts.
4. Meprobamate should not be taken during pregnancy, by nursing mothers or by epileptic patients in whom seizures may be produced.
5. In patients who have taken the drug for prolonged periods, particularly at high dosage, treatment should never be abruptly withdrawn but rather discontinued gradually. Convulsions may follow if the drug is stopped suddenly.

General notes

Tablets should be stored at room temperature. Tablets containing meprobamate and aspirin will deteriorate during storage, particularly if containers are not correctly sealed after use, and this is indicated by the strong 'vinegary' smell produced.

MEPYRAMINE (Anthisan)

Presentation

Tablets—50 mg, 100 mg
Elixir—50 mg in 5 ml
Injection—50 mg in 2 ml
Cream—2%

Actions and uses

Mepyramine is an antihistamine. The actions and uses of antihistamines in general are described in the section dealing with these drugs. In clinical practice Mepyramine is used:

1. To suppress generalised minor allergic responses to allergens such as foodstuffs and drugs.
2. To suppress local allergic reactions i.e. inflammatory skin responses to insect stings and bites, contact allergens, urticaria etc.

Dosage

1. Orally:
   a. *Adults*: 100 mg three times per day increasing as necessary to a total of 1 g per day.
   b. *Children*: 12.5–50 mg three times per day.
2. Parenterally (by intramuscular injection or intravenous infusion): In adults 25–50 mg three times daily.
3. Topically: The cream should be applied two or three times per day.

Nurse monitoring

See the section on antihistamines.

General notes

The drug may be stored at room temperature.

MEQUITAZINE (Primalan)
Presentation
Tablets—5 mg
Actions and uses
Mequitazine is an antihistamine. The actions and uses of antihistamines in general are discussed in the section of these drugs. In clinical practice Mequitazine is used:
1. To suppress local allergic reactions i.e. inflammatory skin responses to insect stings and bites, contact allergens, urticaria etc.
2. As a nasal decongestant e.g. in the treatment of allergic rhinitis and hay fever.

Dosage
Adults: 5 mg twice daily.
Nurse monitoring
See the section on antihistamines.
General notes
The drug may be stored at room temperature.

MERCAPTOPURINE (Puri-Nethol)
Presentation
Tablets—50 mg
Actions and uses
Mercaptopurine is an immunosuppressant and cytotoxic drug which inhibits a number of different enzymes involved in the early stages of purine synthesis. Purines are essential for the formation of DNA and subsequent cell division and if their synthesis is blocked cell division is inhibited.

Dosage
The oral daily dose for adults is usually 2.5–5 mg/kg body weight. Children's doses are as for adults.
Nurse monitoring
1. Bone marrow suppression is an important side effect and may produce anaemia, bleeding due to thrombocytopenia and infection due to suppression of white cell production. Regular blood tests are frequently carried out during treatment to detect the onset of these side effects.
2. This drug commonly causes gastrointestinal side effects including anorexia, nausea, vomiting, diarrhoea and oral ulceration.
3. This drug may also damage the liver and therefore blood tests of liver function should be carried out regularly.
4. The drug Allopurinol (q.v.) which is used in the treatment of hyperuricaemia may alter the body metabolism in such a way that the effect of a particular dose of Mercaptopurine may be markedly increased in patients who are given both drugs. The dose of Mercaptopurine should be reduced to approximately one-quarter of that intended if patients are already on Allopurinol.
5. The nurse should be constantly aware that most cytotoxic drugs are irritant to the skin and mucous surfaces, and are in general very toxic. Great care should therefore be exercised when handling these drugs, and in particular spillage or contamination of personnel or the environment must be avoided. If cytotoxic drugs are handled regularly it is theoretically possible that repeated skin contact or inhalation may produce systemic toxic effects and in nurses who have developed hypersensitivity, severe local and general hypersensitivity reactions.

General notes
1. Mercaptopurine tablets may be stored at room temperature.
2. They should be protected from light and kept dry.

MESTEROLONE (Pro-Viron)
Presentation
Tablets—25 mg
Actions and uses
1. The actions and uses of androgenic hormones and anabolic steroids are discussed in the sections dealing with these drugs.

2. In clinical practice this drug is used primarily for the treatment of hypogonadism in males.

Dosage
The dosage is adjusted according to individual response but is usually in the range of 25 mg two to four times daily.

Nurse monitoring
See the section on androgenic hormones and anabolic steroids.

General notes
The drug may be stored at room temperature.

MESTRANOL (Mestranol (Menophase)

Presentation
The above preparation combines Mestranol with a progestational hormone.

Actions and uses
1. The actions and uses of oestrogenic hormones in general are discussed in the section on these drugs.
2. The actions and uses of the proprietary preparations in which this hormone is included are:
   a. For the treatment of functional uterine bleeding
   b. For the treatment of endometriosis.

Dosage
The doses vary considerably with the indications for use and the individual proprietary preparation.

Nurse monitoring
See the section on combined oestrogen and progestrogenic hormones.

General notes
All the above preparations may be stored at room temperature.

METFORMIN (Glucophage)

Presentation
Tablets—500 mg, 850 mg

Actions and uses
The actions and uses of biguanide drugs are described in the section on these drugs.

Dosage
For adults: 3 × 500 mg or 2 × 850 mg tablets in three or two divided doses respectively with meals.

Nurse monitoring
See the section on biguanide drugs.

General notes
The drug may be stored at room temperature.

METHACYCLINE (Rondomycin)

(See Note 3, p. 310)

Presentation
Capsules—150 mg
Syrup—75 mg in 5 ml

Actions and uses
See the section on tetracyclines.

Dosage
1. *Adults*: The daily oral dosage is 600 mg to 1.2 g taken in 2–4 divided doses.
2. *Children*: The oral dose range is 7.5–15 mg/kg body weight in total daily, usually given in three divided doses.

Nurse monitoring
See the section on tetracyclines.

General notes
The drug may be stored at room temperature.

METHADONE (Physeptone)

Presentation
Tablets—5 mg
Linctus—2 mg in 5 ml
Injection—10 mg in 1 ml

Actions and uses
1. Methadone is a narcotic analgesic and its general actions and uses are described in the section dealing with these drugs.
2. Methadone has an additional specific use in that it is less addictive than other narcotic analgesics such as Morphine and Diamorphine and if used when patients are being weaned off these drugs it may lead to a reduction in the severity of withdrawal symptoms.
3. Methadone is a potent cough

suppressant and the linctus preparation is used for the treatment of severe intractable cough.

Dosage
1. For analgesia:
   Adults should receive 5–10 mg 4-hourly initially increasing if necessary to 30 mg 4-hourly.
2. For the suppression of cough:
   a. *Adults*: 2 mg every 3–4 hours as the linctus preparation
   b. *Children*:
      Under 10 years: 0.25 mg 4-hourly as the linctus preparation.
      Over 10 years: 0.5 mg 4-hourly as the linctus preparation.

Nurse monitoring
See the section on narcotic analgesics.

General notes
1. The drug should be stored in a locked (controlled drug) cupboard.
2. The drug should be stored at room temperature.
3. The linctus is diluted 1 part to 7 parts with syrup when required for administration to children.

METHICILLIN (Celbenin)

(*See Note 3, p. 310*)

Presentation
Injection—1 g vials

Actions and uses
Methicillin is a member of the Penicillin group of drugs with actions and uses similar to those described for Benzylpencillin (q.v.). Methicillin, however, has an important advantage over Benzylpenicillin in that it is more likely to be effective against infections caused by *Staphylococcus aureus* than Benzylpenicillin. In addition therefore to the general recommendations in that section it is specifically indicated for the treatment of infections due to *Staphylococcus aureus*.

Dosage
1. *Adults*:
   a. Intramuscular: 1 g every 4–6 hours
   b. Intravenous: 1 g every 4–6 hours
   c. Intra-articular: 500 mg–1 g once daily
   d. Intrapleural: 500 mg–1 g once daily.
   e. Subconjunctival: 500 mg once per day.
2. *Children*:
   Under 2 years: one-quarter of the adult dose
   Over 2 years: one-half of the adult dose.

Nurse monitoring
See the section on Benzylpenicillin.

General notes
1. Methicillin injection may be stored at room temperature.
2. Once reconstituted, solutions for injection should be used immediately and any unused solution discarded.
3. Solutions should be prepared as follows:
   a. For intramuscular dosage: 1.5 ml Water for Injection should be added to each 1 g vial
   b. For intravenous administration: The vial should be diluted to 20 ml which can then either be given slowly over 3–4 minutes or added to normal saline, 5% dextrose or dextrose/saline mixtures and infused over 4–6 hours
   c. Intra-arterial injections should be prepared in 5 ml of Water for Injection.
   d. Intrapleural injections should be prepared in 10 ml of Water for Injection
   e. Subconjunctival injections should be prepared in 0.5–0.75 ml of water.

METHIXENE (Tremonil)

Presentation
Tablets—5 mg

Actions and uses
The actions and uses of this drug are identical to those described for Benzhexol (q.v.).

Dosage
Adults: 15-30 mg in total daily given in three divided doses.

Nurse monitoring
The Nurse monitoring aspects of Benzhexol (q.v.) apply to this drug.

General notes
The drug may be stored at room temperature.

METHOHEXITONE (Brietal)

Presentation
Injection—100 mg, 500 mg, 2.5 g, 5 g

Actions and uses
Methohexitone sodium is a potent barbiturate (q.v.) with a rapid onset and short duration of action. Its main use therefore is by intravenous injection for the induction of anaesthesia.

Dosage
Methohexitone sodium is administered intravenously as a 1% solution (10 mg/ml) and is given at a rate of 1 ml in five seconds until anaesthesia is induced. If given alone the patient will remain unconscious for 5-7 minutes during which time prolonged anaesthesia using inhalation therapy may be induced if required.

Nurse monitoring
See the section on barbiturates.

General notes
1. Once prepared solutions of Methohexitone sodium should be used immediately. If they are not discarded they rapidly turn cloudy and precipitate free drug rendering them useless.
2. Methohexitone solution for injection should not be mixed with other drugs in the same syringe.

METHOTREXATE

Presentation
Tablets—2.5 mg
Injection—2.5 mg/ml, 5 mg/2 ml, 25 mg/ml, 50 mg/2 ml, 250 mg/10 ml
Powder—50 mg/vial

Actions and uses
The mode of action of methotrexate is as follows:
All cells require for growth a vitamin known as folic acid. Folic acid is converted by a number of enzymatic steps in the cell to its biologically active form, Folinic acid. Methotrexate blocks this conversion and therefore reduces cell growth and multiplication by depriving the cell of Folinic acid. It is used in the treatment of the following conditions:
1. It is used in the treatment of acute lymphoblastic leukaemia. Initial treatment is usually with other drugs but once the leukaemia is under control, Methotrexate is used as maintenance therapy. It is also used for the prevention and treatment of meningeal leukaemia.
2. Other malignancies which have been reported to respond to treatment with Methotrexate include:
   a. Choriocarcinoma and related trophoblastic diseases
   b. Lymphosarcoma
   c. Burkitt's lymphoma
   d. Tumours of the head and neck.
3. Methotrexate is occasionally used in the treatment of severe cases of psoriasis which do not respond to conventional therapy.

Dosage
The drug may be given by oral, intramuscular, intravenous, intra-arterial, intra-articular and intrathecal routes. The doses vary widely according to the route of administration, type of malignant disease under treatment and with the variety of other cytotoxic or immunosuppressant drugs which are used in combination. Because of the wide variety of dosage regimes, none are specifically stated here. However, it should be noted that intrathecal doses are very much smaller than doses given by other routes. Courses of treatment with Methotrexate are very often followed by the administration of

calcium folinate which is a Methotrexate antagonist. This has been found to reduce the incidence of associated toxic effects.

Nurse monitoring
1. The principal toxic effects are suppression of the bone marrow and gastrointestinal disturbance. The former effect leads to leucopenia and thrombocytopenia and a resultant increased risk of severe infection or haemorrhage.
2. One of the earliest manifestations of toxicity is oral soreness frequently progressing to ulceration in the mouth. Other gastrointestinal effects include nausea, vomiting and diarrhoea.
3. Megaloblastic anaemia, skin rashes, alopecia, altered ovarian and testicular function, enteritis with bleeding episodes and intestinal perforation may occur.
4. Damage to specific tissues such as the kidneys, liver, lungs and nervous system have been reported. Liver damage is thought to occur more commonly with long-term oral therapy and renal damage is thought to be more common in intermittent high dose regimes. Intrathecal therapy is the commonest cause of neurotoxicity.
5. The drug has produced abortion and a wide range of fetal abnormalities and must not be taken during pregnancy.
6. The nurse should be constantly aware that most cytotoxic drugs are irritant to the skin and mucous surfaces, and are in general very toxic. Great care should therefore be exercised when handling these drugs, and in particular spillage or contamination of personnel or the environment must be avoided. If cytotoxic drugs are handled regularly it is theoretically possible that repeated skin contact or inhalation may produce systemic toxic effects and in nurses who have developed hypersensitivity, severe local and general hypersensitivity reactions.

General notes
1. Methotrexate should only be diluted with 0.9% sodium chloride injection and should not be mixed with other drugs before administration.
2. Preparations of Methotrexate may be stored at room temperature. Vials containing powder may similarly be stored for up to two weeks after reconstitution.

METHYCLOTHIAZIDE (Enduron)

Presentation
Tablets—5 mg

Actions and uses
See the section on thiazide and related diuretics.

Dosage
The usual adult dose range is 2.5–10 mg which is taken as a single dose since the duration of action is approximately 24 hours.

Nurse monitoring
See the section on thiazide and related diuretics.

General notes
Methyclothiazide tablets may be stored at room temperature.

METHYLCELLULOSE (Celevac, Cologel)

Presentation
Tablet—500 mg
Liquid—450 mg in 5 ml
Granules—64%

Actions and uses
The actions of laxatives are discussed in the section dealing with these drugs. Methylcellulose is a member of group 2, i.e. it swells the volume of faeces and induces a more natural bowel action and increase in frequency of defaecation.

Dosage
1–2 5 ml spoonfuls of granules or 3–6 tablets taken night and morning.
5–15 ml liquid three times daily after meals.

Nurse monitoring
There are no specific problems with this drug. It is worth noting that ingestion of this drug may be associated with a feeling of fullness and it is therefore also used as an aid to dieting.

General notes
1. Preparations containing Methylcellulose may be stored at room temperature.
2. To produce an optimal effect patients should be encouraged to drink plenty of fluid with each dose.

METHYLDOPA (Aldomet)

Presentation
Tablets—125 mg, 250 mg, 500 m
Injection—250 mg in 5 ml

Actions and uses
Methyldopa reduces the blood pressure through a direct action on the centres controlling blood pressure in the brain. It is available for use orally on a regular basis but may be given intravenously in hypertensive emergencies. It has been used for many years safely in obstetrics and is therefore often used for control of hypertension in pregnancy.

Dosage
1. Adult dose: 250 mg two to three times daily, rising to a maximum of 3 g per day in three divided doses.
2. Adult emergency intravenous dose: 250–500 mg 6-hourly as required.
3. Children's dosage:
   Up to 1 year: 6 mg/kg
   1–6 years: 62.5 mg
   7 years plus: 125 mg.
   All these doses should be taken three times per day. The maximum dosage in each age range is four times the dose stated, three times per day. Similar doses are given by intravenous injection if necessary.

Nurse monitoring
Although Methyldopa is a very effective drug in the treatment of hypertension, the major problem with its use is the large number of potentially serious side effects which may occur, and it is in the early detection of these side effects that the nurse can make a major contribution.
1. Neurological side effects: Depression is by far the most important, but paraesthesia, Parkinsonism, involuntary muscle twitching, nightmares, confusion, light-headedness and dizziness may also occur.
2. Cardiovascular: Postural hypotension, fluid retention, worsening of existing angina and bradycardia.
3. Gastrointestinal: Nausea, vomiting, distension, excess flatus, constipation, dry mouth, black tongue and very rarely pancreatitis.
4. Blood: Haemolytic anaemia, leucopenia, granulocytopenia, thrombocytopenia.
5. Other side effects include nasal stuffiness, a raised blood urea, gynaecomastia/galactorrhoea, impotence in makes, loss of libido, skin rashes, drug fever and abnormal liver function tests.

General notes
Methyldopa tablets and injection may be stored at room temperature. The injection is diluted with 100 ml 5% dextrose injection and infused over a period of 30–60 minutes.

METHYLPHENOBARBITONE (Prominal)

Presentation
Tablets—30 mg, 60 mg, 200 mg

Actions and uses
See the section on barbiturates. Methylphenobarbitone has a specific anti-convulsant action and it is used in the treatment of all forms of epilepsy.

Dosage
100–600 mg daily in divided doses.

Nurse monitoring
See the section on barbiturates.

General notes
Tablets containing Methylphenobarbitone may be stored at room temperature.

METHYLPREDNISOLONE (Medrone, Depo-Medrone, Solu-Medrone)

Presentation
Tablets—2 mg, 4 mg, 16 mg
Intravenous or intramuscular injection—40 mg, 125 mg, 500 mg in 1 g
Long-acting intramuscular and intra-articular injection—40 mg in 1 ml, 80 mg in 2 ml, 200 mg in 5 ml
Acne lotion and cream—0.25%

Actions and uses
Methylprednisolone is a corticosteroid drug (q.v.). Its rapid onset of action following intravenous injection makes it particularly useful in the management of severe shock.

Dosage
1. Oral: This varies widely with the nature and severity of the condition being treated.
2. For the treatment of severe shock: Intravenous doses of up to 30 mg/kg body weight daily may be given.
3. Intra-articular injection: Dosages vary between 4 and 80 mg according to the size of the joint under treatment.
4. The lotion is applied sparingly once or twice daily and the cream once to three times daily.

Nurse monitoring
See the section on corticosteroid drugs. It must be remembered that even topical applications may lead to sufficient of the drug being absorbed to produce the systemic effects described in this section.

General notes
Preparations containing Methylprednisolone may be stored at room temperature.

METHYLTESTOSTERONE

Presentation
Tablets—5 mg, 10 mg, 25 mg and 50 mg

Actions and uses
Methyltestosterone is an androgenic hormone. Its actions and uses are discussed in the section on these drugs.

Dosage
The dosage varies according to the indication for its use.

Nurse monitoring
See the section on androgenic hormones.

General notes
The drug may be stored at room temperature.

METHYSERGIDE (Deseril)

Presentation
Tablets—1 mg

Actions and uses
Methysergide has two actions:
1. It constricts blood vessels.
2. It is an antagonist of 5-hydroxytryptamine, a chemical which is released in tissues involved in acute inflammation.

In clinical practice Methysergide has two major uses:
1. For the treatment of the rare carcinoid syndrome where excess production of 5-Hydroxytryptamine leads to attacks of flushing and diarrhoea.
2. It is effective for the prophylactic treatment of migraine but it is now rarely used for this because of toxicity.

Dosage
1. For the treatment of carcinoid syndrome: Up to 20 mg per day may be required according to individual patient response.
2. For the prophylaxis of migraine: 1 or 2 mg three times a day with meals.

Nurse monitoring
1. This drug on rare occasions may cause extensive fibrosis involving the heart, pleura, lung and retroperitoneal tissues. It should, therefore, be given in short courses only and should not be administered for long periods.
2. Common side effects include nausea, epigastric pain, dizziness, drowsiness, restlessness, muscle cramps and psychological effects. Vomiting, muscle weakness, ataxia, weight increase, oedema, tachycardia and postural hypotension may also occur.

3. The vasoconstrictor effect may lead to cold extremities.
4. The drug should be used with great caution in patients with peripheral vascular disease, coronary heart disease, peptic ulceration and reduced kidney or liver function.

General notes
The drug should be stored at room temperature.

METOCLOPRAMIDE (Maxolon)

Presentation
Tablets—10 mg
Syrup—5 mg in 5 ml
Paediatric liquid—1 mg in 1 ml
Injection—10 mg in 2 ml, 100 mg in 20 ml

Actions and uses
Metoclopramide has two major modes of action:
1. It has a direct action on the gut increasing normal gut motility (peristalsis) and increasing gastric emptying time.
2. It has an anti-emetic effect via an action on the central nervous system.

It has the following uses:
1. It can be used to control vomiting associated with gastrointestinal disease, drug therapy (particularly cytotoxic drugs), radiotherapy and postoperative period.
2. In diagnostic radiology Metoclopramide is used to speed the passage of barium through the stomach and also as an aid to duodenal intubation.

Dosage
1. *Adults*:
   a. Oral: 10 mg three times a day.
   b. Parenteral: 10 mg three times a day.
2. *Children*:
   a. Oral: Under 1 year: 1 mg b.d.
   5-15 years: 2.5-5 mg three times daily.
   The total daily dose for children should not exceed 0.5 mg/kg body weight.
   b. Parenteral: as for oral dosage regimes. High dose intravenous infusion using doses of up to 2 mg/kg body weight or more have been administered prior to cytotoxic chemotherapy. This may be repeated every 2 hours up to a maximum dose of 10 mg/kg in 24 hours. Infusions are administered over 15 minutes.
3. For diagnostic procedures a single dose of Metoclopramide is given 9-10 minutes before the examination. Dosage is as follows:
   a. Adults: 10-20 mg.
   b. Children under 3 years: 1 mg.
   c. Children 5-14 years: 2.5-5 mg.

Nurse monitoring
1. It is important to note that Metoclopramide is of little benefit in the prevention or treatment of motion sickness or in the treatment of nausea and vertigo due to Menière's disease or other labyrinthine disturbances.
2. Metoclopramide blocks the action of Dopamine in the central nervous system and produces a range of symptoms and signs similar to those seen in Parkinson's disease. This effect is particularly likely to occur in children and young adults and where higher dosages are used. The effects include facial muscle spasm, trismus, a rhythmic protrusion of the tongue, bulbar speech, muscle spasm around the eyes, rolling of the eyeballs and an unnatural positioning of the head and shoulders.
3. Because drugs of the phenothiazine group (q.v.) also produce similar effects, Metoclopramide and phenothiazines should only be given together with great caution.
4. Metoclopramide stimulates the production of prolactin by the pituitary. This may lead to an increase in breast size in males and galactorrhoea in females.

5. Metoclopramide and anticholinergic drugs (see the section on Poldine and other related compounds) should be avoided as the latter drugs antagonise the effects of Metoclopramide on the gut.

General notes
Preparations containing Metoclopramide may be stored at room temperature. Liquid preparations are sensitive to light and ampoules containing injection solution which show a yellow discolouration should be discarded.

METOLAZONE (Metenix)

Presentation
Tablets—5 mg, 10 mg

Actions and uses
See the section on thiazide and related diuretics.

Dosage
The usual adult dose is 5–20 mg once daily; the duration of action is approximately 18–24 hours.

Nurse monitoring
See the section on thiazide and related diuretics.

General notes
Metolazone tablets may be stored at room temperature.

METOPROLOL (Betaloc, Lopresor)

Presentation
Tablets—50 mg, 100 mg, 200 mg (sustained release)

Actions and uses
Metoprolol is a cardioselective beta-blocker and its actions are described in the section dealing with these drugs.

Dosage
The adult dose range is 100–400 mg per day which is usually given in two equal doses. Sustained release tablets of Metoprolol may be given as a single daily dose.

Nurse monitoring
See the section on beta-adrenoreceptor blocking drugs.

General notes
Metoprolol tablets may be stored at room temperature.

METRONIDAZOLE (Flagyl)

(*See Note 3, p. 310*)

Presentation
Tablets—200 mg and 400 mg
Suppositories—500 mg and 1 g
(for vaginal and rectal administration)
Injection—0.5% for intravenous infusion

Actions and uses
Metronidazole has been found to be effective in the treatment of both bacterial and parasitic infections in man. Its main uses are as follows:
1. Trichomonal vaginitis
2. Amoebiasis
3. Giardiasis
4. Vincent's angina
5. Infections due to anaerobic organisms such as bacteroides species and clostridia
6. Metronidazole is now being used more commonly for the prevention of wound infection and peritonitis after abdominal surgery.

Dosage
1. For the treatment of trichomonal vaginitis:
   a. Adults and children greater than 10 years: 200–400 mg three times a day for 7–10 days or a single dose of 2 g.
   b. Children:
      Less than 3 years: 150 mg per day for 7–10 days
      3–7 years: 200 mg per day for 7–10 days
      7–10 years old: 300 mg per day for 7–10 days.
   This condition may also be treated with 10–20 days' treatment with 500 mg or 1 g as pessaries once per day.
2. a. Acute and chronic hepatic or intestinal amoebiasis:
      i. *Adults*: 2–2.4 g for three days or 400–800 mg three times a day for 5–10 days.
      ii. *Children*: 7.5 mg/kg three times a day for 10 days.
   b. For cyst eradication in symptomless carriers of amoebiasis the same doses apply although shorter courses of treatment are usually effective.

3. For the treatment of giardiasis:
   a. *Adults*: 2 g for three days
   b. *Children*:
      Less than 3 years old: 400 mg for three days
      3–7 years: 600 mg for three days
      7–10 years: 1 g for three days.
4. For the treatment of Vincent's angina: Adult doses are 200 mg three times per day or 400 mg twice a day for a week.
5. For the treatment of serious bacterial infections due to bacteroides or clostridia:
   a. Oral therapy is as follows:
      i. Adult doses vary from 200–400 mg three times a day
      ii. Children and infants should receive 7.5 mg/kg body weight three times daily.
   b. Rectal administration:
      i. Adults and children over 12 years: 1 g suppository 8-hourly.
      ii. Children 5–12 years: 500 mg 8-hourly
      iii. Children 1–5 years: One-half of a 500 mg suppository 8-hourly.
      iv. Children less than 1 year: One-quarter of a 500 mg suppository 8-hourly.
   c. For parenteral treatment:
      i. Adults receive 500 mg eight hourly by i.v. infusion.
      ii. Children under 12 years receive 7.5 mg/kg 8-hourly.
6. For the prevention of wound infection and peritonitis after abdominal surgery the recommended dose for adults is:
   a. 500 mg 8-hourly by i.v. infusion over 20 minutes minutes or
   b. 400 mg three times a day orally or
   c. 1. g three times a day rectally.

Nurse monitoring
1. It is important to note that this drug may cause darkening of the urine and urethral discomfort. The patient should be warned of this possibility to prevent anxiety.
2. Gastrointestinal effects are common. These include anorexia, nausea, an abnormal taste in the mouth and dryness of the tongue.
3. Neurological side effects such as headache are common. More serious neurological side effects such as vertigo, depression, insomnia and drowsiness are less common.
4. Patients with disorders of the blood and disease of the central nervous system should not be given this drug.
5. It is recommended that the drug be avoided in pregnant women.
6. It is noteworthy that some patients may become profoundly sick if they take alcohol when on this drug and they should therefore be warned of this possible effect.
7. It is very important to note that the drug has no effect on diseases caused by *Candida albicans* (thrush).

General notes
1. The drug may be stored at room temperature.
2. Care should be taken to ensure that suppositories are not stored in a warm place e.g. above a radiator, as they might melt.

MEXILETINE (Mexitil)

Presentation
Capsules—50 mg, 200 mg, 360 mg (slow release)
Injection—250 mg in 10 ml

Actions and uses
Mexiletine is an antidysrhythmic drug which is used to abolish or prevent serious ventricular dysrhythmias in patients who have had a myocardial infarction. It is given by intravenous injection initially and subsequently orally for the longterm prophylaxis of these rhythm disturbances.

Dosage
The adult intravenous loading dose is 100–250 mg by bolus injection at a rate of 25 mg/minute. This is

followed by an intravenous infusion containing 500 mg in 500 ml. The first 250 ml is given over 1 hour, the second 250 ml is given more slowly over 2 hours. Further maintenance infusions may be given using 250 mg in 500 ml at a rate of 0.5 mg/minute. For oral maintenance therapy an initial loading dose of 400 mg is followed by 200-250 mg three or four times a day. Alternatively 360 mg twice daily as slow release capsules may be administered.

Nurse monitoring

This drug requires careful monitoring for adverse effects which tend to be dose related. When the drug is being administered intravenously the patient should be observed for light-headedness, confusion, drowsiness, dizziness, diplopia, blurred vision, nystagmus, dysarthria, ataxia, paraesthesias, convulsions, hypotension, bradycardia, atrial fibrillation, nausea, vomiting, dyspepsia, an unpleasant taste and hiccoughs. Such effects are both less frequent and milder with oral therapy.

General notes

Mexiletine capsules and injection may be stored at room temperature. The injection may be added to several infusion solutions including 0.9% sodium chloride injection, 5% dextrose injection, 5% laevulose injection, 1.4% sodium bicarbonate injection and sodium lactate injection.

MEZLOCILLIN (Baypen)

(See Note 3, p. 310)

Presentation

Injection—0.5 g, 1 g, 2 g and 5 g vials

Actions and uses

This drug's actions and uses are identical to those described for Azlocillin (q.v.).

Dosage

1. *Adults*:
   a. By intravenous bolus injection: 2-5 g administered over 2-4 minutes every 6-8 hours.
   b. By rapid intravenous infusion over 15-20 minutes: 2-5 g every 6-8 hours.
   c. By intramuscular injection: 1-2 g every 6-8 hours.
2. *Children*:
   Infants and premature babies less than 3 kg: 75 mg/kg 12-hourly.
   3-5 kg body weight: 0.2-0.4 g 8-hourly.
   5-10 kg body weight: 0.4-0.75 g 8-hourly.
   10-13 kg body weight: 0.75-1 g 8-hourly.
   13-20 kg body weight: 1-1.5 g 8-hourly.
   Over 20 kg body weight: 1.5 g 8-hourly.

Nurse monitoring

See the section on Azlocillin.

General notes

1. The drug may be stored at room temperature.
2. A 10% solution for injection should be prepared immediately before use and any remaining solution discarded.

MIANSERIN (Bolvidon, Norval)

Presentation

Tablets—10 mg, 20 mg, 30 mg

Actions and uses

Mianserin is an antidepressant drug derived from and chemically related to tricyclic antidepressants. Its actions and uses are similar to those described for tricyclic antidepressants (q.v.).

Dosage

For the treatment of depression in adults 30-200 mg is given daily either in divided doses or as a single evening dose taken on retiring.

Nurse monitoring

The Nurse monitoring notes for tricyclic antidepressants (q.v.) are applicable to Mianserin with two possible exceptions:
1. Following acute overdosage there has been a lower incidence of

cardiac side effects, principally tachycardias.
2. Mianserin has less 'anticholinergic' side effects, such as dry mouth, blurred vision, urinary retention, constipation and tachycardia. It is therefore preferable for use in three groups:
   a. Patients with glaucoma
   b. Patients with prostatism
   c. Patients in whom the above side effects are intolerable.

General notes
Tablets containing Mianserin may be stored at room temperature.

MICONAZOLE (Daktarin)

Presentation
Tablets—250 mg
Oral gel, cream and powder—2%
Injection—200 mg in 20 ml
Pessaries and tampons—100 mg

Actions and uses
1. In oral or topical preparations this drug is an effective antifungal agent used in clinical practice for the treatment of disease caused by pathogenic fungi (mainly yeasts and dermatophytes) such as candidiasis.
2. An intravenous solution is available and intravenous infusions of the drug are used to treat systemic infection:
   a. *Candida albicans*
   b. *Candida tropicalis*
   c. *Candida parapsilosis*
   d. *Aspergillus fumigatus*
   e. *Cryptococcus neoformans*
   f. *Coccidioides immites*
   g. *Paracoccidioides brasiliensis*

Dosage
1. *Oral gel*:
   a. *Adults*: 5–10 ml of gel four times daily
   b. Children aged over 6: 5 ml four times daily
   c. Children aged 2–6: 5 ml twice daily
   d. Children less than 2 years: 2.5 ml twice daily.
2. Miconazole tablets: *Adults*: 250 mg four times a day.
3. Pessaries and tampons: One should be inserted into the vagina at night.
4. Topical Miconazole should be applied once or twice daily.
5. Intravenous infusion:
   a. The usual adult dose is 600 mg three times daily as an infusion in 200–500 ml infusion fluid. As a guide clinically effective daily doses have ranged from as low as 600 mg per day to, in a few patients, as high as 3600 mg per day.
   b. In children a daily dose of 40 mg/kg in total is recommended. A dose of 15 mg/kg per infusion should not be exceeded.

Nurse monitoring
1. Miconazole intravenous solution must be diluted with either normal saline or 5% dextrose and administered by slow infusion over at least 30 minutes. Usually a dose of 600 mg would be diluted in 200–500 ml of infusion fluid and lower doses in proportionately lower volumes of fluid.
2. The intravenous infusion can be associated with phlebitis, pruritus, nausea, vomiting, fever, skin rash, drowsiness, diarrhoea, anorexia and flushing.
3. Oral preparations associated with mild gastrointestinal upset.
4. Topical applications have no side effects.

General notes
1. Topical and oral Miconazole preparations may be stored at room temperature.
2. The injection solution should be refrigerated.

MINOCYCLINE (Minocin)

(See Note 3, p. 310)

Presentation
Tablets—50 mg, 100 mg

Actions and uses
General notes on the actions and uses of tetracycline (q.v.) apply to Minocycline. In addition the drug

has been found to be of particular use for the prevention of meningitis due to *Neisseria meningitidis* in the families of carriers of the disease.

Dosage
The adult dose is 50–100 mg every 12 hours. It is worth noting that food appears to have less effect on the absorption of Minocycline than tetracyclines in general and therefore the drug may be taken with food.

Nurse monitoring
1. For general Nurse monitoring notes see the section on tetracyclines.
2. It is worth noting that neurological side effects are particularly prominent with this drug as compared to other tetracyclines. These effects cause light-headedness, dizziness and vertigo.

General notes
The drug may be stored at room temperature.

MITOBRONITOL (Myelobromol)

(Also known as Dibromomannitol)

Presentation
Tablets—125 mg

Actions and uses
Mitobronitol is a cytotoxic drug which is an alkylating agent and has a similar mode of action to Busulphan (q.v.). It is used mainly in the treatment of chronic myeloid leukaemia and occasionally to achieve and maintain remission in the treatment of polycythaemia rubra vera.

Dosage
Adults: initially 250 mg per day is given until white cell count is reduced to less than 20 000/cmm. Thereafter maintenance doses of 125 mg per day or on alternate days are given to maintain the white cell count at an appropriate level.

Nurse monitoring
1. Suppression of bone marrow function may be produced leading to anaemia, haemorrhage due to thrombocytopenia and infection due to suppression of white cell function.
2. Gastrointestinal disturbances, alopecia, skin pigmentation, skin rash and menstrual abnormalities may also occur.
3. The nurse should be constantly aware that most cytotoxic drugs are irritant to the skin and mucous surfaces, and are in general very toxic. Great care should therefore be exercised when handling these drugs, and in particular spillage or contamination of personnel or the environment must be avoided. If cytotoxic drugs are handled regularly it is theoretically possible that repeated skin contact or inhalation may produce systemic toxic effects and in nurses who have developed hypersensitivity, severe local and general hypersensitivity reactions.

General notes
Mitobronitol tablets may be stored at room temperature.

MONOAMINE OXIDASE INHIBITORS

Iproniazid   Phenelzine
Isocarboxazid   Tranylcypromine

Actions and uses
When the enzyme monoamine oxidase, which is present in many tissues in the body, is inhibited by the group of drugs known as monoamine oxidase inhibitors there is a resultant increase in the concentration of 5-hydroxytryptamine and catecholamines in the central nervous system. This leads to marked effects on mental function ranging from feelings of well-being and increased energy to, in some patients, psychosis. This group of drugs therefore is used for the treatment of depression.. However, they have many serious side effects and for this reason are usually only used when other drugs, such as tricyclic antidepressants, have been found to be ineffective.

Dosage
See specific drugs.

Nurse monitoring
1. Severe headache and dangerous hypertensive crisis may be precipitated in patients taking monoamine oxidase inhibiting drugs by the ingestion of certain foodstuffs. These include cheese, yoghurt, pickled herrings, broad beans, yeast extracts, meat extracts (Bovril, Marmite, etc) wines and beers. The nurse may play an important role in both educating patients about food intake and monitoring their diets.
2. The nurse may also play an important role in warning patients that they must never indulge in self-medication of any kind particularly those sold for coughs and colds, as these contain chemicals which may lead to serious hypertension and headache if they are taken at the same time as monoamine oxidase inhibiting drugs.
3. A number of other drugs are extremely dangerous if they are given at the same time as monoamine oxidase inhibitors. The nurse may play an important role in identifying such potential combinations. The major group of drugs contraindicated for concurrent administration with monoamine oxidase inhibitors are as follows:
   a. Other antidepressants: If tricyclic and monoamine oxidase inhibiting drugs are given together mental excitement and hyperpyrexia may occur.
   b. Antihypertensives: Hypertension and excitement may occur with Methyldopa.
   c. Narcotic analgesics: The coincident administration of Pethidine and monoamine oxidase inhibiting drugs may lead to respiratory depression, restlessness, coma and hypotension.
   d. Central nervous system depressants: Barbiturates, tranquillisers, antihistamines, alcohol and anti-Parkinsonian drugs are contraindicated for concurrent administration with monoamine oxidase inhibitor drugs.
   e. Insulin and tolbutamide are contraindicated for concurrent administration with monoamine oxidase inhibiting drugs.
   f. Drugs which stimulate the sympathetic nervous system e.g. Ephedrine, Phenylephrine and the amphetamines may produce serious (and even fatal) rises in blood pressure which result in brain haemorrhage.
4. A common side effect produced by monoamine oxidase inhibiting drugs is hypotension. Symptoms of dizziness on standing, indcating postural hypotension, may occur. It is important to remember that hypertensive crises can still occur in patients who have been rendered hypotensive by the drug.
5. Other side effects include cardiac dysrhythmias, dizziness, headache, anxiety, tremor, convulsions and liver toxicity.
6. It is advisable that all patients receiving monoamine oxidase inhibiting drugs be issued with a warning card which provides a complete list of substances which they may accidentally take and which may lead to the effects described above.

MORPHINE (As Hydrochloride, Sulphate or Tartrate)

Presentation
Morphine sulphate is available in numerous preparations, often in combination with other drugs and in varying strengths. The following are only examples of the many preparations in common use:
Tablets—MST Continus, 10 mg, 30 mg, 60 mg and 100 mg as slow release
Injection—15 mg and 30 mg in 1 ml

Suppositories—15 mg and 30 mg
Mixtures—containing 10, 20, 30 mg in 10 ml
Actions and uses
See the section on narcotic analgesics.
Dosage
N.B. The following doses are given as a guideline only and both initial dosage and maintenance dosage may vary considerably depending on the condition under treatment and the development of tolerance to the drug in the patient.
1. *Adults*:
   a. Orally:
      i. Standard preparations: 10–20 mg 4 to 6-hourly as required
      ii. Slow release tablets (MST Continus) 30–100 mg twice daily
   b. By subcutaneous or intramuscular injection: 15–30 mg 4 to 6-hourly as required for pain.
   c. Intravenous injections may cause a rapid fall in blood pressure. They should be administered slowly and the dosage recommended is 10–20 mg 4 to 6-hourly as required.
2. *Children*: For oral, subcutaneous or intramuscular administration:
   Less than 1 year: 0.15–0.2 mg/kg 8-hourly
   1–7 years: 2–5 mg 8-hourly.
Nurse monitoring
See the section on narcotic analgesics.
General notes
1. Preparations may be stored at room temperature.
2. By law this drug must be kept in a locked (controlled drug) cupboard.

MULTIVITAMINS (Parentrovite)

Presentation
1. There are numerous oral vitamin and multivitamin preparations available either by prescription or direct over-the-counter sales.
2. Parenteral multivitamins are available as Parentrovite, either IMM (intramuscular maintenance), IMHP (intramuscular high potency) or IVHP (intravenous high potency).

Actions and uses
1. Oral Preparations: Vitamins and multivitamin supplements are frequently prescribed and even more frequently purchased directly for use as tonics. There is no real evidence that they are of any benefit for this purpose.
2. In patients who have a documented history and clinical signs of inadequate diet, oral or parenteral preparations may be usefully prescribed to aid physical recovery.
3. In patients with impaired absorption of foodstuffs due either to disease of the gall bladder, pancreas or gut, parenteral vitamin preparations are an essential component of therapy.
4. Parenteral multivitamins have been shown to be useful in the management of delirium tremens, a state of agitated confusion caused by acute cessation of prolonged heavy drinking.

It should be noted that Parentrovite contains primarily a number of the vitamin B complex compounds and vitamin C.

Dosage
1. The dosage of oral preparations varies according to the proprietary brand and nurses are advised to consult manufacturers' literature.
2. Parenteral therapy:
   a. For the treatment of adults with acute psychotic disturbances: Initially 2–4 pairs of intravenous high potency ampoules 4–8 hourly for 48 hours followed by one pair of intravenous or intramuscular high potency ampoules daily for 5–7 days. Maintenance therapy should consist of 1–2 pairs of intramuscular maintenance

ampoules given daily until full health is restored.
  b. *Children*: Parenteral therapy is rarely necessary but when it is indicated children between 6 and 10 years should receive one-third of the adult dose, between 10 and 14 years one-third to one-half of the adult dose, 14 years and over should receive adult doses.

Nurse monitoring
1. The ill-effects caused by administration of an excess of vitamins are discussed more fully under the individual headings (see the sections covering vitamin A, vitamin B complex, vitamin C, vitamin D and vitamin E).
2. Parenteral administration of Parentrovite has a number of problems which are:
   a. With repeated injections anaphylactic shock may occur and appropriate measures such as the injection of adrenaline and soluble glucocorticoids or antihistamines should be readily available during administration of this therapy
   b. Parentrovite contains Pyridoxine and this may antagonise Levodopa therapy for Parkinson's disease
   c. Flushing of the face may rarely occur.
   d. Perhaps the most important point for the nurse to note is that the intramuscular (IMM) preparation should never be given intravenously.

General notes
Ampoules of Parentrovite should be stored in a cool, dry place.

MUSTINE

Presentation
  Injection—10 mg

Actions and uses
Mustine is a cytotoxic drug of the nitrogen mustard group which arrests cell growth by a chemical binding (alkylating) action on substances which are essential for cell division to proceed. Its uses are as follows:
1. In combination with other cytotoxics in the treatment of Hodgkin's disease and other lymphomas.
2. In the treatment of carcinoma of the lung and other solid tumours.
3. By intracavitary injection in the treatment of malignant effusions, particularly pleural effusions.
4. Topically to skin lesions in mycosis fungoides.

Dosage
This varies considerably according to the nature of the malignant disease and the route of administration, and the following is a rough guide only.
1. Intravenous: 400 μg/kg body weight as a single dose or in 4 divided daily doses by slow injection into the tubing of a running sodium chloride 0.9% infusion.
2. Intracavitary: 200–400 μg/kg body weight in 20–50 ml sodium chloride 0.9%.
3. Topical: A solution of 0.02% has been applied to skin lesions.

Nurse monitoring
1. Severe nausea and vomiting are commonly produced within 1 hour of intravenous therapy and last for several hours thereafter.
2. Bone marrow suppression with anaemia, neutropenia and thrombocytopenia is a serious dose-related side effect.
3. Tinnitus, vertigo and deafness may occur.
4. Patients may display hypersensitivity, particularly following topical use, varying from urticaria, other skin reactions to anaphylaxis.
5. The nurse should be constantly aware that most cytotoxic drugs are irritant to the skin and mucous surfaces and are in general very toxic. Great care should therefore be exercised when handling these drugs and in particular spillage or contamination of personnel or the environment must be

avoided. If cytotoxic drugs are handled regularly it is theoretically possible that repeated skin contact or inhalation may produce systemic toxic effects and in nurses who have developed hypersensitivity, severe local and general hypersensitivity reactions.

General notes
1. Mustine injection should be stored under refrigeration and attention is drawn to the provision of an expiry date on labelled vials.
2. After reconstitution, the drug should be used immediately and any remaining drug discarded.

N

NABILONE (Cesamet)

Presentation
Capsules—1 mg

Actions and uses
Nabilone is an anti-emetic drug which is chemically related to substances called cannabinoids which are found in Cannabis resin. It is used in the management of vomiting associated with anticancer therapy.

Dosage
Adults: 1–2 mg taken the night before anti-cancer therapy and repeated 1–3 hours prior to the first dose of anti-cancer drug administered.

Nurse monitoring
1. The major problem with this drug is that it will be liable to misuse since it resembles cannabis and for this reason it is restricted to prescription in hospitals only. The nurse may therefore play a valuable role in ensuring that dosages are taken and that tablets are not allowed to accumulate in the home.
2. Alertness may be impaired and patients should be aware of the risks of impairment of driving skills. This is particularly true if other sedative drugs are taken, particularly alcohol.
3. Patients with a history of psychotic illness may react adversely and should be carefully monitored.

General notes
Nabilone capsules may be stored at room temperature.

NADOLOL (Corgard)

Presentation
Tablets—40 mg, 80 mg

Actions and uses
Nadolol is a non-selective beta-adrenoreceptor blocking drug and its actions and uses are described in the section dealing with these drugs.

Dosage
The usual daily adult dose is 80 mg twice daily.

Nurse monitoring
See the section on beta-adrenoreceptor blocking drugs.

General notes
Nadolol tablets may be stored at room temperature.

NAFTIDROFURYL (Praxilene)

Presentation
Capsules—100 mg
Injection—200 mg in 10 ml

Actions and uses
This drug acts on the cardiovascular system to produce vasodilation. It is used in clinical practice for the following disorders:
1. For the treatment of peripheral vascular insufficiency including Raynaud's phenomenon, intermittent claudication, night cramps and frost bite.
2. It is also used to improve blood supply to the brain in cerebrovascular insufficiency.

Dosage
1. Orally: 100 mg three times per day.
2. Parenterally: By intravenous or intra-arterial infusion: in sodium chloride 0.9%, dextrose 5% or

dextran injection: 200 mg twice daily.

Nurse monitoring
1. It is important to note that this drug must never be administered by intravenous bolus injection.
2. Nausea, epigastric pain, flushing of the skin of the head and neck, tachycardia, postural hypotension, headache and dizziness may occur.

General notes
1. The drug may be stored at room temperature.
2. Solutions should be protected from light.

NALIDIXIC ACID (Negram)

Presentation
Tablets—500 mg
Suspension—300 mg in 5 ml

Actions and uses
This drug has a bactericidal action i.e. it kills the bacteria present in the body. It has been found to be particularly effective against the gram-negative organisms which commonly cause urinary tract infections. These are *E. coli*, Klebsiella, Enterobacter and proteus species. It is important to remember that infections due to *Pseudomonas aeruginosa* are rarely, if ever, effectively treated by Nalidixic acid.

Dosage
1. *Adults*:
   a. For acute urinary tract infections: 1 g four times a day.
   b. For prolonged treatment of chronic infections: 500 mg four times a day.
2. *Children*: Children under three months of age should rarely, if ever, be given this drug as their livers are incapable of metabolising it. Older children should receive 50 mg/kg body weight in total daily, given in divided doses.

Nurse monitoring
1. As noted above the drug should rarely, if ever, be given to children under the age of 3 months.
2. If given to infants, raised intracranial pressure manifest by drowsiness, convulsions and papilloedema may occur.
3. Side effects in older patients may include skin rash, visual disturbance, headache and gastrointestinal symptoms such as nausea, vomiting and abdominal pain.
4. Photosensitivity reactions, urticaria, pruritis, fever and blood disorders may occur in patients who prove to the hypersensitive to the drug.
5. The drug enhances the effect of two other major groups of drugs:
   a. Warfarin, leading to a danger of bleeding unless the dosage is carefully monitored and reduced appropriately.
   b. Oral anti-diabetic drugs where hypoglycaemia may be induced.
6. Nalidixic acid may cause positive reactions to urinary tests with Benidix solution and Clinitest.

General notes
The drug may be stored at room temperature.

NANDROLONE (Durabolin, Deca-Durabolin)

Presentation
Injection—25 mg, 50 mg and 100 mg in 1 ml (as the decanoate salt)
25 mg, 50 mg in 1 ml (as the phenylpropionate salt)

Actions and uses
The actions and uses of anabolic steroids are described in the section dealing with these drugs. In its decanoate form this drug has a duration of action of three weeks while in the phenylproprinate form it has a duration of action of one week.

Dosage
By deep intramuscular injection:
1. *Adults*:
   a. As the phenylproprinate salt: 25 mg to 50 mg once weekly
   b. As the decanoate salt: 25 mg to 50 mg every three weeks

2. *Children*:
   a. Up to 1 mg/kg per month as the phenylpropionate form.
   b. 0.75–1.5 mg/kg every week as the decanoate form.

Nurse monitoring

See the sections on androgenic hormones and anabolic steroids.

General notes

1. The drug may be stored at room temperature.
2. Injection solution should be protected from direct sunlight.

NAPROXEN (Naprosyn)

Presentation

Tablets—250 mg, 500 mg
Suspension—250 mg in 10 ml
Suppositories—500 mg

Actions and uses

See the section on non-steroidal anti-inflammatory analgesic drugs.

Dosage

1. *Adults*:
   a. The initial dosage is usually 250 mg twice per day
   b. Maintenance dosage is usually adjusted to within the range of 370–750 mg in total daily
   c. As an alternative to oral therapy, one suppository (500 mg) may be inserted at night.
2. *Children*: In the treatment of rheumatoid disease a dose of 10 mg/kg per day has been used, although only in children over the age of 5 years.
3. In the treatment of acute gout 750 mg is given initially followed by 250 mg 8-hourly until the attack has clinically resolved.

Nurse monitoring

See the section on anti-inflammatory analgesic drugs, non-steroidal.

General notes

Naproxen tablets, suspension and suppositories may be stored at room temperature.

NARCOTIC ANALGESICS

The narcotic analgesics comprise a group of drugs derived from opium and termed opium alkaloids, and synthetic compounds based on the opium alkaloids. They include the following preparations:

Buprenorphine
Codeine
Dextromoramide
Dextropropoxyphene
Diamorphine
Dihydrocodeine
Dipipanone
Levorphenol
Methadone
Morphine
Papaveretum
Pentazocine
Pethidine
Phenazocine
Piritramide

Actions and uses

1. Narcotic analgesic drugs have a powerful analgesic action mediated by their direct effect on the central nervous system. They are used for the treatment of conditions associated with acute or chronic severe pain such as myocardial infarction, childbirth, postoperative pain and the pain associated with malignant disease. They are also used regularly for pre-operative medication.
2. One of the weaker members of the group, Codeine, is used both as an analgesic and for its cough suppressant and constipating action.

Nurse monitoring

1. The most important point for the nurse to note is that the use of many of the drugs in this group is strictly controlled by law and the legal aspects of prescribing these drugs is further discussed in Appendix 1.
2. The most serious problem encountered with patients who receive these drugs is the production of physical dependence and addiction. Nurses play an important role in giving patients support when such drugs are being withdrawn after short-term use, in identifying patients who may be becoming dependent on these

drugs and in providing support to patients who are being weaned off prolonged use of these drugs.
3. Narcotic analgesics produce a dose-related depression of neurological function resulting in sedation, drowsiness, sleepiness. They may eventually produce profound depression of respiratory function and therefore must be used with great caution in patients who already have poor respiratory function or in those in whom the sedative effect may be enhanced, such as patients with liver cirrhosis.
4. Many analgesics in this group produce severe nausea and vomiting and for this reason they are commonly used in combinations containing anti-emetics.
5. Narcotic analgesics influence the motility of the gut and cause constipation. This may be a major problem which may give rise to great discomfort especially in elderly and bedridden patients.
6. Narcotic analgesics must be used with extreme caution in patients who are also receiving manoamine oxidase inhibitors (q.v.) as the combination of these two types of drug may produce serious cardiovascular reactions.
7. In addition to physical dependence, the phenomenon of tolerance may arise in patients receiving prolonged treatment with these analgesics. The term 'tolerance' basically means that with prolonged treatment patients receive less benefit from doses which were previously effective. This may mean that the frequency of administration and dosage may have to be increased as duration of therapy progresses. As many patients receiving prolonged narcotic analgesia are suffering from chronic pain due to malignant conditions the nurse may play an important role in observing such patients and identifying the relative efficacy of their treatment regimes so that the need for change in therapy may be brought to the attention of the medical staff.

General notes
See specific drugs.

NATAMYCIN (Pimafucin)
Presentation
Pessaries—25 mg
Cream—2%
Oral suspension—1%
Actions and uses
This anti-fungal drug is used most commonly in clinical practice for the treatment of infections due to *Candida albicans*
Dosage
1. Pessaries: One at night.
2. Cream: Apply twice daily.
3. 4 drops after feeds in infants.
Nurse monitoring
No problems are associated with the administration of this drug.
General notes
The drug may be stored at room temperature.

NEFOPAM (Acupan)
Presentation
Tablets—30 mg
Injection—20 mg in 1 ml
Actions and uses
Nefopam is an analgesic drug which acts by a direct effect on the central nervous system. It is chemically unrelated to the narcotic analgesic drugs and it is indicated for the management of moderate to severe pain which is not amenable to treatment with mild analgesics but is not felt to be of sufficient severity to require narcotic analgesia.
Dosage
1. Orally: 30–90 mg three times per day.
2. By intramuscular or intravenous injection: 20 mg four times per day (see Nurse monitoring section for administration procedure).
Nurse monitoring
1. When this drug is given by intramuscular injection care must

be taken to ensure that accidental intravenous injection is avoided. If intravenous injection is contemplated, the drug should be administered slowly the maximum rate of administration recommended being 5 mg/minute. Too rapid intravenous injection may cause syncope.
2. Common side effects include nausea, vomiting, blurred vision, nervousness, light-headedness, dry mouth, drowsiness, sweating, insomnia, headache and tachycardia.
3. Patients with a history of fits should not receive this drug.
4. The metabolism and excretion of Nefopam may be impaired in patients with liver or kidney disease.

General notes
1. The drug may be stored at room temperature.
2. Notes on intramuscular and intravenous administration are included in the Nurse monitoring section.

NEOMYCIN

(See Note 3, p. 310)
Presentation
Tablets—500 mg
N.B. Neomycin is included in a vast range of preparations for topical use including ointments, creams, eye drops and ear drops. It is usually combined with other medicaments particularly other antibiotics and corticosteroids.

Actions and uses
Neomycin is an antibiotic of the aminoglycoside group which resembles Gentamicin (q.v.). It is not absorbed orally and is too toxic for systemic use. It is therefore only useful in the following situations:
1. It may be given in an attempt to sterilise the gut. This is useful before bowel surgery and also may lead to a decrease in protein absorption from the bowel which is useful in patients with cirrhosis of the liver when they develop encephalopathy.
2. It is an effective antibiotic for the treatment of superficial infections of the skin, eye and ear.

Dosage
1. To attempt bowel sterilisation:
   a. *Adults* receive 500 mg–1 g four times per day.
   b. *Children*:
      Less than 1 year: 2 mg/kg four times a day. More than 1 year: 125–250 mg four times a day.

Nurse monitoring
1. Systemic adverse effects are unlikely as very little of the drug is absorbed.
2. Despite the fact that the drug is very poorly absorbed, a large number of patients develop skin rashes due to hypersensitivity.
3. Nurses who are sensitive to the drug develop severe skin rashes if they handle it. Therefore the wearing of protective gloves is advised.

General notes
Neomycin tablets may be stored at room temperature.

NEOSTIGMINE (Prostigmin)

Presentation
Tablets—15 mg Neostigmine Bromide
Ampoules—0.5 mg and 2.5 mg Neostigmine Methylsulphate in 1 ml
Ophthalmic solution—3% Neostigmine Methylsulphate

Actions and uses
Neostigmine prevents the action of the enzyme that destroys acetylcholine in the body. This in effect leads to a prolongation of acetylcholine action which is to stimulate the parasympathetic component of the autonomic nervous system. It has the following uses in clinical practice:
1. For the treatment of myasthenia gravis
2. As an antidote to curariform drugs
3. For the treatment of glaucoma.

4. To restore gut motility in paralytic ileus and post-operative distension and in the treatment of heartburn of pregnancy.

Dosage
1. For the treatment of myasthenia gravis:
   a. *Adults*: A daily dose of 5–20 tablets by mouth or 1–2.5 mg by injection is commonly given but doses higher than these may be needed in some patients.
   b. *Children*: The doses should be decided by the attending physician. A guideline is as follows:
   Neonates: 0.05–0.25 mg by injection or 1–5 mg orally every 4 hours.
   Older children: 0.2–0.5 mg daily by injection or 15–60 mg daily orally.
2. As an antidote to curariform drugs: 1–5 mg intravenously. Atropine 0.4–1.25 mg should normally be given some minutes before this injection.
3. For the treatment of glaucoma: one drop of the 3% ophthalmic solution should be administered every 10 minutes for seven doses and a further five doses may be given if required.
4. To increase gut motility: 1 or 2 tablets taken is required.

Nurse monitoring
1. Side effects include excess salivation, anorexia, nausea, vomiting, abdominal cramp and diarrhoea. Bradycardia and hypotension may occur along with bronchoconstriction and increase in bronchial secretions. Rarely weakness, paralysis, convulsion and coma may occur.
2. It is important to note that the major symptom of overdosage with this drug is increased muscular weakness. When used for the treatment of myasthenia gravis, the patient may become weak and it is then difficult to differentiate whether this is due to inadequate or excessive treatment. In this situation the intravenous administration of Edrophonium chloride (Tensilon) will produce a rapid and short-lived improvement in muscle power if inadequate dosage is the cause of weakness but will not have this effect if overdosage is the cause of weakness.
3. The drug should never be given to patients who are known to suffer from intestinal or urinary obstruction.
4. Patients with bradycardia, bronchial asthma, heart disease, epilepsy, hypotension and Parkinsonism should not receive this drug.

General notes
1. All preparations should be protected from light.
2. Tablets should be stored in well closed containers.

NETILMICIN (Netillin)

(*See Note 3, p. 310*)

Presentation
Injection — 15 mg in 1.5 ml
50 mg in 1 ml
100 mg in 1 ml
150 mg in 1.5 ml

Actions and uses
Netilmicin is a member of the aminoglycoside group of antibiotics and its actions and uses are described in the section on these drugs. It is administered only by injection and is frequently favoured since it produces a lower incidence of adverse effects than do other aminoglycosides.

Dosage
Adults: 4–7.5 mg/kg daily in 2–3 divided doses by intramuscular and intravenous injection or by intravenous infusion.
Children: Higher doses e.g. 6–9 mg/kg daily are used.

Nurse monitoring
See the section on aminoglycoside antibiotics.

General notes
1. Netilmicin injections may be stored at room temperature.
2. The drug should never be mixed with other antibiotics prior to administration.

3. Intravenous infusions are prepared in 100 ml sodium chloride 0.9%, dextrose 5% or dextrose/saline mixtures and infused over 30 minutes to 2 hours.

NICLOSAMIDE (Yomesan)
Presentation
Tablets—500 mg
Actions and uses
This antihelminthic drug is used for the treatment of the following tapeworm infections:
1. Beef tapeworm (*Taenia saginata*)
2. Pork tapeworm (*Taenia solium*)
3. Fish tapeworm (*Diphyllobothrium latum*)
4. Dwarf tapeworm (*Hymenolepis nana*)

Dosage administration
1. For the treatment of beef, pork and fish tapeworm:
   a. Adults and children over 6 years: 2 g
   b. Children from 2–6 years: 1 g
   c. Children under 2 years: 500 mg
2. For the treatment of dwarf tapeworm:
   a. On the first day adults and children over 6: 2 g
      Children over 2–6 years: 1 g
      Children under 2 years: 500 mg
   b. For the subsequent 6 days: adults and children over 6: 1 g daily
      Children from 2–6 years: 500 mg daily
      Children under 2 years: 250 mg daily.

Nurse monitoring
1. A laxative given two hours after treatment with this drug ensures a rapid and complete expulsion of the worm which would otherwise be excreted in pieces during the next few days. It is felt that in the treatment of *Taenia solium* a laxative is essential.
2. The drug may be given without danger to patients with liver, biliary or kidney disease.

General notes
The drug may be stored at room temperature.

NICOFURANOSE (Bradilan)
Presentation
Tablets—250 mg enteric-coated
Actions and uses
This drug dilates peripheral blood vessels and is therefore used in clinical practice to treat the following disorders:
1. Raynaud's syndrome
2. Intermittent claudication
3. Night cramps and chilblains.

Dosage
For adults 500 mg–1 g three times daily.

Nurse monitoring
1. The side effects of all drugs which have vasodilator effect include flushing of the skin of the face and the neck, hypotension, dizziness, faintness (especially on standing up). These side effects may make a reduction in dosage necessary.
2. Gastrointestinal symptoms encountered with this drug include nausea and vomiting.

General notes
The drug may be stored at room temperature.

NICOTINYL ALCOHOL (Ronicol)
Presentation
Tablets—25 mg and 150 mg (slow release)
Actions and uses
The actions and uses of this drug are identical to those described for Nicofuranose (q.v.).

Dosage
Adults: 25–50 mg four times a day or 150–300 mg twice daily as slow release tablets.

Nurse monitoring
The Nurse monitoring section on Nicofuranose (q.v.) applies to this drug.

General notes
The drug may be stored at room temperature.

NICOUMALONE (Sinthrome)

Presentation
Tablets—1 mg and 4 mg

Actions and uses
A number of substances present in blood which play an important part in preventing bleeding by forming clots are produced by the liver from Vitamin K. Nicoumalone inhibits the synthesis of these substances (known as clotting factors) and therefore reduces the ability of the blood to clot. Its principal uses are for the prevention and treatment of thromboembolic states such as deep venous thrombosis and pulmonary embolus. They are also used to prevent the formation of clot in cardiovascular disease either on artificial heart valves or in the atria of patients who have atrial dysrhythmias.

Dosage
1. *Adults*:
   a. Loading dose: Day 1: 8–16 mg; Day 2: 4–12 mg; Day 3: Dosage should be adjusted according to result of blood clotting test.
   b. Maintenance dose: Varies according to individual response and should be decided after reference to the results of blood clotting test.

Nurse monitoring
1. The daily maintenance dose of Nicoumalone is, as noted above, determined by the results of clotting studies. As the effects of bleeding due to overcoagulation or thrombosis due to undercoagulation can be so rapidly catastrophic strict adherence to the recommended dose is mandatory and the nurse may play an important role in ensuring that patients are aware of this.
2. The effects of Nicoumalone may be influenced by a number of factors listed below and the nurse may play an important role by identifying their occurrence and alerting both the patient and medical staff. The following circumstances may lead to a requirement for alteration in dosage:
   a. Acute illness such as chest infection or viral infection
   b. Sudden weight loss
   c. The concurrent administration of other drugs: A number of drugs may affect the patient's dosage requirements. Where drugs are known to interfere with anticoagulant control this has been noted in the Nurse monitoring sections of the drugs in this book.
3. The occurrence of haemorrhage in a patient on Nicoumalone is an indication for immediate withdrawal of the drug and if the haemorrhage is at all serious or repetitive the patient should be referred immediately to hospital for further assessment and, if necessary, they may be given Vitamin K which accelerates a return to normal clotting function.
4. Nicoumalone is relatively contraindicated in patients with severe liver or kidney disease, haemorrhagic conditions or uncontrolled hypertension. It should also be used with great caution immediately after surgery or labour.
5. Nausea, loss of appetite, headache and dizziness may occur.

General notes
The tablets may be stored at room temperature.

NIFEDIPINE (Adalat)

Presentation
Capsules—5 mg and 10 mg
Tablets—20 mg (retard)

Actions and uses
Nifedipine has two main actions
1. It decreases the work done by the heart in two ways.
   a. It directly affects heart muscle, depressing its activity.
   b. It dilates peripheral vessels, reducing the pressure against which the heart has to work.
2. It lowers raised blood pressure by its action on peripheral blood

vessels which results in vasodilatation.
These properties make it useful for the treatment of angina pectoris and hypertension.

Dosage
1. Angina pectoris:
   a. Prophylaxis: 10 mg three times a day initially increasing to a maximum of 20 mg three times a day if necessary.
   5 mg capsules may be useful when carefully tailoring doses to individual need.
   b. Treatment of acute attack: a capsule may be bitten and placed under the tongue to produce a more rapid onset of effect.
2. Hypertension: 20–40 mg usually as 'retard' tablets taken twice a day.

Nurse monitoring
1. Headaches and flushing may be expected in patients on this drug. Lethargy or tiredness may also occur.
2. There is some evidence that occasionally the drug, after an acute myocardial infarction, may divert blood to healthy rather than damaged muscle and so increase the extent of damage.
3. Sometimes angina may be paradoxically exacerbated and require the drug to be stopped.

General notes
The drug may be stored at room temperature. It is light-sensitive but available in foil-wrapped packs to counteract this problem.

NITRAZEPAM (Mogadon)

Presentation
Tablets—5 mg
Capsules—5 mg
Suspension—2.5 mg in 5 ml

Actions and uses
Nitrazepam is a member of the benzodiazepine group (q.v.) which has a pronounced sedative effect and is taken at night as an hypnotic.

Dosage
5–10 mg on retiring.

Nurse monitoring
1. See the section on benzodiazepines.
2. It is essential to re-emphasise that Nitrazepam is particularly likely to cause a hang-over effect with drowsiness and headache the following day. This may be particularly severe when high dosage is used in elderly patients and may lead to frank confusion. It is recommended that the elderly should only very rarely receive a dose exceeding 5 mg of this drug if side effects are to be avoided.

General notes
Preparations containing Nitrazepam may be stored at room temperature.

NITROFURANTOIN (Macrodantin, Furadantin)

Presentation
Tablets—50 mg and 100 mg
Capsules—50 mg and 100 mg
Suspension—25 mg in 5 ml

Actions and uses
Nitrofurantoin is bactericidal i.e. it kills organisms in the body if the concentration of the drug obtained is sufficiently high. At lower concentrations it is bacteriostatic i.e. it inhibits growth and further multiplication of bacterial cells. It is so rapidly excreted from the body that it is only of use in bacterial infections of the bladder. It is debatable whether sufficient concentration is obtained in the kidney for it to be useful in pyelonephritis and it is certianly not useful for infections of other organs of the body. It is usually effective against *E. coli*, Klebsiella and Enterobacter but resistance is a greater problem with proteus and *Pseudomonas aeruginosa*. It is used both in the treatment of urinary tract infections and for prophylaxis against urinary tract infections.

Dosage
1. For the treatment of urinary tract infections:
   a. *Adults*: 100 mg four times a day with meals

b. *Children*:
   Less than 1 year: 2.5 mg/kg body weight four times a day
   1–7 years: 25–50 mg four times a day
   Over 7 years: adult doses are administered.
2. For the prophylaxis of urinary tract infection half of the dose recommended for treatment of acute infections is given.

Nurse monitoring
1. Nausea, vomiting and diarrhoea occur commonly. The incidence and severity of these effects may be reduced if the drug is taken with meals or milk.
2. An uncommon but important side effect is peripheral neuropathy. Patients should be continually asked to report symptoms of numbness or tingling of the feet and if such symptoms occur the drug should be immediately withdrawn before irreversible and more severe changes occur.
3. Other neurological side effects include headache, vertigo, drowsiness, nystagmus and muscle pain.
4. Megaloblastic anaemia is a rare adverse effect.
5. Hypersensitivity reactions including chills, fever, jaundice, liver damage, leucopenia, granulocytopenia and haemolytic anaemia may occur.
6. The drug may rarely damage the lungs especially in elderly patients producing pneumonitis and pulmonary fibrosis.
7. The drug should not be given to patients who have severe renal damage as it may accumulate in the body and produce severe toxic effects.

General notes
The drug may be stored at room temperature.

NOMIFENSINE (Merital)

Presentation
Tablets—100 mg
Capsules—25 mg, 50 mg

Actions and uses
Nomifensine is a tricyclic antidepressant drug. Its actions and uses are described in the section dealing with these drugs.

Dosage
For the treatment of depression in adults 50–200 mg in total per day is administered in one, two or three divided doses.

Nurse monitoring
See the section on tricyclic antidepressant drugs.

General notes
1. Nomifensine tablets and capsules may be stored at room temperature.
2. The capsules should be protected from light.

NORTRIPTYLINE (Aventyl, Allegron)

Presentation
Tablets—10 mg, 25 mg
Capsules—10 mg, 25 mg
Syrup—10 mg in 5 ml

Actions and uses
Nortriptyline is a tricyclic antidepressant drug. Its actions and uses are described in the section on these drugs.

Dosage
For the treatment of depression:
1. *Adult dose ranges vary from 10–25 mg three or four times daily.
2. Children over the age of 12 may be given 10–25 mg three times daily.
3. Children under the age of 12 and the elderly may be given 10 mg three or four times daily.

Nurse monitoring
See the section on tricyclic antidepressant drugs.

General notes
Preparations containing Nortriptyline may be stored at room temperature.

NYSTATIN (Nystan, Mycostatin)

Presentation
Tablets—500 000 units
Suspension—100 000 units in 1 ml

Pessaries—100 000 units
Gel—100 000 units in 1 g
Vaginal cream—100 000 units in 4 g
Cream and ointment—100 000 units in 1 g

Actions and uses

This anti-fungal drug is used most commonly in clinical practice to eradicate infection due to *Candida albicans* either in the gut or the genital tract.

Dosage

1. Orally: One tablet or 1 ml of suspension three or four times daily.
2. Vaginally: One or two pessaries at night.
3. Topical applications should be administered two to four times daily.

Nurse monitoring

1. It is important to note that the drug is not absorbed after oral administration and is not used for systemic infections.
2. The drug does not produce any known side effects.

General notes

The drug may be stored at room temperature.

O

OESTRADIOL VALERATE (Progynova)

Presentation
Tablets—1 mg, 2 mg

Actions and uses
Oestradiol valerate is an oestrogenic substance. The general actions and uses of oestrogens are described in the section on these drugs. Oestradiol valerate in clinical practice is used for the alleviation of menopausal symptoms and the prophylaxis and treatment of post-menopausal sequelae of oestrogen withdrawal such as osteoposrosis and senile vaginitis.

Dosage
For the treatment of menopausal symptoms: 21 day cycles of 1 or 2 mg are administered.

Nurse monitoring
See the section on oestrogenic hormones.

General notes
The drug may be stored at room temperature.

OESTRIOL (Ovestin)

Presentation
Tablets—250 μg

Actions and uses
Oestriol is an oestrogenic substance. The general actions and uses of oestrogens are described in the section on Contraceptives (oral).

Dosage
1. For the treatment of functional dysmenorrhoea: 1 mg daily for 14 days prior to the expected onset of pain.
2. For the treatment of senile vaginitis: 250 μg to 500 μg per day.

Nurse monitoring
See the section on oestrogens.

General notes
The drug may be stored at room temperature.

OESTROGENS, CONJUGATED (Equine) (Premarin)

Presentation
Tablets—0.625 mg, 1.25 mg, 2.5 mg
Injection—25 mg in 5 ml
Vaginal cream—0.625 mg/g

Actions and uses
1. The actions and uses of oestrogenic hormones in general are described in the section on Contraceptives (oral).
2. The oral preparation of this drug has a number of recommended uses:
   a. For the treatment of symptoms due to post-menopausal oestrogen deficiency
   b. For the treatment of senile vaginitis
   c. For the treatment of post-menopausal osteoporosis
   d. For the suppression of lactation
   e. For the treatment of amenorrhoea
   f. For the treatment of prostatic carcinoma
   g. For the treatment of dysfunctional uterine bleeding.
3. The parenteral (intravenous) preparation is used to achieve haemostasis due to capillary bleeding such as in epistaxis or dysfunctional uterine bleeding.
4. The vaginal cream is used for the treatment of atrophic vaginitis.

Dosage
1. Orally:
   a. For the treatment of post-menopausal oestrogen deficiency: 0.625–1.25 mg daily administered cyclically for 21 days every 28 days
   b. For the treatment of senile vaginitis: Cyclical administration for 21 days every 28 days of 1.25–3.75 mg
   c. For the treatment of post-menopausal osteoporosis: cyclical administration for 21 days every 28 days of 1.25–3.75 mg per day
   d. For the suppression of lactation: 3.75 mg every four hours for five doses, or 1.25 mg every four hours for five days
   e. For the treatment of amenorrhoea: 3.75 mg daily in divided doses for 20 days (for the last 5 days progesterone therapy should be added)
   f. For the treatment of prostatic carcinoma: 4.5–7.5 mg daily in divided doses
   g. For the treatment of dysfunctional uterine bleeding:
      i. To achieve haemostasis: 3.75–75 mg daily in divided doses (Haemostasis can usually be expected within 2–4 days)
      ii. For cycle regulation: The daily dose required to produce haemostasis is continued without interruption for 20 days. During each of the last 5–10 days of oestrogen therapy an oral progesterone is given and within 2–5 days of cessation of drugs bleeding should commence.
2. Parenteral administration: To achieve haemostasis:
   a. For adults 25 mg intramuscularly or intravenously
   b. For children 5–10 mg intramuscularly or intravenously
3. Topical application: 2–4 g daily.

Nurse monitoring
See the section on oestrogenic hormones.

General notes
1. Tablets and vaginal cream may be stored at room temperature.
2. Injection vials should be stored in a refrigerator.
3. Once reconstituted with the diluent provided, injections may be kept for up to two months.

ORCIPRENALINE (Alupent)

Presentation
Tablets—20 mg
Syrup—10 mg in 5 ml
Metered aerosol—0.75 mg per dose
Inhalant solution—5%
Injection—0.5 mg in 1 ml, 5 mg in 10 ml

Actions and uses
This drug stimulates the beta component of the sympathetic nervous system. Its useful effects are:
1. It causes relaxation of the smooth muscle in the walls of the large airways (bronchi) and therefore may be used to treat reversible airways obstruction (bronchospasm) due to asthma or other diseases such as bronchitis and emphysema.
2. It inhibits uterine contraction and therefore may be used in obstetric practice for the treatment of premature labour.

Dosage
1. For the treatment of bronchospasm:
   a. Orally:
      i. *Adults*: 20 mg four times a day.
      ii. *Children*:
         3–12 years: 10 mg four times a day to 20 mg three times a day.
         1–3 years: 5–10 mg four times a day.
         0–1 year: 5–10 mg three times a day.

b. Metered aerosol:
   i. *Adults*: 1–2 puffs, a maximum number of 12 puffs in 24 hours with at least 30 minutes between each dosage.
   ii. *Children*:
       6–12 years: 1–2 puffs, a maximum of four doses in 24 hours with at least 30 minutes between each dosage.
       Children under 6 years: 1 puff, a maximum of four puffs in 24 hours with at least 30 minutes between each dosage.
c. By intramuscular injection:
   i. *Adults*: 0.5 mg repeated after 30 minutes if necessary.
   ii. *Children*:
       6–12 years: 0.5 mg repeated after 30 minutes if necessary.
       Children under 6 years: 0.25 mg repeated after 30 minutes if necessary.

Nurse monitoring
1. Patients, as well as being instructed in the correct use of the metered aerosol, must be warned never to exceed the prescribed dosage of this drug.
2. It is worth noting that the beta blocking drugs (q.v.) antagonise the action of Alupent and, therefore, their concurrent administration is undesirable.
3. Transient side effects after administration include palpitation, tachycardia, headache, nausea and abdominal discomfort.
4. The drug should never be given to patients already receiving monoamine oxidase inhibitors.
5. The drug should be used with great care in patients with heart disease, hypertension or thyrotoxicosis.

General notes
1. Preparations containing Orciprenaline may be stored at room temperature.
2. Injection solution and syrup should be protected from light.
3. The pressurised aerosols should never be punctured or incinerated after use.

ORPHENADRINE (Disipal)

Presentation
Tablets—50 mg
Injection—40 mg in 2 ml

Actions and uses
The actions and uses of this drug are identical to those described for Benzhexol (q.v.).

Dosage
In adults:
a. Orally: 150–300 mg in total given in three divided doses.
b. Parenterally: 20–40 mg as a single dose by intramuscular injection.

Nurse monitoring
The Nurse monitoring aspects of Benzhexol (q.v.) apply to this drug.

General notes
This drug may be stored at room temperature.

OXAZEPAM (Serenid-D)

Presentation
Tablets—10 mg, 15 mg
Capsules—30 mg

Actions and uses
Oxazepam is a member of the benzodiazepine group (q.v.). Its principal use is in the treatment of anxiety.

Dosage
10–30 mg three times daily with occasionally an additional 10 or 30 mg dose at night.

Nurse monitoring
See the section on benzodiazepines.

General notes
Tablets and capsules containing Oxazepam may be stored at room temperature.

OXETHAZAINE (Mucaine)

Presentation
Suspension—10 mg in 5 ml.

Actions and uses
Oxethazaine is a local anaesthetic

drug which is taken in an antacid mixture to anaesthetise the lower oesophagus. It is used in the management of oesophagitis, heartburn and hiatus hernia.

Dosage
5–10 ml of suspension four times daily before meals and at bedtime.

Nurse monitoring
The drug is not absorbed and therefore produces no systemic toxic effects.

General notes
Oxethazaine suspension may be stored at room temperature.

OXPENTIFYLLINE (Trental)

Presentation
Tablets—100 mg, 400 mg (slow release)
Injection—100 mg in 5 ml

Actions and uses
Oxypentifylline is a *vasodilatory* which is also said to make red blood cells more able to alter their shape and therefore to penetrate narrowed and damaged vessels improving oxygen supply. It is recommended for use in:
1. Peripheral vascular disease including Raynaud's disease, intermittent claudication, chilblains and night cramps.
2. Cerebrovascular insufficiency.

Dosage
1. Orally: 200 mg three times a day (conventional tablets) or 400 mg two or three times a day (slow-release tablets).
2. Intravenous infusion: 100–400 mg over 90–180 minutes in 500 ml of 0.9% sodium chloride of 5% dextrose.
3. Intravenous injection: 100 mg slowly with the patient in a recumbent position.
4. Intra-arterial injection: 100–300 mg in 20–50 ml of 0.9% sodium chloride over 10–30 minutes.

Nurse monitoring
1. Symptoms which may be experienced during administration of this drug include nausea, gastric upset, dizziness, flushing and malaise.
2. The drug should be used with great caution in patients who already have hypotension or who are receiving antihypertensive drugs or have heart disease.

General notes
The drug may be stored at room temperature.

OXPRENOLOL (Trasicor)

Presentation
Tablets—20 mg, 40 mg, 80 mg, 160 mg (slow release)
Injection—2 mg powder in 2 ml ampoule

Actions and uses
See the section on beta-adrenoreceptor blocking drugs. Oxprenolol is a 'non-selective' drug.

Dosage
1. Intravenous dosage for the management of serious cardiac dysrhythmias is 1–2 mg given over a period of 5 minutes and repeated as necessary every 10–20 minutes to a maximum dosage of 5 mg. The patient's pulse and blood pressure should be carefully monitored during administration and also a continuous ECG monitor must be maintained and injection must be stopped if there is widening of the QRS complex.
2. Intramuscular drug treatment may be given as an alternative to intravenous treatment and the dosage and monitoring is as described for the intravenous administration.
3. Adult oral dosage ranges from 80–480 mg per day usually in three divided doses. For the treatment of hypertension a twice-daily or once-daily dosage regime may be used. A sustained release preparation is available and may be given once per day.
4. For the control of cardiac dysrhythmias in children the drug is given in a dosage of 1 mg/kg body weight usually divided into three doses.

Nurse monitoring
See the section on beta-adrenoreceptor blocking drugs.
General notes
Oxprenolol tablets and powder for injection may be stored at room temperature. Powder for injection should be dissolved in Water for Injections immediately before use.

OXYMETHOLONE (Anapolon)
Presentation
Tablets—50 mg
Actions and uses
1. The actions and uses of anabolic steroids and androgenic hormones in general are discussed in the sections on these drugs.
2. In clinical practice this drug is used for:
   a. The treatment of aplastic and refractory anaemia
   b. As adjunctive therapy in patients with malignant disease where treatment with cytotoxic agents and/or radiotherapy is likely to cause bone marrow depression.

Dosage
For the treatment of aplastic anaemia: 2–5 mg/kg body weight daily for adults and 2–4 mg/kg body weight daily for children in divided doses. The dose should be adjusted within this range according to individual response. Therapy must be maintained for at least three months before a response can be expected and minimum duration of therapy should be six months. After response is obtained it is recommended that that dose be continued for three months and then halved and maintained for at least a further three months. Therapy should be withdrawn gradually.
Nurse monitoring
See the sections on anabolic steroids and androgenic hormones.
General notes
The drug should be stored at room temperature.

OXYTETRACYCLINE (Terramycin, Imperacin)
(*See Note 3, p. 310*)
Presentation
Tablets—250 mg
Capsules—250 mg
Syrup—125 mg in 5 ml
Injection — 100 mg (intramuscular)
250 mg (intravenous)
Ointment—3%
Oxytetracycline is also included in compound eye ointments and drops.
Actions and uses
See the section on Tetracycline.
Dosage
See the section on Tetracycline.
Nurse monitoring
See the section on Tetracycline.
General notes
1. The drug may be stored at room temperature.
2. The syrup should be used within one week of preparation.

OXYTOXIN (Syntocinon)
Presentation
Injection — 2 units in 2 ml
5 units in 1 ml
10 units in 1 ml
50 units in 5 ml
Nasal spray—40 units in 1 ml
Actions and uses
Oxytocin, of which Syntocinon is a synthetic derivative, is a hormone normally found in the posterior lobe of the pituitary gland in the brain. It has two actions which make it useful in clinical practice:
1. It stimulates the milk ejection reflex, i.e. the mechanism by which breast milk passes from its site of production to reach the suckling infant.
2. It stimulates the contraction of the pregnant uterus.

It has the following uses:
1. It may be administered by nasal spray to facilitate breast feeding.
2. It may be administered by intravenous infusion to induce labour.
3. It may be administered by

intravenous infusion (often in combination with Ergometrine as 'Syntometrine') for the treatment of missed abortion or post-partum haemorrhage.

Dosage
1. Intra-nasally for the facilitation of breast feeding: The nasal spray should be administered 2–5 minutes before feeds.
2. Intravenously to induce labour: Most maternity units have a documented procedure for the administration of this drug to induce labour and therefore no specific doses are given here.
3. For the treatment of post-partum haemorrhage or missed abortion: Again the nurse is recommended to acquaint herself with the treatment schedule of the centre to which she is attached.

Nurse monitoring
1. High doses may cause excessive uterine contraction and dosage should therefore be carefully monitored to prevent the potentially disastrous occurrence of a ruptured uterus.
2. When high doses of Syntocinon are given with large volumes of electrolyte free fluid, water intoxication may occur. Initially headache, anorexia, nausea, vomiting and abdominal pain may be the presenting features and this progresses to lethargy, drowsiness, unconsciousness and grand mal type seizures. The concentration of blood electrolytes may be markedly disturbed.

General notes
1. The drug should be stored in a refrigerator.
2. Infusions are generally administered in 5% dextrose solution.

P

PANCREATIN

Presentation
See dosage table

Actions and uses
This preparation is a mixture of enzymes normally produced by the pancreas. In pancreatic disease, where insufficient enzymes are being produced, food cannot be absorbed. Pancreatin, therefore, is used in cases of malabsorption due to pancreatic deficiency.

Dosage

Preparation	Usual Dosage
Combizym tabs	1 or 2 tablets with meals
Combizym composition tabs	1 tablet with meals
Cotazym caps	6 capsules daily, the contents being sprinkled over food
Cotazym B tabs	2 tablets with meals
Enzypan tabs	2–3 with meals
Nutrizym tabs	1–2 tablets with meals
Pancrex powder	5–10 g as powder four times daily before meals
Pancrex V powder	500 mg–2 g as powder four times daily before, or mixed with meals
Pancrex V caps	Contents of 1–3 capsules sprinkled over food four times per day
Pancrex V tabs	5–15 tablets four times per day before meals
Pancrex V Forte tabs	2–6 tablets four times per day before meals

Nurse monitoring
1. When used in very young babies irritation of the skin may occur around the mouth and the anus. Barrier creams will effectively prevent this.
2. Rarely hypersensitivity reactions such as sneezing and skin rash may occur.
3. These preparations are, to say the least, unpleasant. The nurse may play an important supportive role in encouraging the patient to persevere with this treatment.

General notes
Preparations should be stored in a well closed container in a cool place.

PAPAVERETUM (Omnopon)

Presentation
Tablets—10 mg
Injection—10 mg and 20 mg in 1 ml

Actions and uses
The actions and uses of this narcotic analgesic drug are described in the section dealing with these drugs.

Dosage
1. *Adults*: By oral, intramuscular, subcutaneous or intravenous routes 10–20 mg repeated 4–6 hourly as required.
2. *Children*: By oral, intramuscular, subcutaneous or intravenous injection:
   Less than 1 year: 0.2 mg/kg 4 to 6-hourly as required.
   1–7 years: 2–5 mg 4 to 6-hourly as required.

Nurse monitoring
See the section on narcotic analgesic drugs.

211

General notes
1. The drug should be stored at in a locked (controlled drug) cupboard.
2. The drug should be stored at room temperature.

PARACETAMOL (Panadol, Calpol)

Presentation
Tablets—500 mg
Syrup—120 mg in 5 ml

Actions and uses
Paracetamol has both analgesic (pain relieving) and anti-pyretic (temperature reducing) properties. It is used where mild analgesia is indicated for such common complaints as headache and musculoskeletal pain. It is particularly useful for the treatment of mild pain or pyrexia in groups of patients for whom salicylate therapy is contraindicated, such as those with previous gastrointestinal bleeding and also for the treatment of children under one year of age who should not normally be given salicylates.

1. *Adults*: 500 mg–1 g 4 to 6-hourly as required for pain.
2. *Children*:
   Less than 1 year: 120 mg four times a day
   1–5 years: 240 mg four times a day
   5 years and over: Up to 480 mg four times a day.

Nurse monitoring
1. Few if any side effects are associated with the administration of this drug.
2. This drug is widely available for sale without prescription in Great Britain and although it is associated with negligible side effects when taken in normal dosage, it is extremely dangerous if taken as an overdose when severe and fatal liver damage may occur. A specific intravenous treatment regime with N-acetylcysteine is available but its efficacy depends on how quickly the patient receives it after taking the overdose. Thus any patient who has taken such an overdose must be referred to hospital with the utmost speed.
3. As well as liver damage after overdosage, renal and cardiac damage may occur.

General notes
The drug may be stored at room temperature.

PENICILLAMINE (Distamine)

Presentation
Tablets—50 mg, 125 mg, and 250 mg

Actions and uses
Penicillamine has two main actions:
1. It binds heavy metal ions by a process called 'chelation' and therefore may be used in the treatment of the following disorders:
   a. Lead poisoning where it is thought to reduce the absorption of lead
   b. Wilson's disease (hepatolenticular degeneration) where it increases the excretion of copper
   c. Mercury poisoning
   d. Cystinuria where it promotes the excretion of the more soluble form of cystine.
2. It also reduces the inflammatory response in patients with severe rheumatoid arthritis. The reduction in the inflammatory response leads to a subsequent relief of symptoms.

Dosage
1. Lead poisoning and Wilson's disease:
   a. *Adults*: 1–2 g daily in divided doses
   b. *Children*: up to 20 mg/kg daily in divided doses.
2. Rheumatoid arthritis:
   a. *Adults*: Initially 125–250 mg per day is given and gradually increased until a response is obtained. Usually the required do : is in the range of 500–750 mg per day although the response may take several weeks to develop.

After maintaining patients on these high doses for several months it is often possible to reduce the maintenance dose without loss of effect
b. *Children*:
Up to 2 years: 25–50 mg twice a day
2–4 years: 50–100 mg twice a day
4–10 years: 100 mg twice or three times per day.

Nurse monitoring
1. This drug should never be given to patients who are already receiving gold salts or antimalarial treatment such as Chloroquine or Hydroxychloroquine.
2. Routine checks of white cell counts, platelet counts and urine tests for albumin should be performed at weekly intervals in patients on this treatment.
3. Patients may be allergic to Penicillamine. Patients who have already been found to be allergic to Penicillin are particularly at risk from this.
4. Adverse effects include headaches, sore throat, fever, skin rash, nausea, pruritis, muscle and joint pain, altered taste sensitivity, eosinophilia, lymphadenopathy, leucopenia, agranulocytosis, thrombocytopenia, proteinuria and nephrotic syndrome.
5. Patients who have already been found to be allergic to gold injections should never be given Penicillamine.

General notes
Penicillamine tablets may be stored at room temperature.

PENTAERYTHRITOL TETRANITRATE (Myocardol, Peritrate)

Presentation
Tablets — 10 mg, 30 mg
80 mg (sustained release)

Actions and uses
This drug reduces heart work by dilating peripheral blood vessels and lowering peripheral vascular resistance. It is used on a regular basis for the prevention of angina pectoris.

Dosage
The adult dose range is 80–240 mg taken in three or four divided daily doses or 80 mg twice daily as a sustained release tablet.

Nurse monitoring
1. General problems occurring with this drug are similar to those encountered with Glyceryl Trinitrate (q.v.).
2. Common side effects are headache, lethargy and nausea, especially during the early period of treatment.
3. Side effects associated with excessive dose are palpitation, nausea, hypotension, muscular weakness, dizziness, diarrhoea, cyanosis and methaemoglobinaemia.

General notes
Pentaerythritol Tetranitrate tablets may be stored at room temperature.

PENTAZOCINE (Fortral)

Presentation
Tablets—25 mg
Capsules—50 mg
Injection — 30 mg in 1 ml
60 mg in 2 ml
Suppositories—50 mg

Actions and uses
Pentazocine is a derivative of the narcotic analgesic group of drugs but it has a much less potent analgesic effect when compared with Morphine. It is, therefore, used in the management of moderate to severe pain.

Dosage
1. *Adults*:
   a. Orally: 25–100 mg 4 to 6-hourly as required
   b. By intramuscular, intravenous or subcutaneous injection: 30–60 mg 4 to 6-hourly as required
   c. Rectally: 50 mg 4 to 6-hourly as required.
2. *Children*:
   a. Orally:
      Less than 1 year: there are no

dosage recommendations for this age group
1–12 years: It is recommended that if this drug is required in this age group, parenteral therapy be used.
   b. Parenterally:
      i. By intramuscular or subcutaneous injection: 1 mg/kg body weight is the maximum single dose recommended. This should be repeated three to four hourly as required.
      ii. By intravenous injection: 0.5 mg/kg body weight is the maximum single dose recommended, repeated every 3 to 4 hours as required.
   c. By suppository: Suppositories are not recommended as being suitable for administration to children under the age of 12.

Nurse monitoring
1. See the section on narcotic analgesic drugs.
2. Hallucinations and other behavioural abnormalities have been found to be a particular problem with this drug and occur in 10% of patients. The reason they have been reported only rarely is that they tend to be of a pleasant nature.
3. Pentazocine is not subject to the legal requirements associated with 'controlled drugs'.

General notes
The drug may be stored at room temperature.

PENTOBARBITONE (Nembutal)

Presentation
   Capsules—100 mg

Actions and uses
Pentobarbitone is a barbiturate drug (q.v.) which is taken at night as a hypnotic.

Dosage
100–200 mg on retiring.

Nurse monitoring
See the section on barbiturate drugs.

General notes
Capsules containing Pentobarbitone may be stored at room temperature.

PERPHENAZINE (Fentazin)

Presentation
   Tablets—2 mg, 4 mg, 8 mg
   Concentrate—(to be diluted as required with syrup) 8 mg in 4 ml
   Injection—5 mg in 1 ml

Actions and uses
Perphenazine is a phenothiazine drug and its actions and uses are described in the section on these drugs. It is used predominantly for the treatment of severe anxiety and agitation associated with psychotic disorders but it is occasionally, in addition, used for the treatment of nausea and vomiting.

Dosage
1. The usual oral adult dose is 4 mg three times daily increasing to a maximum of 24 mg per day if required.
2. By the parenteral route 5–10 mg intramuscularly is administered followed by further doses at intervals of 6 hours if required.

Nurse monitoring
See the section on phenothiazine drugs.

General notes
1. Preparations containing Perphenazine may be stored at room temperature.
2. Concentrate and solution for injection should be protected from light.
3. Perphenazine injection must never be mixed with other injections in the same syringe.
4. The concentrate is intended to be diluted with syrup to the required concentration before use.

PERHEXILINE (Pexid)

Presentation
   Tablets—100 mg

Actions and uses
The drug has a direct action on the

heart, depressing its activity and therefore reducing work performed. This action makes it useful in the treatment of angina when, if given prophylactically on a regular basis, it may decrease the frequency of anginal attacks.

Dosage
Initially 100 mg twice daily increasing to a maximum of 100 mg four times daily if necessary.

Nurse monitoring
The drug has no effect on the pulse or blood pressure and therefore the nurse's role in this case lies solely with identification of side effects which are:
1. Commonly, giddiness or dizziness.
2. Less commonly, nausea, vomiting or lethargy.
3. Uncommonly, headache, nervousness, lassitude, insomnia; liver damage, abdominal pain; hypoglycaemia; flushing, sweating, skin rashes; peripheral neuropathy.

General notes
Perhexiline tablets may be stored at room temperature.

PERICYAZINE (Neulactil)

Presentation
Tablets—2.5 mg, 10 mg, 25 mg
Syrup—10 mg in 5 ml

Actions and uses
Pericyazine is a neuroleptic drug of the phenothiazine group which is used for its tranquillising or calming effect in severely agitated patients with behavioural disorders such as schizophrenia, senile dementia and mental subnormality. When compared to other major tranquillisers such as chlorpromazine, Pericyazine produces a marked sedative effect, thus it is of particular use in disorders characterised by aggressive or impulsive tendencies.

Dosage
1. *Adults*: Initially 15–75 mg daily in divided doses increased gradually until control of symptoms is achieved. Thereafter the dosage is reduced to the lowest possible daily dose to maintain control in the individual patient.
2. *Elderly adults*: Smaller initial doses are used, e.g. 10 mg daily increased gradually.
3. *Children*: Daily dosages have been calculated on the basis of 0.5 mg for each year of age.

Nurse monitoring
1. The Nurse monitoring section on phenothiazines apply to Pericyazine.
2. It is important to note that Pericyazine has a strong sedative action and may produce marked postural hypotension. It is for this reason that correspondingly low initial doses should be used for elderly subjects who are particularly susceptible to sudden falls in blood pressure and in whom fainting attacks and palpitation may occur.
3. Children are similarly susceptible to the sedative and hypotensive actions of the drug.
4. The unwanted effects of Pericyazine may be less troublesome if the dosage is divided in such a way that the larger portion is administered at night.

General notes
Tablets and syrup preparations of Pericyazide should be stored at room temperature.

PETHIDINE

Presentation
Tablets—25 mg and 50 mg
Injection — 50 mg in 1 ml
 100 mg in 2 ml

Actions and uses
The actions and uses of this narcotic analgesic drug are described in the section on narcotic analgesic drugs.

Dosage
1. *Adults*:
   a. Orally: 50–100 mg 3 to 4-hourly as required
   b. By subcutaneous, intramuscular or intravenous

injection: 50–100 mg 4-hourly as required.
2. *Children*: By oral, intramuscular, subcutaneous or intravenous injection:
Less than 1 year: 1 mg/kg up to three times daily
1–7 years: 12.5 mg up to three times daily
Over 7 years: 25 mg three times daily.

Nurse monitoring
1. The Nurse monitoring aspects of narcotic analgesic drugs in general are described in the section on these drugs.
2. It is worth noting that the side effects experienced with Pethidine are particularly severe in the elderly.

General notes
1. The drug should be stored in a locked (controlled drug) cupboard.
2. The drug should be stored at room temperature.

PHENAZOCINE (Narphen)

Presentation
Tablets—5 mg

Actions and uses
Phenazocine is a narcotic analgesic and its actions and uses are described in the section on these drugs.

Dosage
For adults: 5–20 mg every 4–6 hours as required.

Nurse monitoring
See the section on narcotic analgesic drugs.

General notes
1. The drug should be stored in a locked (controlled drugs) cupboard.
2. The drug should be stored at room temperature.

PHENELZINE (Nardil)

Presentation
Tablets—15 mg

Actions and uses
Phenelzine is a monoamine oxidase inhibiting drug. Its actions and uses are described in the section on these drugs.

Dosage
15 mg three times daily.

Nurse monitoring
See the section on monoamine oxidase inhibitors.

General notes
Phenelzine tablets may be stored at room temperature.

PHENETHICILLIN (Broxil)

(*See Note 3, p. 296*)

Presentation
Tablets—250 mg
Capsules—250 mg
Syrup—125 mg in 5 ml

Actions and uses
Phenethicillin is a member of the Penicillin group of antibiotics. It has actions and uses similar to those described for Phenoxymethylpenicillin (q.v.).

Dosage
1. *Adults*: 250 mg four times per day.
2. *Children*:
Less than 2 years: 62.5 mg four times per day.
Over 2 years: 125 mg four times per day.

Nurse monitoring
See the section on Benzylpenicillin.

General notes
1. Preparations containing Phenethicillin may be stored at room temperature.
2. When reconstituted Phenethicillin syrup should be used within seven days.

PHENINDAMINE (Thephorin)

Presentation
Tablets—25 mg

Actions and uses
Phenindamine is an antihistamine. The actions and uses of antihistamines in general are described in the section on these drugs. In clinical practice Phenindamine is used:
1. To suppress generalised minor allergic responses to allergens such as foodstuffs and drugs.

2. To suppress local allergic reactions i.e. inflammatory skin responses to insect stings and bites, contact allergens, urticaria etc.

Dosage
  Adults: 25–50 mg one to three times per day.

Nurse monitoring
  1. See the section on antihistamines.
  2. It is particularly interesting to note that this drug tends to produce symptoms of C.N.S. stimulation rather than the drowsiness produced by other antihistamines.

General notes
  The drug may be stored at room temperature.

PHENINDIONE (Dindevan)

Presentation
  Tablets—10 mg, 25 mg and 50 mg

Actions and uses
  A number of the substances present in blood which play an important part in preventing bleeding by forming clots are produced by the liver from Vitamin K. Phenindione inhibits the synthesis of these substances (known as clotting factors) and therefore reduces the ability of the blood to clot. Its principal uses are for the prevention and treatment of thromboembolic states such as deep venous thrombosis and pulmonary embolus. It is also used to prevent the formation of clot in cardiovascular disease either on artificial heart valves or in the atria of patients who have atrial dysrhythmias.

Dosage
  Adults:
  a. Loading dose: 200 mg on day 1; 100 mg on day 2. The dosage on day 3 should depend on the result of clotting studies.
  b. Maintenance dosage: depends on the results of blood clotting studies but usuall lies within the range of 50–150 mg per day.

Nurse monitoring
  1. The daily maintenance dose of Phenindione is, as noted above. determined by the results of clotting studies. As the effects of bleeding due to overcoagulation or thrombosis due to undercoagulation can be so rapidly catastrophic strict adherence to the recommended dose is mandatory and the nurse may play an important role in ensuring that patients are aware of this.
  2. The effects of Phenindione may be influenced by a number of factors listed below and the nurse may play an important role by identifying their occurrence and alerting both the patient and medical staff. The following circumstances may lead to a requirement for alteration in dosage:
     a. Acute illness such as chest infection or viral infection
     b. Sudden weight loss
     c. The concurrent administration of other drugs: A number of drugs may affect the patient's dosage requirements. Where drugs are known to interfere with anticoagulant control this has been noted in the Nurse monitoring sections of the drugs in this book.
  3. The occurrence of haemorrhage in a patient on Phenindione is an indication for immediate withdrawal of the drug and if the haemorrhage is at all serious or repetitive the patients should be immediately referred to hospital for further assessment and, if necessary, they may be given Vitamin K which accelerates a return to normal clotting function.
  4. Phenindione is relatively contraindicated in patients with severe liver or kidney disease, haemorrhagic conditions or uncontrolled hypertension. It should also be used with great caution immediately after surgery or labour.
  5. Skin rash, fever, blood dyscrasia, diarrhoea, liver and kidney

damage may all occur with this drug and because of these effects it is now less commonly used than Warfarin.
6. It is important for the nurse to note that metabolites of this drug may impart a pink or orange colour to the urine and this may be mistaken for haematuria. This is particularly important as haematuria is an indication for stopping drug therapy and urgently reassessing blood clotting status.

General notes
The drug may be stored at room temperature.

PHENOBARBITONE

Presentation
Tablets—15 mg, 30 mg, 60 mg, 100 mg
Tablets—30 mg, 60 mg (as sodium salt)
Capsules—60 mg and 100 mg (as slow release)
Elixir—15 mg in 5 ml
Injection—15 mg, 30 mg, 60 mg and 200 mg in 1 ml

Actions and uses
Phenobarbitone is a member of the barbiturate group. Full information is contained in the sections on anticonvulsants and barbiturates. Its major use in clinical practice is in the management of epilepsy, particularly grand mal, petit mal and pscyhomotor seizures. It is additionally occasionally used as a sedative and hypnotic though this is a declining role for barbiturate drugs since safer alternatives exist.

Dosage
1. As an anticonvulsant
   a. Orally:
      i. *Adults*: 90–375 mg (maximum 600 mg) daily taken as a single dose or in divided doses.
      ii. *Children*: 5–10 mg/kg body weight daily as a single dose or in 2 divided doses.
   b. By intramuscular injection:
      i. *Adults*: 50–200 mg single dose
      ii. *Children*: 3–6 mg/kg body weight as a single dose.

N.B. The subcutaneous and intravenous routes may also be used though the strong irritant nature of Phenobarbitone injection should be noted.

2. As a sedative or hypnotic:
   Adults: 15–30 mg 3 or 4 times a day or up to 200 mg at night as a single dose.

Nurse monitoring
See the section on anticonvulsants and barbiturates.

General notes
Preparations containing Phenobarbitone may be stored at room temperature.

PHENOTHIAZINES

Chlorpromazine
Clopenthixol
Flupenthixol
Fluphenazine
Perphenazine
Prochlorperazine
Promazine
Promethazine
Thiethylperazine
Thiopropazate
Thioridazine
Trifluoperazine
Trimeprazine

Actions and uses
The phenothiazine group of drugs possess a wide range of actions. They are used in clinical practice for three main reasons:
1. They have been found to be useful as major tranquillisers (neuroleptics) and are used for treatment of severely anxious patients and to control the marked behavioural abnormality in schizophrenia.
2. A few of this group of drugs possess potent anti-emetic activity and are used in the treatment of conditions associated with vomiting.
3. This group of drugs is used commonly in the routine management of patients with senile dementia, to control behavioural abnormalities.

Dosage
See individual drugs.
Nurse monitoring
1. Contact dermatitis can occur in people handling these drugs regularly. Precautions should therefore be taken against repeated direct contact between the nurse's skin and formulations of these drugs.
2. Solutions of Chlorpromazine cause irritation at injection sites. Injection sites should therefore be varied and discomfort may be relieved by the addition of a local anaesthetic to the injection solution.
3. A common side effect of this group of drugs is postural hypotension. This is especially important in patients who are receiving other anti-hypertensive drugs and should always be borne in mind as a cause of symptoms of dizziness or faintness.
4. Other common side effects include excessive sedation, gastrointestinal upset, photosensitivity and variation in body temperature—more often hypothermia but rarely hyperthermia may occur.
5. Endocrine side effects of this drug include amenorrhoea, failure of ovulation, galactorrhoea and gynaecomastia.
6. Various troublesome neurological side effects may occur in patients, especially those receiving the drug for a prolonged period of time. These are:
   a. A clinical picture similar to Parkinson's disease with a slow shuffling gait, a tremor and a dull expressionless face
   b. Tardive dyskinesia which is manifest as writhing movements of the muscles of the head and neck may occur and may be irreversible.
7. Phenothiazines may produce cholestatic jaundice and should be used with extreme caution in patients with liver disease.
8. Occasionally phenothiazines may affect the production of white blood cells. This makes the patient more susceptible to infection. Any patient presenting with even simple symptoms such as a sore throat should have their white blood cell count checked.

General notes
See individual drugs.

PHENOXYBENZAMINE (Dibenyline)

Presentation
Capsules—10 mg
Injection—100 mg in 2 ml

Actions and uses
Phenoxybenzamine affects the sympathetic nervous system and produces peripheral vascular dilation. It is therefore used for the treatment of diseases where improvement in peripheral blood flow is desired. These include:
1. Raynaud's disease
2. Intermittent claudication
3. Chilblains
4. Frost bite.

It has two further uses in clinical practice:
1. Its ability to block the alpha-receptors of the sympathetic nervous system make it useful in the treatment of phaeochromocytoma (an adrenaline-secreting tumour).
2. The drug has been given by intravenous infusion to attempt to increase tissue perfusion in states of severe shock.

Dosage
1. For the treatment of peripheral vascular disease:
   a. Orally: 20–60 mg per day in 2–4 divided doses.
   b. By intravenous infusion: 0.5 mg– mg/kg in 500 ml of sodium chloride 0.9% infused over one hour.
2. In the treatment of phaeochromocytoma: Up to 200 mg in total per day in divided doses may be necessary.
3. In the treatment of severe shock: An infusion of 0.5 mg–1 mg/kg in 500 ml of

200–500 ml of sodium chloride injection is given over a period of at least one hour.
Nurse monitoring
1. The drug's vasodilator action may produce flushing of the skin of the head and neck, headache, dizziness, tachycardia and postural hypotension.
2. The drug may occasionally cause slight gastrointestinal upset.
3. Inhibition of ejaculation may occur.
4. Other side effects include nasal congestion, dryness of the mouth, constricted pupils, drowsiness and sedation.

General notes
The drug should be stored at room temperature.

PHENOXYMETHYLPENICILLIN

(See Note 3, on p. 310)
N.B. Also referred to as Penicillin V. Several proprietary brands are available.
Presentation
Tablets—125 mg, 250 mg
Syrup, suspension and elixir—
62.5 mg in 5 ml
125 mg in 5 ml
250 mg in 5 ml
Actions and uses
Phenoxymethylpencillin has a mode of action similar to that described for Benzylpenicillin (q.v.). It is usually effective against streptococcus, pneumococcus, meningococcus and gonococcus and rarely effective against staphylococcus. It is therefore indicated for the treatment of diseases caused by these organisms as outlined in Note 3. Phenoxymethylpenicillin has an advantage over Benzylpenicillin in that it is better absorbed and therefore is the drug of choice for oral Penicillin treatment.
Dosage
1. Adults and older children: 500 mg four times a day.
2. Children aged 1–7 years: 125–250 mg four times a day.
3. Children less than one year: 62.5 mg four times a day.

It is important to note that the drug should preferably be given 30 minutes to one hour before meals.
Nurse monitoring
See the section on Benzylpenicillin.
General notes
1. Tablets and powder for preparing oral liquid preparations may be stored at room temperature.
2. Syrup, suspension and elixir should be discarded 7 days after reconstitution or 14 days after reconstitution if refrigerated.

PHENTERMINE (Duromine, Ionamin)

Presentation
Capsules—15 mg and 30 mg
Actions and uses
Anorexogenic drugs abolish hunger by a direct action on the central nervous system. They are thought to have a supplementary effect in that they increase the ability to perform mental and physical work without the need for increased food intake.
Dosage
For adults only: 15 or 30 mg daily at breakfast.
Nurse monitoring
The Nurse monitoring aspects of this drug are identical to those described for Diethylpropion (q.v.).
General notes
The drug may be stored at room temperature.

PHENTOLAMINE (Rogitine)

Presentation
Injection — 10 mg in 1 ml
50 mg in 5 ml
Actions and uses
This drug causes a reduction in blood pressure by dilating peripheral vessels via an effect on the sympathetic nervous system. It is no longer used to treat hypertension but may still rarely be seen in use during the surgical removal of phaeochromocytomata which are tumours associated with the production of excess catecholamines.

Dosage
1. *Adults*: 5–10 mg by intramuscular or intravenous injection.
2. *Children*: 1–5 mg by intravenous injection.

Nurse monitoring
Parenteral Phentolamine frequently produces flushing, dizziness, weakness, tachycardia.

General notes
Solutions should be protected from light and stored in a cool place.

PHENYTOIN (Epanutin)

Presentation
Tablets and capsules—25 mg, 50 mg, 100 mg
Suspension—30 mg in 5 ml
Injection—250 mg in 5 ml

Actions and uses
Phenytoin inhibits the spread of abnormal electrical activity through both the brain and the heart. It therefore has two major uses.
1. It may be given intravenously (or more rarely intramuscularly) to control status epilepticus, and orally to prevent seizures particularly of the grand mal and temporal lobe types.
2. Phenytoin may be given intravenously or more rarely orally to control certain ventricular dysrhythmias, especially when these dysrhythmias are associated with digoxin over-dosage.

Dosage
1. For the treatment of epilepsy:
   a. When given intravenously for status epilepticus the usual adult dose is 150–250 mg. Maximum infusion rate should be 50 mg per minute. Children's dosages are lower than for adults and calculated in proportion to the body weight.
   b. Regular maintenance dose should be between 25–50 mg two or three times daily. It is now accepted that the dosage should be adjusted according to measured blood levels.
2. In the treatment of cardiac arrhythmias, 3.5–5 mg/kg by slow intravenous injection is administered. A second dose may be given if necessary, oral maintenance therapy thereafter would be between 25–50 mg two to three times a day.

Nurse monitoring
The nurse's principal role in the management of patients on these drugs is to contribute to the early detection of either effects of excess dosage or side effects of the drug.
1. The effects of overdosage can be seen:
   a. With too rapid intravenous injection when cardiac arrhythmias may arise. Patients receiving this drug should therefore have pulse, blood pressure and ECG monitoring.
   b. The clinical signs of excess dosage are ataxia, nystagmus, dysarthria and confusion.
2. Side effects include tenderness and hyperplasia of the gums, hirsutism, blood disorders i.e. megaloblastic anaemia, low white cell counts, low platelet counts, pancytopenia and aplastic anaemia. Skin rashes, joint pains, fever and hepatitis can also occur. Finally the nurse should be aware that patients receiving Phenytoin may experience problems if other drugs are added to their regime if these drugs alter liver metabolism. One example of this is Chloramphenicol, which reduces the metabolism of Phenytoin in the liver and may produce toxicity with doses of Phenytoin which previously had produced no unwanted effects.

General notes
All preparations containing Phenytoin may be stored at room temperature. The solution for injection must be given undiluted and never mixed with other drugs. Solutions of Phenytoin should be protected from light.

PHTHALYLSULPHATHIAZOLE (Thalazole)

(See Note 3, p. 310)

Presentation
Tablets—500 mg

Actions and uses
1. The general actions and uses of this sulphonamide drug are described in the section dealing with sulphonamide drugs.
2. The drug has been found to be particularly useful in the treatment of bacillary dysentery.

Dosage
The recommended dose for adults is 5 g daily in divided doses.

Nurse monitoring
See the section on sulphonamide drugs.

General notes
The drug should be stored at room temperature.

PIMOZIDE (Orap)

Presentation
Tablets—2 mg, 4 mg, 10 mg

Actions and uses
Pimozide is a neuroleptic drug which is used for its tranquillising or calming effect in severely agitated patients with a range of behavioural disorders including schizophrenia, hyperactivity and aggressive behavioural disorders. In this respect Pimozide possesses many of the properties of the phenothiazine tranquillisers discussed in the section on phenothiazines.

Dosage
Adults: The dosage varies widely according to the nature and severity of the disorder under treatment. Initially 4–10 mg (increasing to up to 20 mg for acutely agitated patients) is administered. Thereafter the dose is gradually reduced to that which maintains the individual symptom-free.
Children: In children over 12 years of age a dose of 1–3 mg daily has been used.

Nurse monitoring
1. Adverse effects which are associated with the phenothiazine tranquillisers may also occur in patients treated with Pimozide. The nurse monitoring section on phenothiazines thus apply to this drug.
2. Extrapyramidal (Parkinsonian) symptoms and tardive dyskinesia appear to be more common with Pimozide than with the phenothiazines though the occurrence of unwanted sedation is less likely.
3. Other common side effects include skin rashes, glycosuria and altered liver function.

General notes
Pimozide tablets may be stored at room temperature.

PINDOLOL (Visken)

Presentation
Tablets—5 mg, 15 mg

Actions and uses
Pindolol is a non-selective beta-adrenoreceptor blocking drug. Its actions and uses are described under beta-adrenoreceptor blocking drugs (q.v.).

Dosage
The adult dosage regime is usually a daily dose of 15 mg. Alternatively up to 45 mg may be given in two or three divided doses per day.

Nurse monitoring
See the section on beta-adrenoreceptor blocking drugs.

General notes
Pindolol tablets may be stored at room temperature.

PIPERAZINE (Antepar, Pripsen)

Presentation
Tablets—500 mg
Syrup—750 mg in 5 ml
Sachets—4 g (as phosphate)
In preparations of Pripsen, each 10 g sachet contains 4 g of Piperazine phosphate and standardised senna equivalent to 15.3 mg; total sennoside calculated as sennoside B.

Actions and uses
This antihelminthic drug is effective in the treatment of threadworm (enterobiasis) and roundworm (ascariasis).

Dosage
1. Enterobiasis: The dose should be calculated according to age or weight and is given once daily for 7 days.
   Adults (approximate weight over 55 kg): 2 g
   Children over 13 (approximate weight over 40 kg): 2 g
   Children 5–12 (approximate weight 17–40 kg): 1.5 g
   Children 2–4 (approximate weight 13–16 kg): 750 mg
   Children less than 2 (approximate weight below 13 kg): Dose to be recommended by a physician.
2. For the treatment of roundworm:
   Adults (approximate weight over 55 kg): 4 g
   Children 13–16 13–16 years (approximate weight 41–55 kg): 3.75 g
   Children 9–12 years (approximate weight 26–40 kg): 3 g
   Children 2–8 years (approximate weight 13–25 kg): 2.5 g
   Children less than 2 (approximate weight below 13 kg): Dose to be recommended by a physician.

Nurse monitoring
1. When more than one member of the family is affected all affected members should be treated simultaneously.
2. Occasional neurological abnormalities including visual disturbance, dizziness and vertigo may occur.

General notes
The drug may be stored at room temperature.

PIPERAZINE OESTRONE SULPHATE (Harmogen)

Presentation
Tablets—1.5 mg

Actions and uses
1. The actions and uses of oestrogenic substances in general are described in the section on these drugs.
2. In clinical practice this drug is used for oestrogen replacement therapy and the relief of oestrogen deficiency symptoms at or after the menopause and following surgical or radio-therapeutic oophorectomy.

Dosage
The drug is administered in 21–28 day cycles with 5–7 days between each cycle. The dosage varies according to individual response between 1.5 and 4.5 mg per day.

Nurse monitoring
See the section on oestrogenic hormones.

General notes
The drug may be stored at room temperature.

PIRBUTEROL (Exirel)

Presentation
Capsules—10 mg, 15 mg
Syrup—7.5 mg in 5 ml
Inhaler—200 μg per metered dose

Actions and uses
This drug has the actions and uses described for Fenoterol (q.v.)

Dosage
1. Oral:
   a. *Adults and children over 12 years*: 10–15 mg three or four times daily.
   b. *Children 6–12 years*: 7.5 mg four times daily.
2. Inhaler: *Adults and children over 12 years*: 200–400 μg (1–2 metered doses) three or four times a day up to a maximum of 12 inhalations per 24 hours.

Nurse monitoring
See the section on Fenoterol.

General notes
See the section on Fenoterol.

PIRITRAMIDE (Dipidolor)

Presentation
Injection—20 mg in 2 ml

Actions and uses
Piritramide is a narcotic analgesic

drug which is used specifically for post-operative analgesia.
Dosage
This drug is recommended for use in adults only, at dosages of 20 mg by intramuscular injection, repeated as necessary every 6 hours.
Nurse monitoring
See the section on narcotic analgesic drugs.
General notes
1. The drug should be stored in a locked (controlled drug) cupboard.
2. The drug should be stored at room temperature.

PIROXICAM (Feldene)

Presentation
Capsules—10 mg
Actions and uses
See the section on non-steroidal anti-inflammatory analgesic drugs.
Dosage
1. The adult dose is 20 mg once per day.
2. For acute gout 40 mg per day may be prescribed.
Nurse monitoring
See the section on anti-inflammatory analgesic drugs, non-steroidal.
General notes
Piroxicam capsules may be stored at room temperature.

PIZOTIFEN (Sanomigram)

Presentation
Tablets—0.5 mg, 1.5 mg
Actions and uses
Pizotifen inhibits the action of substances which are released within the blood vessels and which cause the vascular changes which lead to the symptoms of severe headache and migraine. In clinical practice it is used for the prophylaxis of migraine.
Dosage
The dose ranges from 0.5–6 mg per day depending on individual patient response.
Nurse monitoring
1. The nurse may play an important role in cautioning patients about the dangers of drowsiness associated with taking this drug, especially in relation to driving vehicles and operating machinery.
2. The drug should never be given to patients who have glaucoma or a predisposition to urinary retention.
3. Apart from drowsiness, common side effects include weight gain and increased appetite. Less frequently dizziness and nausea have occurred.

General notes
The drug may be stored at room temperature.

POLDINE SULPHATE (Nacton)

Presentation
Tablets—2 mg, 4 mg
Actions and uses
Poldine sulphate is an anticholinergic drug which acts by reducing the amount of acid produced by the cells of the stomach. A reduction in gastric and secretion in patients with peptic ulcer may produce symptomatic relief and may aid ulcer healing.
Dosage
For adults the initial dose of 2 mg three times daily and at bedtime may be increased gradually up to a maximum of 4 mg four times a day. The optimum dose is that which provides adequate pain relief without producing troublesome side effects.
Nurse monitoring
Poldine has anticholinergic side effects similar to those described under Hyoscine-N-Butylbromide Buscopan) (q.v.).
General notes
Preparations containing Poldine may be stored at room temperature.

POLYTHIAZIDE (Nephril)

Presentation
Tablets—1 mg
Actions and uses
See the section on thiazide and related diuretics.

Dosage
The adult dose is 0.5–4.0 mg which is taken as a single daily dose. The diuretic action may last up to 48 hours.
Nurse monitoring
See the section on thiazide and related diuretics.
General notes
Polythiazide tablets may be stored at room temperature.

POTASSIUM CLORAZEPATE (Tranxene)

Presentation
Capsules—7.5 mg, 15 mg
Actions and uses
Potassium clorazepate is a member of the benzodiazepine group (q.v.). Its principal use is in the treatment of anxiety.
Dosage
15 mg daily usually administered at night.
Nurse monitoring
See the section on benzodiazepines.
General notes
Capsules containing potassium clorazepate may be stored at room temperature.

POTASSIUM PERCHLORATE (Peroidin)

Presentation
Tablets—200 mg
Actions and uses
Potassium perchlorate prevents the uptake of iodine by the thyroid gland and in this way inhibits the total amount of thyroxine produced by the gland. Its use in the treatment of thyrotoxicosis is limited by the occasional occurrence of severe side effects.
Dosage
1. *Adults*: Initially 800 mg in divided doses daily with maintenance doses reduced to 200–400 mg daily.
2. *Children*: Up to 250 mg daily has been used in children over five years of age.
3. For specialised radioisotope brain scanning, a single dose of 200 mg is given.

Nurse monitoring
1. Hypersensitivity reactions i.e. maculopapular rashes, fever and lymphadenopathy have been reported.
2. The drug can produce gastrointestinal upset and nausea may be severe.
3. Serious adverse effects include aplastic anaemia, pancytopenia, leucopenia and nephrotic syndrome.
4. Some thyrotoxic patients receive prior to operation a short course of potassium iodide. Potassium perchlorate should never be given at the same time as it negates the action of potassium iodide in this situation.

General notes
1. Potassium perchlorate tablets may be stored at room temperature.
2. The tablets should be protected from moisture.

PRAZEPAM (Centrax)

Presentation
Tablets—10 mg
Actions and uses
Prazepam is a benzodiazepine drug (q.v.) which has a long duration of action. It is used in the management of anxiety neurosis.
Dosage
Adults: 5–60 mg daily in 2–3 divided doses with doses in the lower range preferred for elderly patients.
Nurse monitoring
See the section on benzodiazepines.
General notes
Tablets containing prazepam may be stored at room temperature.

PRAZOSIN (Hypovase)

Presentation
Tablets—0.5 mg, 1 mg, 2 mg, 5 mg
Actions and uses
Prazosin lowers the blood pressure by a direct action on the smooth muscle of blood vessels and also by alpha-adrenergic blockade. It is used in the management of hypertension.

Dosage

A significant number of patients suffer from sudden collapse within 30–90 minutes of receiving their first dose of Prazosin. For this reason all patients are commenced on low doses (0.5 mg three times a day) and the dose is increased gradually until the required effect is obtained. The maximum dosage is 20 mg per day usually taken three times a day in divided doses.

Nurse monitoring

1. As noted above sudden collapse may follow initial dose of Prazosin and therefore the initial dose must be small and is usually given on retiring to bed on the first night of treatment.
2. Side effects are numerous and include postural hypotension, drowsiness, headache, lethargy, weakness, palpitations/tachycardia, dry mouth, blurred vision, urinary frequency, nasal congestion, fluid retention, nervousness, depression, vertigo, constipation and diarrhoea, nausea and vomiting, skin rashes, itching, sweating, abdominal pain, paraesthesia, impotence in males, nose bleeds, reddened eyes and tinnitus.
3. Prazosin may exacerbate depression and therefore is relatively contraindicated in patients with such problems.

General notes

Prazosin tablets may be stored at room temperature.

PREDNISOLONE (Precortisyl, Prednesol, Predsol, Deltacortril)

Several other proprietary preparations containing Prednisolone in many different formulations are also available.

Presentation

Tablets — 1 mg, 5 mg, 25 mg
2.5 mg and 5 mg (enteric coated)
Injection—32 mg in 2 ml (intravenous or intramuscular)
Eye/ear drops—0.5%
Suppositories—5 mg
Enema—20 mg in 100 ml

Actions and uses

Prednisolone is a corticosteroid drug and has actions and uses similar to other corticosteroids (q.v.).

Dosage

Dose ranges vary widely depending on the type of illness, the severity of the disease and the route of administration. It is therefore impossible to outline possible dosage regimes in this text.

Nurse monitoring

See the section on corticosteroids.

General notes

1. Preparations containing Prednisolone may be stored at room temperature.
2. In common with other eye drops, containers should not be used for more than seven days for in-patients in a hospital ward or four weeks in the domestic situation or the risk of bacterial contamination becomes too great.

PREDNISONE (Decortisyl, Deltacortone)

Presentation

Tablets—1 mg, 5 mg

Actions and uses

Prednisone is a corticosteroid drug and its actions and uses are described in the section on these drugs. It is worth noting that in the body Prednisone is converted to the active substance Prednisolone.

Dosage

Dose ranges vary widely depending on the type of illness, the severity of the disease and the route of administration. It is therefore impossible to outline possible dosage regimes in this text.

Nurse monitoring

See the section on corticosteroids.

General notes

Prednisone tablets may be stored at room temperature.

PRENYLAMINE (Synadrin)
Presentation
Tablets—60 mg
Actions and uses
Prenylamine dilates peripheral vessels by inhibiting the constricting effect of the sympathetic nervous system on these vessels. Thus the peripheral vascular resistance and therefore heart work is reduced. This action makes the drug useful in the prophylactic treatment of angina pectoris.
Dosage
The usual adult dose is 60 mg three times daily but this may be increased to 60 mg four or five times daily if necessary.
Nurse monitoring
1. Prenylamine produces a slight reduction in the function of the heart muscle and therefore should be used with caution in patients who already have heart failure or who are taking other cardiac depressant drugs such as beta-blockers, Quinidine, Procainamide or Lignocaine.
2. The drug is specifically contraindicated in patients with liver or kidney failure.
3. Adverse effects include gastrointestinal upset, tremor, skin rash, dizziness and hypotension.
4. As it reduces the blood pressure, patients who are also on treatment for hypertension may require to have that treatment reduced if this drug is commenced.

General notes
Prenylamire tablets may be stored at room temperature.

PRILOCAINE (Citanest)
Presentation
Injection—1. Plain: 0.5%, 1% and 4%
2. With adrenaline: 3%
3. With felypressin: 3%
Actions and uses
This drug is a local anaesthetic. Adrenaline and felypressin are vasoconstrictor substances which prolong the duration of its effects.
Dosage
There is considerable variation in the optimum dosage for individual use. It should be noted, however, that the maximum adult dose should not exceed 400 mg.
Nurse monitoring
1. The Nurse monitoring aspects of Lignocaine (local anaesthetic) (q.v.) apply to this drug.
2. At maximum dosage a chemical called methaemoglobin may be produced in the blood. This may lead to an appearance of cyanosis.

General notes
The drug may be stored at room temperature.

PRIMIDONE (Mysoline)
Presentation
Tablets—250 mg
Suspension—250 mg in 5 ml
Actions and uses
Primidone is an anticonvulsant drug which is converted in the body to the active component Phenobarbitone. It is used primarily for the treatment of grand mal epilepsy. In the past combinations of Primidone and Phenobarbitone were used to treat epilepsy but as they are in effect the same drug this practise is now discouraged.
Dosage
As individual doses are extremely variable, the following are simply guidelines for treatment and dosages should always be adjusted to individual requirements. Initiation of treatment is the same for both adults and children. It is recommended that 125 mg be given once daily late in the evening and every three days thereafter the dose should be increased by 125 mg until the daily dosage is 1500 mg in adults and 500 mg in children. Thereafter the dosage should be adjusted until control is obtained or side effects occur. Average daily

maintenance doses are as follows:
1. Adults and children over 9 years: 750–1500 mg.
2. *Children*:
   Up to 2 years: 250–500 mg
   2–5 years: 500–750 mg
   6–9 years: 750–1000 mg.
   It should be noted that although initial treatment is given once daily in the evening, by the time the dosage exceeds 250 mg in total it should be split into a twice daily regime.

Nurse monitoring
1. The Nurse monitoring aspects of anticonvulsant drugs in general are discussed in the section on these drugs.
2. Primidone is converted in the body to Phenobarbitone and therefore further Nurse monitoring aspects of this drug may be found in the section dealing with this drug.

General notes
The drug may be stored at room temperature.

PROBENECID (Benemid)

Presentation
Tablets—500 mg

Actions and uses
Probenecid acts directly on the kidney tubules to produce two main effects:
1. It blocks the excretion of Penicillin and some cephalosporin drugs from the renal tubules and may therefore be used to maintain high blood levels of these drugs.
2. It promotes the excretion of uric acid and urate from the renal tubules and may therefore be used to reduce the blood urate concentration in hyperuricaemia and gout.

Dosage
1. Hyperuricaemia and gout: Adults usually receive 250 mg twice daily initially. The dose is increased after a week to 500 mg twice daily. Up to 2 g per day may be given in 2–4 divided doses where necessary.
2. Adjunct therapy with Penicillin and cephalosporins:
   a. *Adults*: 2 g daily in divided doses
   b. *Children*:
      i. Children under 50 kg: 25 mg/kg daily in divided doses
      ii. Children over 50 kg should receive the adult dose.

Nurse monitoring
1. The nurse may play a major role in preventing the occurrence of renal stone formation or renal colic in patients on this drug by continually monitoring their fluid intake and encouraging them to take an adequate amount of fluid each day as this reduces the incidence of such side effects.
2. Aspirin blocks the effect of Probenecid and as patients may frequently be taking this drug in addition to prescribed medication the nurse may contribute to the management of such patients by ensuring that they know that they should never take Aspirin when taking Probenecid.
3. Common side effects include anorexia, nausea, vomiting, headache and frequency of micturition.
4. More rarely allergic reactions may occur when patients are given this drug. They include anaphylactic shock, dermatitis, pruritis, fever, sore gums and occasionally haemolytic anaemia.
5. Rare serious side effects include nephrotic syndrome, liver damage and aplastic anaemia.
6. Probenecid must be used with caution in patients with a history of peptic ulcer disease.
7. Probenecid must never be given to patients receiving Methotrexate as it may induce Methotrexate toxicity.
8. As Probenecid reduces the level of blood urate it may at the onset of treatment include acute attacks of gout and it is common

practise for the patient to receive a course of Indomethacin or Phenylbutazone at the beginning of treatment.

General notes
Probenecid tablets may be stored at room temperature.

PROCAINAMIDE (Pronestyl)

Presentation
Tablets—250 mg, 500 mg (durules or sustained release)
Injection—1 g in 10 ml (multidose vials)

Actions and uses
Procainamide has a depressant action on the heart and reduces contractility and excitability of heart muscle and conductivity of the electrical conducting tissues. It is therefore useful in the treatment of ventricular and supraventricular dysrhythmias. It may be given in an emergency either intravenously or intramuscularly and for long-term treatment it may be given orally.

Dosage
1. *Adults*:
   a. Intravenously: 25–50 mg per minute up to a total of 1 g with continous ECG and blood pressure monitoring.
   b. Intramuscularly: 250 mg as a single intramuscular dose.
   c. Oral dosage: With oral treatment a serum concentration of between 4 and 8 μg/ml has been found to be effective. Two oral preparations are available:
      i. 250 mg of Procainamide every 4–6 hours; or
      ii. 1–1.5 g of the sustained release durule preparation three times per day.
2. *Children*: The suggested dosage for children is 50 mg/kg body weight divided into 4–6 doses per day.

Nurse monitoring
1. The nurse will rarely see Procainamide given intravenously outwith the hospital setting. Rapid intravenous dosage of this drug can lead to hypotension, ventricular fibrillation and cardiac arrest. Constant monitoring of blood pressure and ECG monitoring is essential when the drug is given by the intravenous route.
2. Side effects from Procainamide occur most frequently after high dosage or in patients with heart failure or renal failure. The commonest side effects are anorexia, diarrhoea, nausea and vomiting.
3. When patients have been on Procainamide for a prolonged period of time, they may develop a syndrome similar to systemic lupus erythematosus with joint pains, skin lesions, pleuritic chest pain and the other features of this disease. The development of such symptoms in a patient on Procainamide is an indication for blood tests to be carried out on the patient to detect LE cells and if these are present the drug should be stopped and if necessary an alternative anti-dysrhythmic drug should be substituted. This syndrome characteristically resolves after withdrawal of the drug.
4. Because Procainamide depresses cardiac contractility it may lead to the development of heart failure. The nurse should therefore monitor the patient for symptoms of heart failure such as breathlessness on exertion or on lying flat in bed and ankle oedema.
5. Flushing, skin rash and pruritis, depression, psychotic reaction and hallucinations, bitter taste in the mouth, muscle weakness, leucopenia and agranulocytosis are other side effects which have been encountered with this drug.

General notes
Procainamide tablets and solution for injection may be stored at room temperature.

PROCAINE PENICILLIN G (Depocillin)

(See Note 3, p. 310)

Presentation
Injection—300 mg (300 000 units) in 1 ml

Actions and uses
The combination in one vial of Benzylpenicillin (Penicillin G) and Procaine gives this preparation a prolonged action. It therefore may be given once or twice daily. Other than this, its actions and uses are identical to those described for Benzylpenicillin (q.v.).

Dosage
N.B. Procaine Penicillin G is given by intramuscular injection only.
1. Adults and children over 25 kg: 300 mg once or twice daily
2. *Children*:
   Less than 1 year: 15 mg (15 000) per kg body weight once per day
   Over 1 year: 150 mg (150 000)–300 mg (300 000) once per day

Nurse monitoring
See the section on Benzylpenicillin.

General notes
The drug should be stored in a refrigerator.

PROCARBAZINE (Natulan)

Presentation
Capsules—50 mg

Actions and uses
The mode of action of Procarbazine remains unclear but it would appear to prevent cell division by interfering with one of the basic biochemical steps necessary for this process. Its main use is in the treatment of Hodgkin's disease, although very rarely it may be indicated for the management of solid tumours.

Dosage
1. *Adults*: 50–200 mg orally divided in up to three doses daily.
2. *Children*: 100 mg per m² body surface area.

Nurse monitoring
1. Nearly all patients suffer from anorexia, nausea and vomiting. These symptoms may become less troublesome as treatment continues.
2. Bone marrow depression may produce thrombocytopenia and leucopenia. Regular blood counts are carried out during treatment to monitor this but should these effects arise the patient would be at an increased risk of severe infection or haemorrhage.
3. The drug should not be given to patients with severe liver or kidney disease.
4. Procarbazine is derived from the hydrazines which is one group of monoamine oxidase inhibitors which are used in the treatment of depression. This relationship leads to a number of important points:
   a. It has an action as a weak monoamine oxidase inhibitor and may produce hypertension if certain drugs and foodstuffs are taken concurrently (see the section on monoamine oxidase inhibitors). Patients should carry an appropriate monoamine oxidase inhibitor warning card while treated with Procarbazine.
   b. Its mild monoamine oxidase inhibitor action may lead to side effects of somnolence, confusion and ataxia.
5. It should not be given concurrently with other monoamine oxidase inhibitors.
6. The nurse should be constantly aware that cytotoxic drugs are highly dangerous and therefore must be handled with great care. Spillage and contamination of the skin of the patient or nurse may lead to a degree of absorption of the drug which, if chronically repeated, may cause damage and the skin may also be sensitised to the drug making it, in some cases, impossible for the nurse to continue working with the drug.

General notes
Procarbazine capsules may be stored at room temperature.

PROCHLORPERAZINE (Stemetil, Vertigon)

Presentation
Tablets—5 mg, 25 mg
Capsules—10 mg, 15 mg (both as slow release)
Syrup—5 mg in 5 ml
Injection — 12.5 mg in 1 ml
25 mg in 2 ml
Suppositories—5 mg, 25 mg

Actions and uses
Prochlorperazine is a member of the phenothiazine group and its actions and uses are described in the section on these drugs. As this is a very widely used drug it is worth detailing its specific uses which are:
1. For the treatment of severe anxiety states.
2. For the treatment of behavioural disorders in schizophrenia and other psychotic states.
3. For the treatment of nausea and vomiting, particularly when this is due to other drug therapy.
4. For the symptomatic relief of vertigo and vomiting in neurological disorders such as Menière's disease.

Dosage
1. Psychosis: 75–100 mg in total daily is given in 2–3 divided doses by the oral, rectal or intramuscular route.
2. Nausea and vomiting:
   a. The oral dose is 10–20 mg
   b. The rectal dose is 25 mg
   c. The intramuscular dose is 12.5 mg.
3. For the treatment of vertigo and nausea associated with neurological disorders such as Menière's disease: 10–15 mg as slow release capsules once or twice daily is given.
4. Children's doses are as follows:
   Less than 1 year:
   Orally 0.125 mg/kg three times per day
   Children over 1 year:
   i. Orally 2.5–5 mg three times per day
   ii. Rectally 2.5–5 mg once or twice per day.

Nurse monitoring
The Nurse monitoring aspects of this drug are described under phenothiazines (q.v.).

General notes
1. Preparations containing Prochlorperazine may be stored at room temperature but they should be protected from direct sunlight.
2. Prochlorperazine injection must not be mixed with other drugs.

PROCYCLIDINE (Kemadrin)

Presentation
Tablets—5 mg
Injection—10 mg in 2 ml

Actions and uses
The actions and uses of this drug are identical to those described for Benzhexol (q.v.).

Dosage
For adults:
  a. Orally: 20–30 mg in three or four divided doses daily
  b. Parenterally (by intravenous or intramuscular injection): 10–20 mg

Nurse monitoring
The Nurse monitoring aspects of Benzhexol (q.v.) apply to this drug.

General notes
The drug may be stored at room temperature.

PROGESTERONE (Cyclogest)

Presentation
Vaginal/rectal suppositories—200 mg and 400 mg

Actions and uses
The actions and uses of progestational hormones are discussed under Hormones (2). In clinical practice Progesterone is used most commonly for the treatment of premenstrual symptoms.

Dosage
200–400 mg rectally or vaginally once or twice daily from the 12th–14th day of the menstrual cycle or until menstruation recommences.

Nurse monitoring
See the section on progestational hormones.
General notes
The drug may be stored at room temperature.

PROMAZINE (Sparine)

Presentation
Tablets—25 mg, 50 mg, 100 mg
Suspension—50 mg in 5 ml
Injection — 50 mg in 1 ml
100 mg in 2 ml

Actions and uses
Promazine is a member of the phenothiazine group of drugs and its actions and uses are described in the section dealing with these drugs.

Dosage
1. *Adults*:
   a. Orally: 25–100 mg three to four times per day
   b. Intramuscularly: 25–50 mg repeated after 6–8 hours as required to a maximum of 100 mg per day.
2. Children's doses are usually calculated according to body weight.

Nurse monitoring
The Nurse monitoring aspects of this drug are described under phenothiazines (q.v.).

General notes
Preparations containing Promazine may be stored at room temperature.

PROMETHAZINE (Phenergan, Avomine)

Presentation
Tablets—10 mg, 25 mg (as hydrochloride)
25 mg (as theoclate)
Elixir—5 mg in 5 ml
Injection—25 mg in 1 ml

Action
Promethazine is a member of the phenothiazine group of drugs but is unusual in that it has little if any appreciable tranquillising activity. It is, however, found to be very useful for its anti-emetic, sedative and antihistaminic effects. It is particularly useful in the prevention and treatment of motion sickness and in the treatment of irradiation sickness, postoperative vomiting, the nausea and vomiting of pregnancy, drug-induced nausea and vomiting and for the symptomatic relief of nausea and vertigo in Menière's disease and other labyrinthine disturbances.

1. For the treatment of nausea and vomiting:
   a. *Adults*: Adult doses are as follows:
      i. Orally: 25–75 mg at night with two or three additional day time doses of 10–20 mg
      ii. Intramuscularly: Up to 100 mg may be given
      iii. Intravenously: Up to 100 mg may be given. The drug must be diluted to 10 times its volume with Water for Injection and administered very slowly.
   b. *Children*:
      Less than 1 year old: Doses of 1.5 mg/kg are given. In older children 15–25 mg is administered in a single dose as necessary.
2. For the prevention of motion sickness, Promethazine theoclate is administered in a dose of 25 mg on the night prior to undertaking a journey and a further 25 mg one to two hours prior to commencing the journey.

Nurse monitoring
1. Promethazine is a phenothiazine drug but in the dosages recommended and when used for the treatment of conditions described above, the problems encountered with phenothiazine drugs in general (q.v.) are rarely encountered.
2. It is important to remember that sedation may commonly occur and patients must be warned about the dangers of taking this drug while operating heavy machinery or driving.

General notes
Preparations containing Promethazine may be stored at room temperature.

PROPANTHELINE (Pro-Banthine)
Dosage
Tablets—15 mg
Injection—30 mg
Actions and uses
1. It has an anticholinergic effect similar to Poldine (q.v.) and is therefore useful for the symptomatic relief and healing of peptic ulceration.
2. One of this drug's side effects is to produce urinary retention and for this reason it is used occasionally in the treatment of enuresis.

Dosage
1. Peptic ulcer:
   a. *Adults*: The usual oral dose is 15 mg three times a day and at bedtime. By intravenous injection 30 mg in 10 ml sodium chloride injection 0.9 is given at a rate not exceeding 6 mg per minute. 30 mg in 1 ml of water may be given by the intramuscular route.
2. Enuresis: In children 15–45 mg may be taken at night as a single dose.

Nurse monitoring
The Nurse monitoring notes on this drug are identical to those for Hyoscine-N-Butylbromide (Buscopan) (q.v.).

General notes
Preparations containing Propantheline may be stored at room temperature.

PROPRANOLOL (Inderal)

Presentation
Tablets—10 mg, 40 mg, 80 mg, 160 mg
Capsules—160 mg slow release
Injection—1 mg in 1 ml

Actions and uses
Propranolol is a non-selective beta-adrenoreceptor blocking drug. Its actions and uses are described under Beta-adrenoreceptor blocking drugs (q.v.).

Dosage
1. By intravenous injection in an emergency situation, up to 1 mg may be given over 1 minute. Pulse, blood pressure and cardiac (ECG) monitoring must be continuous during the period of injection and injection must be stopped if profound bradycardia, hypotension or widening of the QRS complex occurs.
2. Adult oral maintenance dosage ranges from 80–480 mg per day. In the treatment of hypertension slow release capsules are available and total dosage is given once daily. In the treatment of dysrhythmias and angina the dosage is usually divided and given twice, three or four times a day.
3. The dosage for children is as follows:
   Up to 1 year: 1 mg/kg
   1–6 years: 10 mg
   7 year plus: 20 mg
   These oral doses may be doubled if necessary.
4. Dosage for intravenous injection in children is as follows:
   The intravenous dosage for the treatment of acute cardiac dysrhythmias is:
   Age 1–5: 0.3 mg
   Age 6–12: 0.5 mg
   Note: The intravenous dose should be halved if a patient is anaesthetised.

Nurse monitoring
See the section on beta-adrenoreceptor blocking drugs.

General notes
Propranolol tablets, capsules and injection may be stored at room temperature. Injection solution may be diluted for ease of administration with 5% dextrose, 0.9% sodium chloride or dextrose/saline mixtures immediately before use but no other drugs should be mixed in the same syringe.

PROSTAGLANDIN E_2 (Prostin E_2, Dinoprostone)

Presentation
Tablets—0.5 mg
Sterile solutions—1 mg in 1 ml alcohol (0.75 ml ampoule)
10 mg in 1 ml alcohol (0.5 ml ampoule)

Actions and uses
Prostaglandin E_2 has the capacity to induce contraction of the uterus. It, therefore, has the following uses:
1. The induction of labour
2. Termination of pregnancy
3. The induction of labour in missed abortion
4. Treatment of hydatidiform mole.

Dosage
1. For the induction of labour:
   a. Orally: 0.5 mg initially and thereafter 1 mg at hourly intervals until an adequate uterine response has been achieved. Thereafter the dose may be reduced to 0.5 mg hourly.
   b. Intravenously: 1 mg/ml solution in alcohol is diluted with 0.9% sodium chloride or 5% dextrose to produce a solution containing 1.5 μg/ml. This is infused intravenously at a rate of 0.25 μg/minute for 30 minutes, the dose being subsequently maintained or increased according to patient response.
2. For the termination of pregnancy or treatment of missed abortion or hydatidiform mole: A solution containing 5 μg/ml is infused intravenously at a rate of 2.5 μg/minute for 30 minutes and then maintained or increased to 5 μg/minute. This higher concentration should be administered for at least four hours before further increases are made.
3. For the termination of pregnancy: 1 ml of a solution containing 100 μg/ml may be instilled extra-amniotically through a suitable Foley catheter. Subsequent doses of 1 or 2 ml of the same concentration solution should be given at intervals usually of two hours according to uterine response.

Nurse monitoring
1. Nausea, vomiting and diarrhoea occur commonly at doses required to terminate pregnancy by the intravenous route but are less common after the extra-amniotic route for termination. Such symptoms are rare when the concentrations administered by the intravenous route for induction of labour are used.
2. Transient cardiovascular symptoms have been noticed including flushing, shivering, headache, dizziness.
3. Very rarely convulsions and changes in the electro-encephalogram have occurred.
4. Local tissue irritation or erythema may follow intravenous infusion. This will disappear within 2–5 hours of stopping the infusion.
5. Infusion of this compound may occasionally lead to pyrexia.
6. Uterine rupture has occurred only rarely with this substance.
7. The drug should be used with caution in patients who have glaucoma or suffer from asthma.

General notes
1. Prostaglandin preparations should be refrigerated.
2. Once diluted the solutions should be used within 24 hours.

PROSTAGLANDIN F_2 alpha (Dinoprost)

Presentation
Sterile solutions—5 mg/ml: 1.5 ml, 4 ml and 5 ml ampoules

Actions and uses
The actions and uses of prostaglandin F_2 alpha are identical to those described for prostaglandin E_2 (q.v.).

Dosage
1. For the induction of labour: The drug is administered intravenously. It is diluted in normal saline or 5% dextrose to a concentration of 15 μg/ml and administered initially in a dosage

of 2.5 µg/minute. This regime is maintained for at least 30 minutes and subsequent dose changes depend on patient response.
2. For the induction of labour after fetal death: An initial infusion concentration of 5 µg/minute may be given and increases should be at intervals of not less than one hour.
3. For the termination of pregnancy, missed abortion or hydatidiform mole: A solution containing the equivalent of 50 µg/ml is infused intravenously at a rate of 25 µg/minute for at least 30 minutes, then maintained or increased to 50 µg/minute according to response. This raae should be maintained for at least four hours before further increases are made.
4. For the termination of pregnancy by extra-amniotic administration: A solution containing 375 µg may be injected via a catheter.
5. For intra-amniotic termination of pregnancy: 40 mg may be injected slowly into the amniotic sac.

Nurse monitoring
The Nurse monitoring aspects of this drug are identical to those described for prostaglandin E_2 (q.v.).

General notes
1. The drug may be stored at room temperature.
2. Diluted solutions should be used within 24 hours if the intravenous or intra-amniotic route is contemplated. Solutions may be retained for up to 48 hours if they are to be given by the extra-amniotic route.

PROTRIPTYLINE (Concordin)

Presentation
Tablets—5 mg, 10 mg

Actions and uses
Protriptyline is a tricyclic antidepressant drug. Its actions and uses are described in the section on these drugs.

Dosage
For the treatment of depression in adults the total daily dose is 15–60 mg given in three divided doses.

Nurse monitoring
See the section on tricyclic antidepressant drugs.

General notes
Tablets containing Protriptyline may be stored at room temperature.

PYRAZINAMIDE (Zinamide)

Presentation
Tablets—500 mg

Actions and uses
Pyrazinamide has been found to be effective against the organism *Mycobacterium tuberculosis* and is therefore used for the treatment of tuberculosis. It is rarely used as the first choice for treatment of this disease and is reserved for cases where resistance develops to the more commonly used drugs, or where severe side effects are experienced with more commonly used drugs.

Dosage
The recommended dosage is 20–35 mg/kg body weight in total per day given in divided doses. The maximum daily dose should not exceed 3 g.

Nurse monitoring
1. Patients undergoing treatment for tuberculosis receive their drugs for considerable periods of time. The nurse may play an important role in reminding patients that their drug therapy must be taken regularly for as long as recommended by medical staff, whether or not they themselves feel that they have recovered.
2. Common side effects experienced by patients on this drug include anorexia, nausea, vomiting, fever, tiredness, difficulty with micturition and arthralgia which may be due to gout (see below).
3. Photosensitivity and skin rash may occur.

4. The drug may effect concentration in the blood of uric acid and may precipitate attacks of joint pain due to gout.
5. The main drawback to the drug's use is that it may cause serious disturbance of liver function.
6. The drug should be used with caution in patients with diabetes as loss of control has occurred when the drug has been introduced.
7. The drug may occasionally cause some impairment of renal function.

General notes
The drug may be stored at room temperature.

PYRIDOSTIGMINE (Mestinon)

Presentation
Tablets—60 mg
Injection—1 mg in 1 ml

Actions and uses
The actions of Pyridostigmine are identical to those described for Neostigmine (q.v.). In clinical practice its principal use is in the management of myasthenia gravis, where it has the advantage over Neostigmine of having a longer duration of action. It may also be given intramuscularly in the treatment of paralytic ileus or postoperative urinary retention.

Dosage
1. For treatment of myasthenia gravis:
   a. *Adults*: 60–240 mg 4 to 6-hourly according to individual response
   b. *Children*: Up to 7 mg/kg body weight in total per day is given in six divided doses.
2. For the treatment of paralytic ileus or post-operative urinary retention: A dose of 1–2 mg may be given intramuscularly.

Nurse monitoring
1. The nurse monitoring aspects of Pyridostigmine are identical to those described for Neostigmine (q.v.).
2. It is worth noting that in practice there are fewer problems with gastrointestinal upset with Pyridostigmine as compared with Neostigmine.

General notes
The drug may be stored at room temperature.

PYRIMETHAMINE (Daraprim)

Presentation
Tablets—25 mg

Actions and uses
Pyrimethamine is an antimalarial used, normally in combination with other drugs, in the prevention of malaria. It also possesses useful action against other parasitic organisms and is used in combination with a sulphonamide in the control of toxoplasmosis.

Dosage
1. For antimalarial prophylaxis (in combination with other drugs).
   Adults: 25 mg taken once per week.
   Children: Over 5 years should receive half the adult dosage.
2. For the treatment of toxoplasmosis:
   Adults: 50–75 mg daily (in combination with sulphonamide) reduced according to the patient's response after 1–3 weeks. Treatment is then continued for a further 4–5 weeks.

Nurse monitoring
1. Once weekly administration for the suppression of malaria is not usually associated with side effects.
2. Patients undergoing malaria prophylaxis must ensure that regular weekly doses are taken. It should be stressed that treatment must be continued for a period of 4 weeks after return from an area where malaria is endemic.

3. With larger doses used in the treatment of toxoplasmosis, side effects may arise. These include megaloblastic anaemia, leucopenia, thrombocytopenia and aplastic anaemia. Very high doses have produced vomiting, convulsions and respiratory failure.

General notes
Tablets may be stored at room temperature.

Q

QUINALBARBITONE (Seconal)

Presentation
Capsules—50 mg, 100 mg

Actions and uses
Quinalbarbitone is a barbiturate drug (q.v.) which is taken at night as a hypnotic.

Dosage
50–100 mg on retiring.

Nurse monitoring
See the section on barbiturate drugs.

General notes
Quinalbarbitone capsules may be stored at room temperature.

QUINESTRADOL (Pentovis)

Presentation
Capsules—250 μg

Actions and uses
1. The actions and uses of oestrogens in general are described in the section on these drugs.
2. Quinestradol exerts an oestrogenic effect on the lower segment of the genital tract and is indicated for the treatment of post-menopausal vaginitis and senile vaginitis.

Dosage
For the treatment of senile vaginitis: 500 μg twice daily.

Nurse monitoring
1. This compound appears to be free of the side effects commonly associated with other oestrogenic hormones (q.v.).
2. Prolonged exposure to any oestrogen may increase the risk of the development of endometrial carcinoma.
3. Patients with known or suspected oestrogen-dependent carcinomata should not be given the compound.
4. The drug is not recommended for use in pre-pubertal patients.

General notes
The drug may be stored at room temperature.

QUINESTROL (Estrovis)

Presentation
Tablets—4 mg

Actions and uses
Quinestrol is an oestrogenic substance. The actions and uses of oestrogens in general are described in the section on these drugs. Quinestrol is used in clinical practice for the inhibition of lactation and suppression of established lactation.

Dosage
1. For the inhibition of lactation: 4 mg is given within 6 hours of delivery. A second dose of 4 mg should only be administered should symptoms of lactation subsequently develop. This is most likely to occur 4 to 6 days after the first dose.
2. For the suppression of lactation: 4 mg should be given immediately after the decision to suppress lactation has been taken, followed by a second dose of 4 mg 48 hours later.

Nurse monitoring
1. The Nurse monitoring aspect of oestrogens in general are discussed in the section on these drugs.
2. It should be noted that as most patients receive only one or two

doses of this drug, they are very unlikely to suffer side effects. The commonest side effect noted is when two doses are prescribed—the subsequent menstrual period is likely to be heavier than usual.

General notes
The drug may be stored at room temperature.

QUINIDINE (Kinidin)

Presentation
Tablets—200 mg
Sustained release tablets equivalent to 200 mg Quinidine base

Actions and uses
Quinidine depresses heart function by reducing the excitability of the heart muscle and prolonging its refractory period. It is therefore useful in the treatment of cardiac dysrhythmias. Conventional tablets require to be taken in large and frequent dosage to maintain an effective blood level and it is therefore advantageous to use the sustained release tablet to guarantee effectiveness of the drug.

Dosage
1. *Adults*: 400 mg–1 g taken twice daily as sustained release tablets.
2. *Children*: The recommended dosage of Quinidine Sulphate is 6 mg/kg body weight five times daily.

It should be noted that to avoid hypersensitivity (as mentioned below) all patients should be given a small test dose prior to commencement of the above regimes.

Nurse monitoring
1. As mentioned above, it is essential to give a minute dose of Quinidine to all patients prior to commencement of normal therapy to detect those who may be likely to suffer a hypersensitivity reaction. Symptoms which have been found to be associated with such hypersensitivity are as follows: tinnitus, vertigo, visual disturbance, headache, confusion, erythematous skin rashes, anorexia, nausea, vomiting, diarrhoea, chest pain, abdominal pain, fever, respiratory distress, cyanosis, hypotension and shock. Thrombocytopenic purpura has also occurred.
2. Side effects which may occur in patients not hypersensitive to the drug include tinnitus, deafness, blurred vision, headache, dizziness and vomiting.
3. Excess dosage of the drug may lead to cardiac arrhythmias including heart block, paroxysmal ventricular tachycardia, ventricular fibrillation and cardiac arrest. As symptoms described in section (2) may precede these serious cardiac arrhythmias, the nurse may play a vital role in their prevention by detecting such symptoms in patients on the drug and advising medical staff accordingly.

General notes
Quinidine tablets may be stored at room temperature.

QUININE (Sulphate and Bisulphate)

Presentation
Tablets—200 mg and 300 mg

Actions and uses
This drug was originally used for the treatment of malaria. It is now rarely used as an anti-malarial drug as more effective preparations have been developed. However, it was noted that when Quinine was used it was effective in reducing painful night cramps suffered by a fair proportion of the older population. Its use nowadays is limited to the treatment of this condition.

Dosage
200–600 mg as a single dose on retiring.

Nurse monitoring
1. Perhaps the most important point to note about Quinine Sulphate is that it must not under any circumstances be confused with Quinidine which is a drug that is used for the treatment of serious abnormalities in cardiac rhythm.

2. Certain individuals may prove hypersensitive to this drug and may suffer the following symptoms:
   a. Tinnitus, headache, visual disturbance and blindness
   b. Nausea and abdominal pain
   c. Skin rash
   d. Blood disorders including haemolytic anaemia and thrombocytopenia.
3. It is recommended that the drug be avoided or used with extreme caution in patients with optic neuritis, heart disease or abnormalities of blood coagulation.
4. The drug may enhance the effect of oral anticoagulants (q.v.) producing an increased bleeding tendency.

General notes
The tablets may be stored at room temperature.

R

RANITIDINE (Zantac)

Presentation
Tablets—150 mg
Injection—50 mg in 5 ml

Actions and uses
Ranitidine is a recently developed drug with H_2 receptor antagonist activity similar to that of Cimetidine. Its uses therefore are identical to those of Cimetidine. Ranitidine has a longer action and therefore fewer daily doses need be taken.

Dosage
Adults:
  a. Orally
    i. Initial treatment to promote ulcer healing 150 mg twice per day
    ii. to maintain long-term remission of symptoms 150 mg may be given each evening.
  b. Parenteral
    i. a slow intravenous bolus injection of 50 mg over 1 minute may be given every 8 hours
    ii. alternatively an intravenous infusion at the rate of 25 mg per hour over 2 hours repeated every 6–8 hours may be given.

Nurse monitoring
1. As Ranitidine is a recently introduced drug, it is important that the nurse vigilantly monitor all patients in case problems arise which may be in fact side effects of the drug. Should any problems be noticed in patients on the drug, they should be reported to the appropriate authorities.
2. At present Ranitidine does not appear to produce the wide range of adverse effects associated with Cimetidine.
3. Diarrhoea and skin rashes are occasionally encountered.

General notes
1. Ranitidine tablest may be stored at room temperature.
2. Injection solutions should be stored in a cool place i.e. away from sources of heat such as radiators.
3. Infusions should not be prepared in 0.9% Sodium Chloride.

RAZOXANE (Razoxin)

Presentation
Tablets—125 mg

Actions and uses
Razoxane is a cytotoxic drug which prevents growth of malignant cells by interfering with the processes involved in cellular division. It is used in the treatment of acute myeloid leukaemia and sarcomata.

Dosage
1. In acute myeloid leukaemia: Three-day courses of 125 mg three times daily are used.
2. For the treatment of sarcomata: 125 mg once or twice daily is given in combination with radiotherapy.

Nurse monitoring
1. Common symptoms encountered with this drug include nausea, vomiting and diarrhoea.
2. Skin rashes and alopecia may occur with this drug.
3. When used in combination with radiotherapy, subcutaneous fibrosis, oesophagitis and pneumonitis may be produced.

4. The nurse should be constantly aware that most cytotoxic drugs are irritant to the skin and mucous surfaces, and are in general very toxic. Great care should therefore be exercised when handling these drugs, and in particular spillage or contamination of personnel or the environment must be avoided. If cytotoxic drugs are handled regularly it is theoretically possible that repeated skin contact or inhalation may produce systemic toxic effects and in nurses who have developed hypersensitivity, severe local and general hypersensitivity reactions.

General notes
1. Razoxane tablets may be stored at room temperature.
2. They should be protected from moisture and light.

REPROTEROL (Bronchodil)

Presentation
Tablets—20 mg
Elixir—10 mg in 5 ml
Inhaler—500 µg per dose of metered aerosol

Actions and uses
This drug has a highly selective action on receptors in bronchial smooth muscle, causing relaxation of muscle tone. It is used, therefore, for the treatment of reversible airways obstruction (bronchospasm) in asthma and other conditions such as bronchitis and emphysema.

Dosage
1. By inhalation: *Adults and children*: One or two inhalations three times daily. More frequent, 3–6 hourly administration may be required to treat an acute attack.
2. Oral: *Adults*: 10–20 mg three times daily (doses in the lower range are used for children).

Nurse monitoring
1. Rarely, this drug may cause palpitation, tachycardia, headache and fine muscle tremor.
2. The drug should be used with caution in patients with heart disease manifest by rhythm disturbances, angina, hyperthyroidism and hypertension.

General notes
1. Preparations of Reproterol may be stored at room temperature.
2. Aerosols should never be punctured or incinerated after use.

RESERPINE (Serpasil)

Presentation
Tablets—0.1 mg, 0.25 mg

Actions and uses
Reserpine reduces the action of the sympathetic nervous system on blood vessel walls and in the heart and leads to a reduction in blood pressure. It has been used in the past as a treatment for hypertension but because of its troublesome side effects it is now less frequently used. Small doses of Reserpine have also been used to treat depression but more effective and safer drugs are now available and it is therefore rarely used for this purpose.

Dosage
The usual adult daily dose is 0.5 mg once per day.

Nurse monitoring
1. The major reason for the discontinuation of the use of Reserpine in the treatment of hypertension has been because of the frequently encountered side effect of depression.
2. Common side effects include nasal stuffiness, diarrhoea, drowsiness, sedation, bradycardia, postural hypotension, fluid retention, increased appetite and weight gain.
3. The drug is contraindicated in patients with peptic ulceration or ulcerative colitis.

General notes
Reserpine and related substances may be stored at room temperature in tablet form. An injection of Reserpine was formerly available

and can be prepared in some Pharmacy Departments, though its stability is a major problem.

RIFAMPICIN (Rifadin, Rimactane)
Presentation
Capsules—150 mg, 300 mg
Syrup—100 mg in 5 ml
N.B. Rifampicin is available in combination with Isoniazid as Rifinah or Rimactazid.

Actions and uses
1. Rifampicin is anti-bacterial drug which is particularly effective against the tubercle bacillis (*Mycobacterium tuberculosis*). It has a bacteriostatic action inhibiting further growth and replication of the organism at low dose, and a bacteriocidal action (killing the organisms) at high dosage. The drug is usally used in combination with other anti-tuberculous agents (q.v.) for the prophylaxis and treatment of tuberulosis.
2. The drug is used less commonly for the treatment of other infections which include brucellosis, gastroenteritis, gonorrhoea, histoplasmosis, leprosy and leishmaniasis.
3. The drug is effective in the eradication of the organism *Neisseria meningitidis* (which causes bacterial meningitis) from the nasopharynx of carriers of the organism, and it is also used to prevent the occurrence of meningococcal meningitis in patients who have been in close contact with a case or carrier.

Dosage
1. *Adults*: 8–12 mg/kg body weight may be taken daily in a single dose. In practise 600 mg has been found to be well tolerated, effective and safe in most adult patients'. To ensure rapid and complete absorption, the drug should preferably be taken before meals. It is recommended that in frail or elderly patients, or patients with impaired liver function, dosage should be calculated on the basis of 8 mg/kg body weight per day.
2. *Children*:
Less than 1 year: 15 mg/kg. 1–7 years: 15–20 mg/kg to a maximum of 300 mg per day. Over 7 years: Up to 20 mg/kg body weight per day to a maximum of 600 mg.

Nurse monitoring
1. Patients undergoing treatment for tuberculosis receive their drugs for considerable periods of time. The nurse plays an important role in reminding patients that their drug therapy must be taken regularly for as long as recommended by medical staff, whether or not they themselves feel that they have recovered.
2. As noted above, it is important that the drug should be administered prior to meals as it is rapidly and better absorbed if taken in this way.
3. The drug is usually well tolerated but occasionally patients experience gastrointestinal upset which may be manifest as anorexia, nausea, vomiting or diarrhoea.
4. Rarely abnormal liver or kidney function may be detected in patients on this drug and regular blood tests are usually performed to detect the occurrence of this side effect.
5. This drug may cause a reddish discolouration of urine, sputum and tears, and to avoid potential worry and distress, patients should be warned to expect such an effect.
6. Skin rashes and blood dyscrasias (leucopenia, thrombocytopenia or haemolytic anaemia) occasionally occur.
7. Other rare side effects felt by the patient include dizziness, confusion, drowsiness, ataxia, peripheral neuropathy, blurred vision, hearing loss and menstrual disturbance.

General notes
The drug may be stored at room temperature.

RIMITEROL (Pulmadil)

Presentation
Inhaler—200 µg/dose as a pressurised aerosol or 'breath activated' auto-inhaler.

Actions and uses
Rimiterol stimulates the beta$_2$ adrenergic sites in the smooth muscle of the airways. This causes relaxation of muscle tone and alleviation of bonchospasm. In clinical practice it is used for the prevention and treatment of asthma and other conditions producing bronchospasm.

Dosage
One to three inhalations three or four times a day for both adults and children (a maximum of eight treatments of three puffs in any 24-hour period is recommended).

Nurse monitoring
1. Occasionally palpitations, tachycardia, headache and muscle tremor may be produced as side effects.
2. The drug should be administered with great caution in patients who also suffer from hypertension, coronary artery disease or thyrotoxicosis.

General notes
1. Preparations may be stored at room temperature.
2. Aerosols must never be punctured or incinerated after use.

RITODRINE (Yutopar)

Presentation
Tablets—10 mg
Injection—10 mg in 1 ml

Action and uses
Ritodrine has a direct action on the uterine smooth muscle causing it to relax and therefore reducing contractions. It is used to prevent labour in the management of:
1. Uncomplicated premature labour.
2. Fetal asphyxia in labour when relaxation is required to improve the condition of the baby before planned, assisted delivery.

Dosage
1. For the treatment of uncomplicated premature labour: Ritodrine is administered as soon as possible at the onset of labour as follows:
   a. Initially, 50 µg/minute by intravenous infusion in Sodium Chloride 0.9% injection, Dextrose 5% Injection or Dextrose/Saline mixtures. The infusion rate is increases gradually by 50 µg/minute every 10 minutes until the required response is obtained or the heart rate reaches 140 beats/minute. This level of dosage is generally in the range, 150–350 µg/minute. Intravenous infusions are continued for 12–48 hours after uterine contractions have ceased. If intravenous therapy is not possible, 10 mg Ritodrine every 3–8 hourly may be given by intramuscular injection and continued for 12–48 hours as above.
   b. Maintenance oral Ritodrine is started about 30 minutes before intravenous therapy is completed. Up to 10 mg every 2 hours is given for the initial 24 hours and reduced thereafter to 10–20 mg or less, 4–6 hourly depending upon response or the presence of troublesome side effects. The total oral dose must not exceed 120 mg/day. Oral therapy is continued for as long as it is required to prolong pregnancy.
2. The treatment of fetal asphyxia prior to planned assisted delivery: Initially, 50 µg/minute by intravenous infusion increased rapidly until uterine activity is suppressed or the maternal heart rate reaches 140 beats/minute. The required dose level is usually of the order 350 µg/minute or less. Delivery of the baby is carried out 15 minutes to 1 hour after infusions are started depending upon fetal scalp blood pH.

Nurse monitoring

1. The drug may affect maternal pulse rate leading to tachycardia and palpitations. The nurse may play an important role in titrating intravenous infusion dosage and preventing excess administration of the drug. It is important to note that a maternal trachycardia of up to 140 beats/minute is generally acceptable in a healthy patient.
2. Other side effects seen with this drug are flushing, sweating, tremor, nausea and vomiting.
3. Extremely careful patient monitoring is essential in patients who have heart disease or for those who are receiving other drugs which may increase or reduce the response to Ritodrine e.g. monomine oxidase inhibitors, tricyclic antidepressants, and other drugs which stimulate the sympathetic nervous system and beta-adrenoreceptor blockers.
4. It should be noted that the drug should be used with great care in patients on co-incident treatment with corticosteroid drugs as pulmonary oedema may occur in the mother.
5. The drug should be avoided or used with great caution in the following situations:
    a. Antepartum haemorrhage requiring immediate delivery
    b. Intra-uterine fetal death
    c. Chorioamniolitis
    d. Maternal cardiac disease
    e. Cord compression
    f. Diabetes mellitus
    g. Hypertension
    h. Hypertenthyroidism
6. It is important to note that the drug is much less effective if the membranes have been ruptured or if the cervix has dilated greater than 4 cm.

General notes

1. Ritodrine tablets and injection solution may be stored at room temperature though they should be protected from light.
2. Deterioration of the injection is evident if the solution is discoloured or else a precipitate may appear in the solution. Solutions with any evidence of deterioration should be immediately discarded.

S

SALBUTAMOL (Ventolin)

Presentation
Tablets—2 mg, 4 mg and 8 mg (slow release)
Syrup—2 mg in 5 ml
Injection — 0.5 mg in 1 ml
 0.25 mg in 5 ml
 5 mg in 5 ml (for intravenous infusion)
Inhalation—100 μg/dose of metered aerosol
 200 μg and 400 μg as Rotacaps
 0.5% as respirator solution
Nebules for inhalation—2.5 mg in 2.5 ml unit

Actions and uses
1. This drug stimulates receptors known as beta$_2$ adrenergic receptors. The effect of this stimulation is to relax bronchial muscle and relieve bronchospasm. Salbutamol is, therefore, used for the acute and chronic relief of bronchospasm in asthma and other condition such as chronic bronchitis, where reversible airways obstruction has been shown to exist.
2. It has an additional use in that it may be given by intravenous infusion for the management of premature labour. In this case the beta$_2$ adrenergic stimulant action reduces contraction of uterine muscle.

Dosage
1. For the treatment of asthma:
   a. By inhalation:
      i. Using a metered aerosol: 2 inhalations 3 or 4 times a day
      ii. Using rotacaps: 200–400 μg three or four times a day
      iii. For acute severe conditions the respirator solution is administered by intermittent positive pressure using oxygen rich air or via a suitable nebuliser.
      iv. Alternatively, in acute severe conditions 1 or 2 'nebules' may be inhaled via a nebuliser 4 or 5 times daily.
   b. Orally:
      i. *Adults*: 2–8 mg three or four times a day
      ii. *Children*:
       2–6 years: 1–2 mg three or four times daily
       6–12 years: 2 mg three or four times daily
       Over 12 years: 2–4 mg three or four times daily
   c. Parenteral:
      i. By subcutaneous or intramuscular injection for adults: 0.5 mg 4-hourly as required
      ii. By slow intravenous injection for adults: 4 μg/kg body weight
      iii. By intravenous infusion: 3–20 μg/minute.
2. For the treatment of premature labour: An intravenous infusion is administered at a rate of 10–45 μg/minute and adjusted to control uterine contractions. It is usual to commence with a rate of 10 μg/minute and increase accordingly. Once uterine contractions have ceased the infusion rate should be maintained for one hour and then

reduced by 50% decrements at 6-hourly intervals. Treatment may be continued orally with Ventolin tablets, 4 mg given three or four times daily.

Nurse monitoring
1. Common side effects include fine muscle tremor, palpitations, tachycardia, flushing and headache.
2. The drug should be used with caution in patients who have heart disease manifest by rhythm disturbance or angina, hyperthyroidism and hypertension.
3. When intravenously administered elevation of blood glucose may be caused and care, therefore, should be exercised when diabetic patients are being treated.
4. Intramuscular use of the undiluted injection produces slight pain and stinging.
5. In the management of premature labour intravenous infusion of Salbutamol has occasionally caused nausea, vomiting and headache.

General notes
1. Preparations of Salbutamol may be stored at room temperature.
2. Preparations should be protected from light.
3. Solutions for injection can be diluted using Water for Injections.
4. Intravenous infusions are prepared in 0.9% sodium chloride or dextrose 5% or dextrose/saline injections.
5. Aerosols should never be punctured or incinerated after use.

SALSALATE (Disalcid)

Presentation
Tablets—500 mg
Capsules—500 mg

Actions and uses
1. See the section on Aspirin.
2. Salsalate is converted to Aspirin in the blood following absorption.

It may therefore be used as an alternative to Aspirin in patients who have experienced intolerable gastrointestinal upsets caused by that drug.

Dosage
1. *Adults*: The dose range is 2–4 g daily in three or four divided doses which are usually taken with meals and at bed-time.
2. *Children*: It is not recommended that children receive this form of Aspirin.

Nurse monitoring
1. See the section on Aspirin.

General notes
Salsalate tablets and capsules may be stored at room temperature.

SELEGILINE (Eldepryl)

Presentation
Tablets—5 mg

Actions and uses
Selegiline, by a complex actions in the brain, potentiates the action of Levodopa (in Madopar and Sinemet) in the treatment of Parkinson's disease and it is used in conjunction with these drugs.

Dosage
Adults: Initially 5 mg once daily, increased to 10 mg if necessary.

Nurse monitoring
Selegiline is used in conjunction with Madopar or Sinemet (or Levodopa alone) and it should be noted that a reduction in dosage of these drugs is often possible. The nurse must therefore be vigilant for the occurrence of Levodopa side effects which indicate the need to reduce Levodopa dosage.

General notes
Selegiline tablets may be stored at room temperature.

SENNOSIDE (Senokot, X-prep)

Presentation
Tablets—7.5 mg
Granules—5.5 mg in 1 g
Syrup—15 mg in 10 ml

Actions and uses
See the section on laxatives for general discussion. Sennoside acts by action 1, i.e. it has an irritant effect on the gut wall. It is used for the treatment of constipation.

Dosage
1. *Adults*: 15–30 mg or 1–2.5 ml spoonsfuls of granules taken as a single dose at bedtime.
2. *Children*:
   Under 2 years: Up to 5 mg
   2–6 years: One-quarter of the adult dose
   Over 6 years: One half of the adult dose.
3. X-prep is a single dose of Sennoside (142 mg in 71 ml of fluid) which is taken between 2 and 4 p.m. on the day prior to radiographic procedures involving the bowel.

Nurse monitoring
1. The granular form of this drug may be stirred into hot milk, sprinkled on food or eaten plain and as it is more acceptable to the patient, better compliance may be achieved.
2. Because of its irritant effect on the bowel it may produce cramping abdominal pain.

General notes
1. Preparations containing Sennoside may be stored at room temperature.
2. Liquid preparations are sensitive to light and should be kept in amber bottles.
3. Granules should be kept in a closed, air-tight container since they may absorb moisture from the air.

SINEMET

Presentation
Sinemet 110 containing 10 mg of Carbidopa and 100 mg of Levodopa
Sinemet 275 containing 25 mg of Carbidopa and 250 mg of Levodopa
Sinemet Plus containing 25 mg of Carbidopa and 100 mg of Levodopa

Actions and uses
Sinemet contains Levodopa: See the description of the actions and uses of this drug. It is used in clinical practice principally for the treatment of Parkinsonism. The advantages of combining Carbidopa with Levodopa are thought to be improved control throughout the day and a reduced overall dose of Levodopa.

Dosage
N.B. Dosages for individual patients are carefully titrated using low initial dosages with gradual increments. The following is only one example of such a scheme using Sinemet 275
1. Patients not receiving Levodopa: Initially a half tablet of Sinemet 275 is given once or twice a day. This is subsequently increased by half a tablet every day or every other day until optimum response is achieved.
2. Patients receiving Levodopa: At least 12 hours before Sinemet is started (or 24 hours if slow release preparations of Levodopa are used), all Levodopa containing medication should be discontinued. The starting dose of Sinemet should be equivalent to 20% of the previous Levodopa dose. The dosage should be gradually increased and most patients can be maintained on a dosage of 3–6 tablets of Sinemet 275 per day. It is recommended that no patient should receive more than eight tablets of Sinemet 275 per day.

Nurse monitoring
The Nurse monitoring aspects of Levodopa (q.v.) apply to this drug.

General notes
The drugs may be stored at room temperature.

SODIUM AMINOSALICYLATE (P.A.S., Paramisan)

Presentation
Powder for oral use is available although sodium aminosalicylate is almost always used in combination

with Isoniazid in the preparation 'Inapasade'.

Actions and uses
Sodium aminosalicylate is an antibacterial drug which is of use only for the treatment of tuberculosis caused by the organism mycobacterium tuberculosis. Its action may be either bacteriostatic (inhibining growth replication of the organism) or bacteriocidal (killing the organism), depending on the concentration achieved in the tissues. If used on its own for the treatment of tuberculosis it will be, in a large number of cases, ineffective as the organism gradually develops resistance to it and therefore it usually is used in combination with other antituberculous drugs (q.v.).

Dosage
1. *Adults*:
   a. As a single drug: 10–20 g daily in divided doses
   b. In combination with Isoniazid: the recommended P.A.S. dosage is 6 g twice per day.

Nurse monitoring
1. Patients undergoing treatment for tuberculosis receive their drugs for considerable periods of time. The nurse may play an important role in reminding patients that their drug therapy must be taken regularly for as long as recommended by medical staff, whether or not they themselves feel that they have recovered.
2. Gastrointestinal side effects are common and include nausea, vomiting and diarrhoea. These may be minimised if the drug is taken with meals. This may lead to some confusion for patients if they are receiving this drug with Rifampicin which is recommended to be taken before meals and the nurse may contribute greatly by ensuring that the patient understands when to take the various preparations and by helping to educate the patient so that they understand why it is necessary to take the tablets in such a manner.
3. Fever, skin rash, jaundice, hypokalaemia (manifest as weakness) and liver damage may also occur.
4. Rare but severe side effects include:
   a. Renal damage which may be manifest by the appearance of albuminuria or haematuria
   b. Psychotic reactions
   c. Blood disorders including haemolytic anaemia and throbocytopenia.
5. Prolonged courses of treatment interfere with iodine metabolism in the body and may produce an enlarged thyroid (a goitre) or thyroid under-activity.
6. The toxic effects of sodium aminosalicylate and salicylates such as Aspirin are additive and therefore patients should be warned against taking Aspirin whilst on this treatment.
7. It is recommended that the drug should be used with great caution or preferably avoided in patients who have previously been found to have impaired renal function.

General notes
The drug may be stored at room temperature.

SODIUM AUROTHIOMALATE (Myocrisin)

Presentation
Injection—0.5 ml ampoules containing 1 mg, 5 mg, 10 mg, 20 mg and 50 mg

Actions and uses
This drug is a gold salt and is used in the treatment of chronic rheumatoid disease which has not responded adequately to conventional anti-inflammatory analgesic therapy. It is not in itself an analgesic but by modifying the auto-immune inflammatory process involved in the disease, it may lead to a reduction in pain.

Dosage
1. *Adults*: A course of injections each of 50 mg is usually given at

weekly intervals to a total dose of 1 g. For the first few weeks less than 50 mg may be given so that patients who suffer severe side effects may be detected before they have received large doses.

2. *Children*: This drug is only used for the treatment of Still's disease. Graded doses at weekly intervals are used up to a maximum which is based on body weight i.e. less than 25 kg–10 mg; 25–50 kg—20 mg; 50 kg or over—50 mg.

Nurse monitoring
1. Early side effects from this drug may precede the more serious life-threatening side effects and the nurse may play an important part in managing these patients by helping to detect the early side effects which include skin rashes, pruritis, a metallic taste in the mouth, a painful throat or tongue, mouth ulcers, bruising, bleeding gums, menorrhagia, nose bleeds, dry cough or progressive breathlessness.
2. Serious side effects include skin eruptions, pulmonary fibrosis, renal toxicity, blood dyscrasia such as agranulocytosis, thrombocytopenia and aplastic anaemia.
3. The drug should never be given to patients with liver or kidney disease, diabetes, history of toxaemia during pregnancy, blood dyscrasias or exfoliative dermatitis.
4. Laboratory tests such as blood counts, urine tests for protein and chest X-rays are carried out regularly during a course of treatment. It is essential that these tests are performed regularly and the nurse may again contribute by emphasising the importance of having these tests done to the patient.
5. During treatment the details of the course of treatment and laboratory results are usually recorded together on a pre-designed 'gold card'. The nurse may contribute by ensuring such cards are fully and accurately filled out.

General notes
1. Sodium Aurothiomalate injection may be stored at room temperature.
2. As the solution is light sensitive any darkening in the usual straw colour indicates degradation and such solutions must be discarded.

SODIUM CROMOGLYCATE (Intal, Lomusol, Nalcrom, Opticrom, Rynacrom)

Presentation
Spincaps for Inhalation—20 mg plain 20 mg compound (with isoprenaline 0.1 mg)
Capsules—100 mg
Nasal Spray and Drops—2%
Nasal Insufflation—capsules containing 10 mg
Nebuliser Solution—20 mg in 2 ml
Eye Drops—2%

Actions and uses
1. This drug binds to cells present in the airways which under certain conditions would normally release chemicals which would cause an increase in muscle tone in the airways causing bronchospasm manifest as dyspnoea and wheezing. It is, therefore, useful for the prophylactic treatment of conditions associated with bronchospasm.
2. The drug has been postulated to be effective orally in the management of ulcerative colitis, proctitis, proctocolitis and food allergy.
3. When rhinitis and conjunctivitis is caused by an allergic reaction, the cells which release the chemicals causing the symptoms may be prevented from releasing these chemicals by the application of this drug directly to the nasal or conjunctival surfaces.

Dosage
1. For the treatment of bronchospasm: For adults and

children the normal dose is 1 spincap (contents of each capsule are inhaled through a spinhaler) at intervals ranging from 3-6 hours.
2. For the treatment of ulcerative colitis, proctitis, proctocolitis and food allergy:
   a. *Adults*: 200 mg orally four times a day before meals
   b. *Children* (over 2 years): Up to 100 mg orally four times daily before meals.
3. For the treatment of allergic rhinitis instil into the nostrils 6 times daily.
4. For conjunctivis, 1 or 2 drops into the eye 4 times daily using 2% eye drops.

Nurse monitoring
1. It is essential to note that this drug is only useful for the prophylaxis i.e. prevention of attacks of bronchospasm, and it is no use in the acute attack.
2. A special whistle type spinhaler is available to encourage proper use of spincaps in young children.
3. Administration of the drug as noted above does not produce any immediate effect, patients may therefore come to the conclusion that the drug is doing them no good and may stop taking it. The nurse may play an important role in educating the patient on the benefits of continuing with treatment.
4. When the drug is taken orally for the management of ulcerative colitis, proctitis, proctocolitis or food allergy it may be either swallowed whole or taken in a solution. It is worth noting that when food allergy is being treated, administration in a solution is preferred.
5. As with other eye drops, the drug itself may produce slight irritation to the eyes.
6. Eye drops should be discarded 4 weeks after opening.

General notes
1. Preparation containing sodium cromoglycate may be stored at room temperature.
2. Capsules and solutions should be stored in moisture-proof containers and protected from light.
3. It should be clearly understood that the spincaps are for inhalation and should not be swallowed.

SODIUM IRON EDETATE (Sytron)

Presentation
Liquid—55 mg of elemental iron in 10 ml

Actions and uses
See the section on Irons (oral).

Dosage
1. For the treatment of iron deficiency anaemia:
   a. *Adults*: 10-20 ml per day
   b. *Children*:
      Less than 1 year: 5-10 ml per day
      1-7 years: 10-15 ml per day
      7-12 years: 15-20 ml per day
      Over 12 years: adult doses apply.
2. For the prevention of iron deficiency anaemia in pregnancy: 10 ml twice a day.

Nurse monitoring
See the section Irons (oral).

General notes
The drug may be stored at room temperature.

SODIUM NITROPRUSSIDE (Nipride)

Presentation
Injection—50 mg ampoules

Actions and uses
Sodium nitroprusside has a direct action on blood vessels causing peripheral vasodilation and a reduction in peripheral resistance. It is therefore useful in the management of hypertension. It is available for intravenous infusion only and has been found to be of use in the treatment of hypertensive crises.

Dosage
The drug is usually given by continuous infusion of a 0.01 or

0.05% solution in dextrose. The initial rate is between 0.5 and 8 μg/kg body weight per minute. Maintenance dosage depends on the control obtained but 3 μg/kg per minute has been found to be the average infusion required to maintain the blood pressure at 30–40% below the pre-treatment blood pressure. The maximum recommended rate of infusion is 11 μg/kg per minute.

Nurse monitoring
1. Once Sodium nitroprusside has been diluted in dextrose for infusion it will deteriorate, if exposed to sunlight. Some of the products of deterioration are harmful and therefore it is essential that the nurse ensures that the infusion bottle and as much of the infusion apparatus as possible is completely shielded from exposure to light.
2. During the initial period of treatment the blood pressure must be monitored on an almost continuous basis.
3. Sodium nitroprusside has a very short duration of action and therefore infusions must be constantly monitored to ensure that accidental reduction or increase in infusion rate does not occur as drastic effects may ensue.
4. Prolonged therapy may be associated with cyanide intoxication. This is characterised by tachycardia, sweating, hyperventilation, cardiac dysrhythmia and metabolic acidosis.
5. Common side effects with this drug include nausea, vomiting, anorexia, abdominal pain, apprehension, restlessness, muscle twitching, retrosternal chest pain, palpitations and dizziness.

General notes
Sodium nitroprusside ampoules may be stored at room temperature. The injection solution is prepared by first mixing with dextrose 5% in ampoules which are usually provided, then the required amount is added to dextrose 5% for infusion. Any unused solution should be immediately discarded. The drug is sensitive to sunlight and during infusion the bottle should be covered by a protective opaque bag.

SODIUM PICOSULPHATE (Laxoberal)

Presentation
Syrup—5 ml in 5 ml

Actions and uses
The actions and uses of laxative drugs are described in the section on these drugs. Sodium Picosulphate falls into group 1. It is converted by bacterial action into an active substance in the gut and tends to produce bowel evacuation 10–14 hours after administration.

Dosage
1. *Adults*: 5–15 ml
2. *Children*:
   0–5 years: 2.5 ml
   5–10 years: 2.5–5 ml
In all cases a single night-time dose is taken.

Nurse monitoring
1. In common with most laxatives, excessive doses may produce abdominal discomfort.
2. As the drug requires the presence of gut bacteria to convert it to its active component its effectiveness may be lost in patients who are taking broad-spectrum antibiotics.

General notes
1. Sodium Picosulphate may be stored at room temperature.
2. It should be protected from light.
3. For ease of administration the syrup should be diluted with water.

SODIUM VALPROATE (Epilim)

Presentation
Tablets—100 mg, 200 mg and 500 mg (enteric-coated)
Syrup—200 mg in 5 ml

Actions and uses
The actions and uses of anticonvulsant drugs are discussed in the section on these drugs.

Dosage
N.B. Individual dosage requirements vary greatly. The following doses are given as a guideline only.
1. *Adults*: An initial dose of 600 mg is given increasing each day until an optimum response is achieved. The usual dose range is 1000–2000 mg per day.
2. *Children*:
Over 20 kg body weight: 400 mg daily initially increasing to maintenance doses usually in the range 20–30 mg/kg body weight per day in total.
Under 20 kg body weight: 20–50 mg/kg body weight per day in total.

Nurse monitoring
1. The Nurse monitoring aspects of anticonvulsant drugs in general are discussed in the section on these drugs.
2. This drug should preferably be taken with or immediately after food in order to minimise the common side effect of gastrointestinal irritation. Enteric-coated tablets may have to be used if gastric upset still occurs.
3. Metabolites of Sodium Valproate are excreted in the urine and may give false positive results for ketones. It is especially important that this effect be recognised in diabetic patients where the presence of ketonuria usually leads to hospital referral.
4. As this drug may reduce the number of platelets circulating in the blood, unexplained bruising or haemorrhage should always be taken as an indication to check the patient's blood and if thrombocytopenia (reduced platelets) has been produced, the drug should be stopped.
5. Liver damage may occasionally occur.
6. A few patients suffer from hair loss.
7. When the drug is used in high dosage tremor may be a problem.

General notes
1. The drug should be stored at room temperature.
2. If for ease of administration dilution of Sodium Valproate syrup is necessary, syrup BP should be used and the diluted preparation discarded after 14 days if not used.

SOTALOL (Beta-Cardone, Sotacor)

Presentation
Tablets—40 mg, 80 mg, 160 mg, 200 mg
Injection—10 mg in 5 ml

Actions and uses
Sotalol is a non-selective beta-adrenoreceptor blocking drug. Its actions are described in the section on these drugs.

Dosage
1. It may be given intravenously in emergency situations for cardiac dysrhythmias in a dosage of 10–20 mg. This is usually given over five minutes and is repeated as necessary. Careful monitoring of pulse, blood pressure and electrocardiogram is necessary during administration (see equivalent section for Propranolol, q.v.).
2. The oral daily adult maintenance dose range is 120–640 mg and it may be given as a single dose or in three or four divided doses.

Nurse monitoring
See the section on beta-adrenoreceptor blocking drugs.

General notes
Sotalol tablets and injection may be stored at room temperature.

SPIRONOLACTONE (Aldactone, Spiroctan)

Presentation
Tablets—25 mg, 100 mg
Injection—200 mg in 20 ml (as Canrenoate potassium).

Actions and uses
Spironolactone inhibits the adrenal hormone aldosterone and thus is a 'potassium-sparing' diuretic which prevents excessive potassium loss. It is usually given together with

other diuretics to prevent the devleopment of hypokalaemia (excessive blood potassium loss) which often occurs in patients treated with diuretic drugs. It is usually unnecessary for patients treated with Spironolactone to be given potassium supplement tablets such as Slow K or Sando K.

Dosage
1. Oral:
   The usual adult dose range of Spironolactone is 50–500 mg daily; it is occasionally given in divided daily doses though a single dose is usually adequate. It takes about 3 days of treatment before the maximum effect of Spironolactone is achieved and this effect may persist for 2–3 days after therapy is discontinued.
   Children's doses are:
   Up to 1 year: 0.6 mg/kg four times daily
   1–6 years: 6.25 mg four times daily
   7 years plus: 12.5 mg four times daily.
2. Injection:
   Adults may receive up to 800 mg daily by slow intravenous injection either as a single dose or in divided dosage. The injection period should be at least 2–3 minutes per 200 mg dose.

Nurse monitoring
Patients receiving Spironolactone should be observed for the occasional occurrence of excessive potassium retention (hyperkalaemia). This is particularly important in patients with renal failure. This may be manifest by confusion, drowsiness, anorexia, nausea, vomiting and other features of uraemia. Less common side effects include breast enlargement in the male (gynaecomastia), milk secretion in the female (galactorrhoea) and skin rashes.

General notes
Spironolactone tablets may be stored at room temperature.

STANOZOLOL (Stromba)
Presentation
Tablets—5 mg
Injection—50 mg in 1 ml
Actions and uses
1. See the section discussing the actions and uses of anabolic steroids.
2. This drug is occasionally used to aid recovery from prolonged and debilitating illness or following major surgery.

Dosage
1. By the oral route: 5 mg daily with food
2. By deep intramuscular injection: 50 mg every 2–3 weeks.

Nurse monitoring
See the sections on adrogenic hormones and anabolic steroids.

General notes
The drug may be stored at room temperature.

STILBOESTROL (Tampovagan)
Presentation
Tablets—0.5 mg, 1 mg and 5 mg
Pessaries—0.5 mg
Actions and uses
Stilboestrol is an oestrogenic substance which has the following uses in clinical practice.
1. For the treatment of menopausal symptoms.
2. For the treatment of secondary amenorrhoea due to ovarian insufficiency.
3. For the inhibition of lactation.
4. For palliative treatment of malignant neoplasm.
5. For post-coital contraception.

Dosage
1. For the treatment of menopausal symptoms: 0.1–1 mg by mouth daily.
2. For the treatment of secondary amenorrhoea: 0.25–1 mg daily during the proliferative phase of the menstrual cycle.
3. For the inhibition of lactation: 5 mg is given twice or thrice daily initially with subsequent reduction in dosage.

4. For the palliative treatment of malignant neoplasm of the breast: 10–20 mg is usually given daily. For carcinoma of the prostate between 1 and 3 mg is given daily.
5. For post-coital contraception: 25 mg is given twice daily for five days starting within 72 hours of intercourse.

Nurse monitoring
See the section on oestrogenic hormones.

General notes
The drug may be stored at room temperature.

STREPTOKINASE (Kabikinase)

Presentation
Vials for intravascular administration contain either 600 000 or 250 000 or 100 000 i.u.

Actions and uses
This enzyme stimulates the action of the fibrinolytic system in man and, therefore, promotes the dissolution of clots. In clinical practice it has been used as a thrombolytic agent in:
1. Venous thrombosis
2. Pulmonary embolism
3. Acute arterial thromboembolism
4. Clotted haemodialysis shunts
5. Occlusion of the retinal vessels.

Dosage
1. *Adults*: An initial dose of 600 000 i.u. over a period of 30–60 minutes is given followed by maintenance doses of 100 000 i.u. hourly for three or more days. The initial and maintenance doses may be titrated by measuring the anti-streptokinase antibody level of the individual.
2. *Children*: There are no absolute recommendations on dosage for children other than that the adult scheme should be used and reduced according to the size of the patient.

Nurse monitoring
1. If other anticoagulants have been given (Heparin or oral anticoagulants such as Warfarin), they should be stopped prior to the administration of Streptokinase.
2. Allergic reactions ranging from fever to anaphylactic shock may occur.
3. The drug should not be used in patients with severe hypertension, defects of blood coagulation, peptic ulceration and during menstruation.
4. The nurse should note that the preparation normally has a faint straw colour and such discolouration does not indicate degeneration of the preparation.

General notes
1. Vials of Streptokinase should be stored below 25°C before reconstitution.
2. The vial containing a prepared concentrated solution may be stored for 24 hours in a refrigerator.
3. Diluted solution should be used within 12 hours of preparation.
4. The diluents of choice are physiological saline and 5% dextrose but other diluents should not be used.

STREPTOKINASE/STREPTODORNASE (Varidase)

Presentation
Vials containing Streptokinase 100 000 units, Streptodornase 250 000 units
Oral tablets each containing 10 000 units of Streptokinase and 2500 units of Streptodornase

Actions and uses
1. The combination of these two enzymes in solution is suitable for use by local application to help in the dissolution of clotted blood and fibrinous or purulent accumulations.
2. Oral treatment is recommended for use for its generalised anti-inflammatory effect thereby relieving the symptoms of inflammation, pain, swelling and tenderness in such conditions as thrombophlebitis, cellulitis, sinusitis, contusions, skin ulcers, sprains and fractures.

Dosage

1. For local administration: The dosage depends on the condition under treatment. Some examples are as follows:
   a. For treatment of a pneumothorax or thoracic empyema: An initial dose of 200 000 units of Streptokinase and 50 000 units of Streptodornase is suggested. This amount should be applied to single or multiple sites as the case warrants.
   b. For treatment of maxillary sinus empyema: Recommended doses would be from 10 000 to 15 000 units of Streptokinase and 2500 to 3750 units of Streptodornase in a volume of 2–3 ml.
2. For local administration: The usual dose is one tablet four times daily.

Nurse monitoring

1. It is essential to note that vials of Varidase powder are for local application only and should never be administered parenterally.
2. Occasional allergic skin reactions may occur.
3. This drug should be administered orally with great caution in patients who have abnormalities of blood coagulation or abnormal liver function.

General notes

1. Varidase topical:
   a. Must be kept in its original pack in a refrigerator
   b. Once reconstituted, solutions are stable for one week
   c. For reconstitution Water for Injections or sterile physiological saline should be used.
2. Oral preparations: The drug should be stored in a cool, dry place in containers which prevent access of moisture.

STREPTOMYCIN

(See Note 3, p. 310)

Presentation

Injection—1 g

Actions and uses

This aminoglycoside antibiotic is primarily reserved for the treatment of tuberculosis and more rarely for the treatment and prevention of chronic respiratory infections and bacterial endocarditis.

Dosage

1. For the treatment of tuberculosis:
   a. Adults receive 0.75–1 g per day by a single intramuscular injection
   b. Children receive 30 mg/kg daily by a single intramuscular injection
   c. In the treatment of tuberculous meningitis intrathecal doses of 50 mg for adults or 1 mg/kg for children may be given daily.
2. Non-tuberculous infections:
   a. *Adults*: Intramuscular doses of 0.75–1 g per day are administered
   b. Children receive 25 mg/kg daily.

Nurse monitoring

1. The most important toxic effect of this drug is damage to the auditory nerve with resultant deafness and loss of balance. The risk of this increases with high dosage, prolonged duration of treatment, or when the patient is over 40 years of age. Recovery may occur over weeks or months but is often incomplete. The development of any symptoms suggestive of damage to the auditory nerve is an indication immediately to stop treatment.
2. Allergic reactions may occur, including rash and fever.
3. Vague feelings of paraesthesia of the lips, headache, lassitude, and dizziness may occur after each injection. They are less common if the patient is kept at rest after an injection. This is because with muscular activity absorption from the intramuscular injection site is increased and high plasma concentrations may occur.
4. These injections are particularly painful and the patient may usefully receive support and

encouragement from the attending nurse.
5. It is essential that the nurse notes that Streptomycin is a potent skin sensitiser and severe skin reactions may occur in nurses who handle the drug if they are sensitive to it. The wearing of protective gloves during handling of the drug is therefore advised.

General notes
1. Streptomycin powder and vials may be stored at room temperature.
2. After reconstitution the solutions may be kept for several days in a refrigerator.
3. Streptomycin is for deep intramuscular injection and occasionally intrathecal injection only.

SUCCINYLSULPHATHIAZOLE (Sulfasuxidine)

(See Note 3, p. 310)
Presentation
Tablets—500 mg
Actions and uses
This sulphonamide drug is used principally for the treatment of ulcerative colitis.
Dosage
1. *Adults*: 2.5–3 g six times per day.
2. *Children*:
   12–16 kg: 500–750 mg six times per day.
   16–36 kg: 750–1.5 g six times per day.
   36–56 kg: 1.5–2.5 g six times per day.

It is important to note that the above doses are maintenance doses and higher doses may be used for the treatment of acute exacerbations of ulcerative colitis.
Nurse monitoring
See the section on sulphonamide drugs.
General notes
1. Succinylsulphathiazole tablets may be stored at room temperature.

2. The drug should be kept in a dry place and maintained in tightly closed containers to protect from moisture.

SUCRALFATE (Antepsin)

Presentation
Tablets—1 g
Actions and uses
Sucralfate is used in the treatment of gastric and duodenal ulcer when it exerts an action which is similar to that of Tri-potassium Di-citrato Bismuthate (De-Nol). Briefly, the drug binds to protein in the ulcer crater, thereby forming a protective layer of a chemically complex substance which resists further digestion of the ulcer by gastric acid and pepsin and therefore aids healing.
Dosage
Adults: 1–2 g four times a day for up to 6 weeks.
Nurse monitoring
1. Patients should be instructed to take dosages 1 hour before meals with a single dose at bedtime.
2. The absorption of Tetracycline drugs may be impaired by the presence of Sucralfate and such combination should be avoided or, if necessary, doses of Tetracycline drugs should not be given within 2 hours of Sucralfate administration.
3. The drug should be used with caution in patients with kidney impairment due to the possibility of aluminium retention. However, it is interesting to note that Sucralfate has been administered to a patients with renal failure in an attempt to bind phosphate in the gut and so reduce hyperphosphataemia.
4. The only side effect of note is constipation.

General notes
Tablets may be stored at room temperature.

SULINDAC (Clinoril)

Presentation
Tablets—100 mg, 200 mg

Actions and uses
See the section on non-steroidal anti-inflammatory analgesic drugs.

Dosage
The usual adult dose is 100–200 mg twice daily usually taken with fluids at mealtimes.

Nurse monitoring
See the section on anti-inflammatory analgesic drugs, non-steroidal.

General notes
Sulindac tablets may be stored at room temperature.

SULPHACETAMIDE (Albucid)

(See Note 3, p. 310)

Presentation
Eye drops—10%, 20% and 30%
Eye ointment—2½%, 6% and 10%

Actions and uses
Sulphacetamide is a sulphonamide drug (q.v.) which is administered in solution or ointment directly on to the eye for the treatment of infections including styes and conjunctivitis and for the prevention of infection following ulceration of the cornea.

Dosage
1. The ointment is applied 2–4 times daily.
2. Drops may be applied as frequently as two hourly.

Nurse monitoring
Some slight irritation of the conjunctiva may be produced by the higher concentration of the drug especially in eye drops. This may itself cause some pain, redness and grittiness.

General notes
The drug may be stored at room temperature.

SULPHADIMIDINE (Sulphamezathine)

(See Note 3, p. 310)

Presentation
Tablets—500 mg
Injection—1 g in 3 ml
Paediatric mixture—500 mg in 5 ml

Actions and uses
1. For general actions and uses see the section on sulphonamide drugs.
2. Sulphadimidine has been found to be especially useful in the treatment of:
   a. Meningococcal meningitis
   b. Urinary tract infection
   c. Bacillary dysentery.

Dosage
1. *Adults*:
   a. For the treatment of acute infection: Oral, intramuscular and intravenous doses are the same and are up to 3 g initially followed by 0.5–1.5 g 6-hourly.
   b. For the prophylaxis of urinary tract infection: 500 mg to 1 g orally each day is recommended.
2. Children's doses are as follows:
   Less than 1 year: 25 mg/kg four times per day
   1–7 years: 250–500 mg four times per day
   Over 7 years: Adult doses are given.

Nurse monitoring
See the section on sulphonamide drugs.

General notes
1. The drug may be stored at room temperature.
2. Injection solutions must be protected from light.

SULPHADIMETHOXINE (Madribon)

(See Note 3, p. 310)

Presentation
Tablets—500 mg

Actions and uses
See the section on sulphonamide drugs.

Dosage
For adults: 2 g is administered initially followed by 1 g once per day.

Nurse monitoring
See the section on sulphonamide drugs.

General notes
The drug may be stored at room temperature.

SULPHAFURAZOLE (Gantrisin)

(See Note 3, p. 310)

Presentation
Tablets—500 mg
Syrup—500 mg in 5 ml

Actions and uses
See the section on sulphonamide drugs.

Dosage
1. *Adults*: 2 g initially followed by 1 g 4–6 hourly
2. *Children*: 30 mg/kg initially followed by 15 mg/kg 4–6 hourly.

Nurse monitoring
See the section on sulphonamide drugs.

General notes
The drug may be stored at room temperature.

SULPHAMETHOXYPYRIDAZINE (Lederkyn)

(See Note 3, p. 310)

Presentation
Tablets—500 mg

Actions and uses
See the section on sulphonamide drugs.

Dosage
The adult oral dosage is 1 g initially followed by 500 mg once daily.

Nurse monitoring
See the section on sulphonamide drugs.

General notes
The drug may be stored at room temperature.

SULPHAMETOPYRAZINE (Kelfezine W)

(See Note 3, p. 310)

Presentation
Tablets—2 g
Suspension—100 mg in 1 ml

Actions and uses
See the section on sulphonamide drugs.

Dosage
1. *Adults*: 2 g once per week
2. *Children*: 30 mg/kg once per week.

Nurse monitoring
See the section on sulphonamide drugs.

General notes
The drug may be stored at room temperature.

SULPHAPHENAZOLE (Orisulf)

(See Note 3, p. 310)

Presentation
Tablets—500 mg

Actions and uses
See the section on sulphonamides.

Dosage
Adults: 500 mg—2 g per day.

Nurse monitoring
See the section on sulphonamide drugs.

General notes
The drug may be stored at room temperature.

SULPHAPYRIDINE (M & B 693)

(See Note 3, p. 310)

Presentation
Tablets—500 mg

Actions and uses
Although a member of the sulphonamide group of drugs, Sulphapyridine is restricted in its use to two main clinical situations both of which are rare—namely dermatitis herpetiformis and pyoderma gangrenosa.

Dosage
1. For the treatment of dermatitis herpetiformis: 3–4 g in total per day initially. After the blisters have gone 0.5–1 g per day maintenance dose is then continued.
2. For the treatment of pyoderma gangrenosa: 1–2 g three to four times a day has been found to be effective.

Nurse monitoring
1. The Nurse monitoring notes for sulphonamide drugs apply to this drug.
2. Haemolytic anaemia has been caused in patients with glucose 6 phosphatase dehydrogenase deficiency.

General notes
The drug may be stored at room temperature.

SULPHASALAZINE (Salazopyrin)
Presentation
Tablets—0.5 g plain and enteric coated
Suppositories—0.5 g
Enema—3 g in 100 ml
Actions and uses
Sulphasalazine is a combination of two drugs:
1. An anti-inflammatory salicylic acid derivative
2. An anti-infective sulphonamide derivative, sulphapyridine.

It is used for the induction and maintenance of remission in ulcerative colitis, distal proctocolitis, stump proctitis and Crohn's disease.
Dosage
1. *Adults*: 1–2 g four times per day initially orally. Once remission of the disease has been obtained lower daily dosages i.e. 1.5–2 g in total per day may be sufficient.
2. *Children*: 40–60 mg/kg body weight daily initially, reducing to a maintenance dose of 20–30 mg/kg body weight.

The drug may also be given for a local effect via suppositories. These should be given morning and night after defaecation. An alternative local treatment is one enema given daily usually at bed time.
Nurse monitoring
1. It is important to note that Sulphasalazine is a combination of a salicylate and sulphonamide and therefore is contraindicated in patients with a history of allergy to sulphonamide drugs or salicylates.
2. The salicylate component may give any of the side effects described in the section on non-steroidal anti-inflammatory analgesic drugs (q.v.).
3. The sulphonamide component of Sulphasalazine can produce any of the side effects associated with sulphonamides (q.v.).

General notes
Preparations containing Sulphasalazine may be stored at room temperature. It is important that suppositories are not stored in a warm place e.g. near or above a radiator since they will readily melt.

SULPHINPYRAZONE (Anturan)
Presentation
Tablets—100 mg, 200 mg
Actions and uses
Sulphinpyrazone has two important actions:
1. It increases the urinary excretion of uric acid and urate and is therefore useful for the treatment of hyperuricaemia and gout. It has no analgesic properties and is therefore only useful for reducing blood urate in the long term.
2. It has an additional quite separate action in that it inhibits platelet breakdown, adhesion and aggregation and thus reduces the tendency for blood to clot. In clinical practice this action has led to it being given to patients after myocardial infarction to reduce the incidence of reinfarction or sudden death.

Dosage
1. Hyperuricaemia and gout: The initial dose of Sulphinpyrazone is 100–200 mg daily taken with meals or milk. The dosage is gradually increased over a week until the daily dosage of 600 mg is reached. After the blood urate concentration has been controlled the maintenance dose may be reduced to as low as 200 mg.
2. Following myocardial infarction: 200 mg four times daily is the prescribed dose. It is usual to commmence this about one month after the initial myocardial infarction.

The above doses are for adults only.
Nurse monitoring
1. The nurse may play an important role in helping to prevent the serious side effect of urate stone formation by monitoring carefully

patients' fluid intake and encouraging them to drink large quantities of fluid daily.
2. As Aspirin antagonises the uricosuric action of this drug the nurse may play an important role in detecting patients who are taking this drug in addition to prescribed medicines and advising them to stop, and also by educating all patients as to the necessity to avoid taking Aspirin at the same time as Sulphinpyrazone.
3. The drug may occasionally produce gastrointestinal upset and gastric bleeding and therefore must be used with caution in patients with a history of peptic ulcer disease.
4. Rare side effects for which withdrawal of treatment is necessary include skin rashes and blood dyscrasias (aplastic anaemia, leucopenia and thrombocytopenia).

General notes
Sulphinpyrazone tablets may be stored at room temperature.

SUPHONAMIDES

(See Note 3, p. 310)
Presentation
See individual compounds.
Actions and uses
The sulphonamide group of drugs although cemically unrelated to antibiotics are used for the prevention and treatment of a wide variety of diseases due to bacterial infection. The following sulphonamides are in current use:
Phthaylsulphathiazole
Succinylsulphathiazole
Sulphacetamide
Sulphadimethoxine
Sulphadimidine
Sulphafurazole
Sulphamethoxazole (in Cotrimoxazole)
Sulphamethoxypyridazine
Sulphametopyrazine
Sulphaphenazole
Sulphapyridine
Sulphasalazine

All bacteria require folic acid in order to be able to grow and multiply. This folic acid is usually synthesised by bacteria themselves within cells. Sulphonamides act by preventing the production of folic acid in bacterial cells. The sulphonamides have a bacteriostatic rather than bactericidal action. The former term means that they prevent further growth and reduplication of cells whereas the latter term implies that the drug actually kills cells already present in the body. In practice many organisms are found to be resistant to sulphonamides. This is because these organisms have developed alternative means of synthesising folic acid to the pathway of synthesis that is blocked by the drug. Sulphonamides have a wide range of action against both Gram-positive and Gram-negative organisms (see the section on antibiotics). They are used to treat a wide range of infections including bacterial diarrhoea, urinary infection, chest infection, bacterial meningitis, venereal disease and various dermatological infections.

Dosage
See individual drugs.
Nurse monitoring
1. Unless a high fluid intake and urine output is achieved there is a danger that patients receiving these drugs may suffer kidney damage due to crystallisation of the drug in the renal tract. The nurse may play an important role in both encouraging a high fluid intake and in monitoring urine output so that early warning of inadequate fluid intake may be obtained.
2. There are two important instances in which Sulphonamides may affect the action of other drugs concurrently being administered to patients:
   a. In diabetic patients on oral anti-diabetic drugs the sulphonamides may precipitate hypoglycaemia with dizziness, sweating, tachycardia, fainting and

eventually coma. Such patients should be carefully observed and warned of the dangers of this potential complication.
   b. In patients receiving the drug Warfarin for the purpose of anticoagulation the coincident administration of sulphonamides may lead to an increase in Warfarin's action with the resultant danger of severe haemorrhage. Regular checks on clotting function should therefore be made when sulphonamides are instituted in such cases.
3. Hypersensitivity reactions to sulphonamides may occur and these include skin rash, fever, joint pains and the more severe erythema multiforme and Stevens-Johnson syndrome.
4. As well as the danger of the drug precipitating into the kidney substance when fluid intake is poor, sulphonamides may have a direct damaging action on the kidney.
5. Sulphonamides may exert a wide range of toxic effects on the blood and bone marrow leading to megaloblastic anaemia, haemolytic anaemia, thrombocytopenia and aplastic anaemia. More rarely agranulocytosis (complete absence of white cells) with resultant risk of overwhelming infection may occur.
6. Liver damage and jaundice may occasionally occur. Jaundice is specially likely to occur in very young children, and may be dangerous. Such patients should not, therefore, receive sulphonamides.

SULTHIAME (Ospolot)
Presentation
Tablets—50 mg and 200 mg
Suspension—50 mg in 5 ml
Actions and uses
The actions and uses of anticonvulsant drugs in general are discussed in the section on these drugs.
Dosage
N.B. Individual dosage requirements vary greatly. The following doses are given as a guide only.
1. *Adults*: An initial dose of 100 mg twice per day is recommended. The optimum dose is usually 200 mg three times per day but should be tailored to individual needs.
2. *Children*: Recommended doses vary according to body weight as follows:
   a. Initial dose: 3–5 mg/kg daily in equal divided doses
   b. Maintenance dosage: This falls within the range of 10–15 mg/kg body weight daily in total, given in equal divided doses.
Nurse monitoring
1. The Nurse monitoring aspects of anticonvulsant drugs in general are discussed in the section on these drugs.
2. Side effects are usually mild and subside after 7–14 days of treatment. The nurse may play an important role, therefore, in encouraging the patient to continue treatment despite sometimes unpleasant side effects which include paraesthesia of the limbs and face giving symptoms of numbness and tingling, gastrointestinal upset, headache and dizziness.
3. If this drug is added to the regime of a patient already receiving Phenytoin, then toxicity due to Phenytoin may be produced. Phenytoin dosages should, therefore, be monitored and altered accordingly after the introduction of this drug.
General notes
The drug should be stored at room temperature.

SUPROFEN (Suprol)

Presentation
Capsules—200 mg

Actions and uses
Suprofen is a non-steroidal anti-inflammatory analgesic drug which is used primarily for its analgesic action, i.e. for the treatment of acute pain such as that occurring post-operatively, following dental surgery, etc. Since it also possesses an action which reduces inflammation, it is particularly useful for painful inflammatory conditions such as osteoarthritis and other skeletal-muscular disorders.

Dosage
Adults: 200 mg 3 or 4 times daily.

Nurse monitoring
See the section on anti-inflammatory analgesics, non-steroidal.

General notes
Suprofen capsules may be stored at room temperature.

SYNTOMETRINE (A combination of Ergometrine and Oxytocin)

Presentation
Syntometrine is available as a parenteral solution containing 500 µg of Ergometrine maleate and 5 units of Oxytocin in 1 ml.

Actions and uses
The combination of these two drugs is effective by intramuscular injection in the stimulation of uterine contraction. In clinical practice it is used mainly to stimulate uterine contraction and it may also be given to prevent or treat post-partum haemorrhage and to stimulate uterine contracture in labour.

Dosage
1. To stimulate uterine contraction and cessation of bleeding after birth of the placenta: An intramuscular injection of 1 ml is usually administered.
2. When used for the other reasons described above dosage varies according to the clinical practice of the centre concerned and the nurse is advised to seek advice from her local obstetric unit.

Nurse monitoring
1. High doses may cause excessive uterine contraction and dosage should therefore be carefully monitored to prevent the potentially disastrous occurrence of a ruptured uterus.
2. When high doses of Syntometrine are given with large volumes of electrolyte-free fluid, water intoxication may occur. Initially headache, anorexia, nausea, vomiting and abdominal pain may be the presenting features and this progresses to lethargy, drowsiness, unconsciousness and grand mal type seizures. The concentration of blood electrolytes may be markedly disturbed.

General notes
1. The drug should be protected from light.
2. The drug should be stored at room temperature.

T

TALAMPICILLIN (Talpen)

(*See Note 3, p. 310*)

Presentation
Tablets—250 mg
Syrup — 125 mg in 5 ml
250 my in 5 ml

Actions and uses
After absorption from the gastrointestinal tract, Talampicillin is converted to Ampicillin. Its actions and uses are therefore identical to Ampicillin (q.v.).

Dosage
1. *Adults*: 250 mg three times per day
2. *Children*:
   Less than 2 years: 3–7 mg/kg three times per day
   2 years and older: 125–250 mg three times per day.

Nurse monitoring
See the section on Ampicillin.

General notes
1. Preparations containing Talampicillin may be stored at room temperature.
2. Once reconstituted Talampicillin syrup should be used within seven days.

TAMOXIFEN (Nolvadex)

Presentation
Tablets—10 mg, 20 mg

Actions and uses
Tamoxifen is an oestrogen antagonist which has two major uses:
1. It is used in the treatment of breast cancer.
2. It is used to stimulate ovulation in patients suffering from infertility.

Dosage
1. For the treatment of breast cancer: 10–20 mg is given twice daily.
2. For the treatment of infertility: 10 mg is given twice daily on the second, third, fourth and fifth days of the menstrual cycles if patients are menstruating regularly. In women who are not menstruating the initial course may begin on any day.

Nurse monitoring
1. Because of its oestrogen antagonist action it frequently produces hot flushing, vaginal bleeding and pruritis vulvae.
2. Gastrointestinal upset, light headedness and fluid retention may occur.
3. Thrombocytopenia has been rarely reported.
4. When used for the treatment of breast cancer it may produce pain at the site of the tumour.

General notes
1. Tamoxifen tablets may be stored at room temperature.
2. The drug should be protected from light.

TEMAZEPAM (Normison, Euhypnos)

Presentation
Capsules—10 mg, 20 mg

Actions and uses
Temazepam is a benzodiazepine drug (q.v.). It has a marked sedative effect and is therefore taken at night as an hypnotic. It is particularly interesting to note that this drug has

a very short action. It therefore tends to produce less hang-over effect the following day and is particularly useful in treating insomnia in elderly patients where day time confusion can be avoided.

Dosage
10–60 mg taken on retiring. It is recommended that as low a dose as possible be used for elderly patients.

Nurse monitoring
See the section on benzodiazepines.

General notes
Preparations containing Temazepam may be stored at room temperature.

TERBUTALINE (Bricanyl)

Presentation
Tablets—5 mg, 7.5 mg sustained release
Syrup—0.3 mg in 1 ml
Inhalation—250 μg/dose of metered aerosol or 'spacer' inhaler.
2.5 or 10 mg/ml as respirator solution
Injection—0.5 mg in 1 ml

Actions and uses
1. This drug stimulates receptors known as beta$_2$ adrenergic receptors in the smooth muscle of the airways with the result that the airways dilate. It is used in clinical practice for the prevention and treatment of conditions such as asthma and chronic bronchitis which produce bronchospasm.
2. The drug may be administered to reduce uterine contraction in the management of premature labour.

Dosage
1. For the treatment of bronchospasm:
   a. By inhalation:
      i. Via metered aerosol: 1 or 2 inhalations three or four times a day.
      ii. For acute severe conditions respirator solution is administered via a suitable nebuliser.
   b. Orally: 5 mg two or three times daily for adults. Infants and children: 0.75—2.5 mg three times per day.
   c. Parenteral:
      i. By subcutaneous intramuscular and slow intravenous injection: 0.2–0.5 mg four times daily for adults. 0.01 mg/kg to a maximum dose of 0.3 mg in children.
      ii. By intravenous infusion: For adults 1.5–2.5 mg should be dissolved in 500 ml and administered at a rate of 10 to 20 drops per minute for 8–10 hours.
2. For the management of premature labour:
   10–25 μg/minute by intravenous infusion is recommended.

Nurse monitoring
1. Common side effects produced are muscle tremor, palpitation, tachycardia, flushing and headache.
2. The drug should be used with great caution in patients who have heart disease manifest by rhythm disturbance or angina, thyrotoxicosis and hypertension.

General notes
1. Preparations may be stored at room temperature.
2. Syrup may be diluted with water.
3. Injections may be diluted with Water for Injections, sodium chloride or dextrose.
4. Aerosols must not be punctured or incinerated after use.

TERFENADINE (Triludan)

Presentation
Tablets—60 mg
Suspension—30 mg in 5 ml

Actions and uses
Terfenadine is an antihistamine. The actions and uses of antihistamines in general are described in the antihistamine section. Terfenadine is used specifically:
1. To suppress generalised minor allergic responses to allergens such as foodstuffs and drugs.
2. To suppress local allergic reactions i.e. inflammatory skin

responses to insect stings and bites, contact allergens, urticaria, etc.
3. Orally for other allergic conditions e.g. hay fever and allergic rhinitis.

Dosage
1. *Adults*: 60 mg twice daily
2. *Children*: 6–12 years only should receive half the adult dose.

Nurse monitoring
1. See the section on antihistamines.
2. Studies with this drug indicate that sedation is less of a problem than with other antihistamines.

General notes
The drug may be stored at room temperature.

TESTOSTERONE (Sustanon, Testoral, Primoteston)

Presentation
Sublingual tablets—10 mg
Sustanon 100 contains—
Testosterone proprionate BP 20 mg, Testosterone Phenylproprionate 40 mg and Testosterone isocaproate 40 mg
Primoteston contains—250 mg of Testosterone enanthate

Actions and uses
The actions and uses of this androgenic hormone are discussed in the section dealing with these drugs.

Dosage
1. For the treatment of hypogonadism in males:
   a. 10–30 mg daily sublingually
   b. By depot administration dosages are administered at variable intervals according to patient response.
2. For the treatment of mammary carcinoma in females: 250 mg of the enanthate or 1 ml of Sustanon 100 or 250 every 2–6 weeks.

Nurse monitoring
See the section on androgenic hormones.

General notes
1. Preparations may be stored at room temperature.
2. Preparations should be protected from light.

TETRACYCLINE (Achromycin)

(*See Note 3, p. 310*)

Presentation
Tablets—250 mg
Capsules—250 mg
Syrup—125 mg in 5 ml
Injection—250 mg and 500 mg (intravenous). 100 mg (intramuscular)
Ointment—3%
Eye/ear ointment and eye drops—1%

Actions and uses
1. For general notes on actions and uses see Tetracyclines (q.v.).
2. Topical applications are available for use in skin, eye and ear infections. The drug is effective against local infections caused by both Gram-positive and Gram-negative organisms including streptococci, staphylococci and coliform organisms.

Dosage
1. *Adults*:
   a. Orally: 1–2 g daily in total taken in four divided doses half an hour before meals.
   b. By intramuscular injection: 200–300 mg in total daily administered in divided doses either 8 or 12-hourly.
   c. By intravenous injection: 1–2 g daily in total administered in divided doses either 8 or 12-hourly. When administered intravenously the drug should be dissolved in sodium chloride 0.9% or dextrose 5% injections, and infused over 6–12 hours. See Nurse monitoring notes below.
2. *Children*:
   Less than 1 year:
   i. Orally: 6.25 mg/kg four times a day
   ii. Intramuscularly: 2.5 mg/kg three times daily
   1–7 years:
   i. Orally: 62.5–125 mg four times a day

ii. Intramuscularly: 25–50 mg three times a day
iii. Intravenously: 62.5–125 mg four times a day.

Children over 7 years should receive half the adult doses described above

Nurse monitoring
1. See the section on Tetracyclines.
2. It should be noted that intramuscular tetracycline injections contain procaine (a local anaesthetic) to reduce pain at the injection site.
3. When given intravenously, the injections should be reconstituted by adding 5 ml of Water for Injections to the 250 mg vial or 10 ml to the 500 mg vial. The solution should then be diluted to a concentration not exceeding 500 mg in 500 ml with normal saline or 5% dextrose or sodium lactate compound injection B.P. The infusion should then be given over 6–12 hours to provide the dosage required.

General notes
1. The drug may be stored at room temperature.
2. Syrups should be used within one week of preparation.
3. Reconstituted injections for intravenous administration are stable at room temperature for 12 hours only.

TETRACYCLINES

(See Note 3, p. 310)
This group of antibiotic includes:
Chlortetracycline
Demethylchlortetracycline
Doxycycline
Methacycline
Minocycline
Oxytetracycline
Tetracycline

Actions and uses
The tetracycline group of antibiotics are bacteriostatic i.e. they prevent further growth and multiplication of bacteria but do not kill them. The mechanism of action is by interfering with the synthesis of proteins necessary for growth and division of bacterial cells.
Tetracyclines have a broad spectrum of activity against both Gram-positive and Gram-negative organisms. It is important to note that infections due to proteus and *Pseudomonas aeruginosa* are usually not sensitive to Tetracyclines. They are used for the following conditions:
1. They are frequently used to treat acute exacerbations of chronic bronchitis and upper and lower respiratory tract infections.
2. They are effective in the treatment of the following specific infections:
   a. Brucellosis
   b. Q-fever
   c. Infections due to rickettsia (typhus)
   d. Non-specific urethritis
   e. Sinusitis
   f. Pustular acne vulgaris
   g. Pneumonia due to mycoplasma and psittacosis
   h. Trachoma.
3. Topical applications for skin, eye and ear infections due to staphylococcal, streptococcal and coliform organisms are available.

Dosage
See specific drugs.

Nurse monitoring
1. Gastrointestinal upsets including heartburn, anorexia, nausea and vomiting may commonly occur with this drug. It is important to note that if the drug is given with milk or food to try to reduce these symptoms, the actual concentration absorbed may be reduced and therefore the treatment may be rendered ineffective. The nurse may play an important role in discouraging the patient from taking the tablets with milk or especailly antacids.
2. Diarrhoea may sometimes occur. This may be due to a change in the flora of the gut caused by tetracyclines but it may also be due to superinfection with proteus, pseudomonas or staphylococcus or *Clostridium*

difficile (the latter organism causing pseudomembranous enterocolitis). It is therefore recommended that the drug be discontinued if patients develop severe and persistent diarrhoea.
3. If the drug is taken during late pregnancy or administered to young children (less than 12 years of age), permanent staining of the teeth and bones may occur. This is because tetracyclines have been found to be taken up by growing bones and teeth. This group of drugs is therefore, for this reason, contraindicated in pregnant women and young children.
4. The drug is not recommended for administration to pregnant women for the following reasons:
   a. Their children's teeth may be permanently stained
   b. There is a risk of liver and pancreatic damage. Liver damage is especially likely if tetracyclines are given during pregnancy by the intravenous route.
5. Patients with impaired renal function should not given tetracyclines as they may worsen the degree of renal failure by inhibiting body protein synthesis.
6. Other adverse effects include photosensitivity reactions and hypersensitivity producing urticaria, asthma, dyspnoea, itching, oedema and hypotension.
7. Tetracyclines affect blood clotting function and therefore if they are given to patients already on anticoagulants, the anticoagulant dose may have to be altered.
8. The coincident administration of antacids, iron tablets and milk will all reduce the amount of tetracycline absorbed from the gut and may render its administration ineffective.
9. Superinfection with fungi i.e. oral candidiasis, or proteus, pseudomonas and staphylococcus may occur.

General notes
See specific drugs.

THEOPHYLLINE (Neulin, Pro-Vent, Slo-Phyllin, Theo-Dur, Theorgrad, Theosol, Uniphyllin)

Presentation
Tablets—125 mg
Tablets (slow release)—175 mg, 200 mg, 250 mg, 300 mg, 350 mg and 400 mg.
Capsules, slow release—60 mg, 125 mg, 250 mg and 300 mg.
Syrup—60 mg in 5 ml
Suppositories—300 mg

Actions and uses
Theophylline has the actions and uses described for Aminophylline though it is not water soluble and cannot therefore be produced in an injectable form.

Dosage
1. *Adults*:
   a. Oral: 125–250 mg (conventional tablets) taken 3 or 4 times daily. In most cases, slow release tablets or capsules are taken twice daily (one daily in the case of Uniphylline); the usual dose is one or two slow release tablets or capsules.
   b. Rectal: One or two suppositories, usually inserted at night for nocturnal wheeze.
2. *Children*:
   Oral: Initially a dose of up to 5 mg/kg body weight is given followed by maintenance doses of 2.5 mg/kg or more every 6 hours. Children aged 3–5 years or more should if possible take slow release preparations e.g. one or two tablets or capsules twice daily. For this purpose Slo-phyllin capsules may be preferred since they can be opened and taken as small pellets to facilitate administration.
3. *Premature infants*:
   Oral: For the management of apnoea, 3 mg/kg body weight is taken every 8 hours.

Nurse monitoring
See the section on Aminophylline.

General notes
See the section on Aminophylline.

THIABENDAZOLE (Mintezol)

Presentation
Tablets—500 mg

Actions and uses
Thiabendazole is an antihelminthic drug which is used both in the United Kingdom and in tropical countries for the treatment of:
1. Threadworm disease (enterobiasis)
2. Roundworm disease (Ascariasis)
3. Hookworm disease (due to *Necator americanis* or *Ankylostoma duodenale*)
4. Whipworm disease (Trichiniasis).

Dosage
Each dose given is dependent on body weight. The number of doses given is dependent on the disease under treatment.
Dosage with respect to weight is as follows:
 10 kg: 250 mg
 20 kg: 500 mg
 30 kg: 750 mg
 40 kg: 1 g
 50 kg: 1.25 g
 60 kg or over: 1.5 g
1. For the treatment of threadworm: Two doses are given on one day and again one week later.
2. For the treatment of strongyloidiasis, roundworm and hookworm disease and whipworm disease two doses are given each day for two successive days. Alternatively a single dose of 50 mg/kg may be given but this produces a higher incidence of side effects.
3. For the treatment of cutaneous larva migrans two doses per day for two successive days.
4. For the treatment of trichinosis two doses a day for 2–4 successive days.

Nurse monitoring
1. Patients should be reminded that tablets should be chewed prior to swallowing.
2. There is no need for dietary restriction, complementary medication or cleansing enemata.
3. Side effects are common especially with high single dosage treatment regimes and include anorexia, nausea, vomiting, dizziness, diarrhoea, epigastric pain, pruritis, weariness, giddiness, headache and drowsiness.
4. Hypersensitivity to the drug may result in fever, facial flushing, chills, angioneurotic oedema and more rarely anaphylactic shock.

General notes
The drug may be stored at room temperature.

THIAZIDE AND RELATED DIURETICS

 Bendrofluazide
 Chlorothiazide
 Chlorthalidone
 Cyclopethiazide
 Hydrochlorothiazide
 Hydroflumethiazide
 Mefruside
 Methyclothiazide
 Metolazone
 Polythiazide
 Xipamide

Actions and uses
Most of the plasma passing through the kidney is reabsorbed at various sites along the tubules of the kidney. Thiazide diuretics decrease the ability of the kidney to reabsorb sodium and water in the distal part of the tubules, thus increasing urine output. They are therefore useful in diseases where fluid accumulates in the form of oedema i.e. heart failure, nephrotic syndrome, and liver cell failure. In addition they have a direct action on blood vessel walls which leads to a reduction in blood pressure, and they may therefore be used in the treatment of hypertension.
Onset of action is within one to two hours and duration of action tends to be for some hours. They therefore produce a more gentle and long lasting diuresis than 'loop' diuretics, such as Frusemide (q.v.).

Dosage
See individual drugs.

Nurse monitoring
This group of drugs can cause important side effects which must

be detected as early as possible to prevent their potentially serious consequences.

1. Hypokalaemia: The patient may become apathetic and confused and may develop muscle weakness or abdominal distension. If these signs are noticed more serious effects of hypokalaemia such as potentially fatal cardiac arrhythmias in patients on Digoxin and coma in patients with liver cell failure, may be prevented. (In patients on Digoxin or with liver cell failure coincident administration of potassium supplements or a potassium-sparing diuretic such as Spironolactone is recommended.)
2. Dehydration may occur causing postural hypotension and collapse.
3. An increase in blood urate may occur causing gout. Joint pains in patients on these drugs should always make the nurse suspect this complication.
4. The drugs may alter glucose metabolism leading to hyperglycaemia and glycosuria. Thus any diabetic patient receiving these drugs should be followed up closely in case change in treatment is required.
5. Thrombocytopenia may occur very rarely. This may be detected initially by observing small haemorrhages or bruises in the skin and if confirmed by checking the platelet count the drug should be stopped.

THIETHYLPERAZINE (Torecan)

Presentation
Tablets—10 mg (expressed as the maleate salt)
Injection—10.86 mg (as maleate) in 1 ml (equivalent to 6.5 mg base)
Suppositories—Each equivalent to 6.5 mg base

Actions and uses
Thiethylperazine is a member of the phenothiazine group and its actions and uses are described in the section on these drugs. The drug is almost exclusively used for its antiemetic properties in the control of nausea and vomiting associated with drug therapy, radiotherapy, the post-operative period, etc. In addition, Thiethylperazine is of value for the symptomatic relief of vertigo and vomiting in neurological disorders such as Menière's disease.

Dosage
Adults (thiethylperazine is not recommended for use in children):
Oral: 10 mg (as maleate) two or three times a day
Injection: 6.5 mg (as base) by the intramuscular route
Suppositories: One suppository inserted morning and night.

Nurse monitoring
The Nurse monitoring aspects of this drug are described under phenothiazines (q.v.).

General notes
1. Prepartions containing Thiethylperazine may be stored at room temperature but they should be protected from direct sunlight.
2. Thiethylperazine injection must not be mixed with other drugs.

THIOGUANINE (Lanvis)

Presentation
Tablets—40 mg

Actions and uses
Thioguanine is a cytotoxic drug which is used for the treatment of acute leukaemia and chronic myeloid leukaemia.

Dosage
Adults and children: A single oral daily dose of 2–2.5 mg/kg body weight is usually given. Treatment courses may last from 5–20 days.

Nurse monitoring
1. Bone marrow suppression with resultant increased risk of haemorrhage, anaemia and infection is the most serious adverse effect from this drug. Frequent blood counts are

usually performed during treatment courses.
2. Symptoms commonly produced include nausea, vomiting, anorexia.
3. Stomatitis and jaundice due to altered liver function may occur with this drug.
4. Hyperuricaemia occasionally resulting in gout and impairment of renal function may be produced.

General notes
Thioguanine tablets may be stored at room temperature.

THIOPENTONE (Intraval)

Presentation
Injection—500 mg, 1 g, 2.5 g, 5 g vials for preparation of 2.5 or 5% solutions
Rectal—Thiopentone sodium solution has been administered rectally to produce sleep within 10–12 minutes.

Actions and uses
Thiopentone sodium is a barbiturate drug (q.v.) with a rapid onset and short duration of action. It has the following uses:
1. It may be administered intravenously to induce anaesthesia. The anaesthesia produced is of short duration when the drug is given alone.
2. It may be administered rectally to produce sleep, its onset of action being approximately 10–12 minutes.

Dosage
1. For induction of anaesthesia: A 2.5% or more occasionally a 5% solution is used and injected very slowly into a superficial vein. The total dosage administered is that required to induce anaesthesia and in general is not likely to be more than 500 mg. Doses in excess of 500 mg may be associated with an unnecessarily prolonged recovery time and other complications (see the section on barbiturates).
2. The dosage required for rectal administration to induce sleep is calculated on the basis of 1 g per 23 kg body weight. The required quantity is dissolved in 25 ml of water and instilled through a rectal catheter.

Nurse monitoring
See the section on barbiturates.

General notes
1. Vials containing Thiopentone sodium as dry powder may be stored at room temperature. When reconstituted however solutions readily break down producing cloudiness and precipitation or crystallisation. Solutions are therefore not suitable for prolonged storage and should be discarded immediately after use.
2. Solutions are strongly alkaline and therefore should not be mixed with other drugs in the same syringe.

THIOPROPAZATE (Dartalan)

Presentation
Tablet—5 mg, 10 mg

Actions and uses
Thiopropazate is a member of the phenothiazine group of drugs and its actions and uses are described in the section on these drugs.

Dosage
The recommended oral adult dose is 5–10 mg three times daily.

Nurse monitoring
See the section on phenothiazines.

General notes
The drug should be stored at room temperature.

THIORIDAZINE (Melleril)

Presentation
Tablets—10 mg, 25 mg, 50 mg, 100 mg
Syrup/suspension—25 mg in 5 ml. 100 mg in 5 ml

Actions and uses
Thioridazine is a member of the phenothiazine group of drugs and its actions and uses are described in

the section dealing with these drugs.

Dosage
1. *Adults*: According to individual requirements and the reason for treatment. The adult oral dose ranges from 30–600 mg daily in total. It is administered in three or four divided doses.
2. *Children*:
Under 5 years: 1 mg/kg body weight.
Over 5 years: one-quarter to one-half of the adult dose is administered.

Nurse monitoring
See the section on phenothiazines.

General notes
1. The drug should be stored at room temperature.
2. The drug should be protected from direct sunlight.

THYMOXAMINE (Opilon)

Presentation
Tablets—40 mg.
Injection—5 mg in 1 ml.
30 mg in 2 ml.

Actions and uses
Thymoxamine acts on the sympathetic nervous system and produces peripheral vasodilation. It is used in the treatment of peripheral vascular disease including Raynaud's disease, intermittent claudication, chilblains and frost bite.

Dosage
In adults:
1. Orally: 40 mg four times a day.
2. By intravenous bolus or intra-arterial bolus: 0.1 mg/kg four times daily.
3. By intravenous infusion: 30 mg in 500 mg sodium chloride 0.9% 6-hourly by continuous infusion.

Nurse monitoring
1. Nurse monitoring aspects of vasodilator drugs discussed under Nicofuranose apply to this drug.
2. The drug should be used with great caution in patients who have had a recent myocardial infarction, those who are at present on anti-hypertensive therapy and in diabetics (when insulin requirements may be altered).

General notes
1. Tablets should be stored at room temperature.
2. Injection solution should be stored in a refrigerator.

THYROID

Presentation
Tablets—60 mg

Actions and uses
Thyroid is a crude extract from the thyroid gland. Its actions and uses are similar to Thyroxine (q.v.), but it is very important to note that this is now an out-dated method of giving Thyroxine replacement and is not as reliable as administering pure Thyroxine.

Dosage
60 mg of thyroid extract is thought to be equivalent in activity to 0.1 mg of pure Thyroxine.

Nurse monitoring
See the section on Thyroxine.

General notes
Thyroid tablets may be stored at room temperature.

THYROXINE (Eltroxin)

Presentation
Tablets—25 μg (0.025 mg), 50 μg (0.05 mg), 100 μg (0.1 mg)

Actions and uses
Thyroxine is the hormone released by the thyroid gland which is essential for maintaining a normal metabolic rate. Deficiency leads to obesity, coarse skin and hair, hoarseness, constipation, impairment of intellect, an inability to tolerate cold temperatures and in severe cases it may lead to psychosis or coma. Thyroxine's primary use is in the treatment of disorders associated with under production of thyroid hormone.

Dosage
1. Replacement therapy may be taken orally once daily in the morning. It is not essential to take the drug any more than once a day as it takes a particularly long time for it to be metabolised and multiple daily dosages are of no benefit.
2. The actual dose necessary for patients is variable and is usually adjusted by observing clinical improvement and measuring thyroid hormone in the blood. Normal adult replacement doses vary between 0.05 and 0.2 mg per day.
3. It is essential that replacement therapy should be commenced at very low dosages and very cautiously in elderly patients and patients with ischaemic heart disease (see below).

Nurse monitoring
1. Any patient receiving Thyroxine is likely to be on this drug for life. As the effects of stopping taking the drug take some time to manifest themselves, patients may come to believe that the drug is unnecessary. As hypothyroidism has many effects on physical and mental function and in the long term may lead to death due to ischaemic heart disease, it is essential that all patients be encouraged to take replacement dosage regularly and the nurse may play a major role in encouraging patients to do this.
2. Thyroxine has no adverse effects when given in appropriate dosage. However, if too much is given too quickly, especially to elderly patients or patients with angina, severe angina or myocardial infarction may be precipitated. Such patients should receive initially as low doses as 0.025 mg on alternate days for the first 1-2 months followed by cautious increases in dose over the next six months or so to a full replacement regime.
3. Excessive dosage may produce anginal pain, cardiac dysrhythmias, palpitations, cramps, tachycardia, diarrhoea, restlessness, excitability, headache, flushing, sweating, weight loss and muscle weakness.
4. Any patients who have hypothyroidism due to inadequate pituitary function (hypopituitarism should always have steroid replacement treatment commenced before Thyroxine is commenced. Failure to do this may lead to death.

General notes
1. Tablets containing Thyroxine may be stored at room temperature.
2. The tablets should be protected from light.

TIAPROFENIC ACID (Surgam)

Presentation
Tablets—200 mg, 300 mg

Actions and uses
Tiaprofenic acid is a member of the propionic acid group of non-steroidal anti-inflammatory drugs. It therefore has the actions and uses of drugs described under anti-inflammatory analgesics, non-steroidal.

Dosage
Adults: 600 mg daily in divided doses

Nurse monitoring
The nurse monitoring notes for anti-inflammatory analgesics, non-steroidal, apply to this drug.

General notes
Tiaprofenic acid tablets may be stored at room temperature.

TICARCILLIN (Ticar)

(*See Note 3, p. 310*)

Presentation
Injection—1 g and 5 g vials

Actions and uses
Ticarcillin is a derivative of the Penicilling group of antibiotics. It has a much wider spectrum of activity than the parent drug Benzylpenicillin and is effective against many Gram-positive and Gram-negative organisms. Its mode of action is

identical to that described for Benzylpenicillin (q.v.). The indications for its use are for the treatment of infection at any site in the body where it is caused by an organism sensitive to Ticarcillin. It is of particular interest to note that Ticarcillin is often effective in the treatment of serious infections due to pseudomonas species which are commonly resistant to other antibiotics.

Dosage
1. *Adults*:
   a. For severe infection: 15–20 g at intervals of 6–8 hours
   b. For urinary tract infection: 4 g 6-hourly.
2. *Children*:
   a. For serious infection: 200–300 mg/kg body weight in total per day given in divided doses either 6 or 8-hourly
   b. For the treatment of urinary tract infection: 50–100 mg/kg body weight in total daily given in divided doses.

Nurse monitoring
See the section on Benzylpenicillin.

General notes
1. Ticarcillin injection may be stored at room temperature.
2. For intramuscular injection: 1 g vials are reconstituted with 2 ml of Water for Injections.
3. For intravenous bolus injection: Vials are prepared initially with 2 ml Water for Injections and diluted to 20 ml solution. They should be given over 3–4 minutes.
4. For intravenous infusion: The vials are diluted in the diluent provided. It is interesting to note that the solution warms as Ticarcillin dissolves. Rapid intravenous infusion should be given over 30–40 minutes.

TIMOLOL (Betim, Blocadren)

Presentation
Tablets—10 mg

Actions and uses
Timolol is a non-selective beta-adrenoreceptor blocking drug and its actions are described in the section on these drugs.

Dosage
The adult oral range is 15–60 mg daily in 2 or 3 divided doses.

Nurse monitoring
See the section on beta-adrenoreceptor blocking drugs.

General notes
Timolol tablets may be stored at room temperature.

TOBRAMYCIN (Nebcin)

(*See Note 3, p. 296*)

Presentation
Injection — 40 mg in 1 ml
20 mg in 2 ml
80 mg in 2 ml

Actions and uses
Tobramycin is an aminoglycoside antibiotic. Its actions and uses are described in the section on these drugs. It may occasionally be effective for the treatment of micro-organisms resistant to Gentamicin.

Dosage
The dosage for adults and children is calculated on the basis of 2–5 mg/kg in total per day usually given in three or four divided doses by the intramuscular or intravenous route. For the treatment of severe infection in neonates 4 mg/kg per day in total given in two divided doses may be used.

Nurse monitoring
1. The Nurse monitoring notes on aminoglycoside antibiotics (q.v.) apply to this drug, other than that Tobramycin may be administered by intravenous infusion.
2. When given by intravenous infusion the drug is diluted with 50–100 ml of normal saline or 5% dextrose in adults, and appropriately lower volumes in children. The infusion is administered over a period of 20–60 minutes.

General notes
The drug may be stored at room temperature.

TOCAINIDE (Tonocard)

Presentation
Tablets—400 mg and 600 mg
Injection — 750 mg in 5 ml (bolus injection)
— 750 mg in 75 ml (infusion)

Actions and uses
Tocainide has an antidysryhythmic action which resembles Lignocaine. It is administered intravenously in the treatment of serious ventricular dysrhythmias complicating myocardial infarction and thereafter for long term oral prophylaxis against recurrence.

Dosage
1. Intravenous: 500–750 mg by slow intravenous injection or by intravenous infusion over 15–30 minutes.
1. Oral: 600–800 mg administered immediately after injection then followed 8 hours later with a maintenance dose of 1200 mg in total daily in 2 or 3 divided doses.

Nurse monitoring
See the section on Lignocaine.

General notes
Preparations containing Tocainide are stored at room temperature.

TOLAZAMIDE (Tolanase)

Presentation
Tablets—100 mg, 250 mg

Actions and uses
See the section on oral hypoglycaemic drugs (1).

Dosage
100 mg—1 g daily in 2–3 divided doses.

Nurse monitoring
See the section on oral hypoglycaemic drugs (1).

General notes
Tablets may be stored at room temperature.

TOLBUTAMIDE (Rastinon, Pramidex)

Presentation
Tablets—500 mg

Actions and uses
See the section on oral hypoglycaemic drugs (1).

Dosage
500 mg to 1.5 g daily in 2–3 divided doses is recommended.

Nurse monitoring
See the section on oral hypoglycaemic drugs (1).

General notes
Tablets may be stored at room temperature.

TOLMETIN (Tolectin)

Presentation
Tablets—200 mg

Actions and uses
See the section on anti-inflammatory analgesic drugs, non-steroidal.

Dosage
The adult dose is 400 mg three times daily increased if necessary up to 900 mg daily in divided doses.

Nurse monitoring
See the section on non-steroidal anti-inflammatory analgesic drugs.

General notes
Tolmetin tablets may be stored at room temperature.

TRANEXAMIC ACID (Cyklokapron)

Presentation
Tablets—500 mg
Injection—500 mg in 5 ml

Actions and uses
The actions and uses of Tranexamic acid are identical to those described for Aminocaproic acid (q.v.).

Dosage
1. *Adults*:
   a. Orally: 1–1.5 g two or three times per day
   b. Intravenously: 500 mg–1 g by slow intravenous injection (at a rate of 1 ml per minute)
   c. As a bladder washout: 1 g in 1 litre of 0.9% sodium chloride irrigated at a rate of 1 ml per minute.
2. *Children*: Orally, 25 mg/kg two or three times per day.

Nurse monitoring
1. Common symptoms include gastrointestinal upset (nausea, vomiting and diarrhoea), postural hypotension and dizziness.
2. There is an increased incidence of thrombosis with this drug.
3. The risk of thrombosis is markedly increased if patients have reduced renal function or are concurrently receiving oral contraceptive medication.

General notes
The drug may be stored at room temperature.

TRANYLCYPROMINE (Parnate)
Presentation
Tablets—10 mg
Actions and uses
Tranylcypromine is a monoamine oxidase inhibiting drug. Its actions and uses are described in the section on these drugs.
Dosages
10 mg two or three times daily.
Nurse monitoring
See the section on monoamine oxidase inhibiting drugs.
General notes
Tranylcypromine tablets may be stored at room temperature.

TRAZIDONE (Molipaxin)
Presentation
Capsules—50 mg and 100 mg
Liquid—50 mg in 5 ml
Actions and uses
Trazidone is an anti-depressant drug which is derived from and is closely related chemically to tricyclic antidepressants. Its actions and uses are similar to those described for tricyclic antidepressants.
Dosage
Adults: 200–600 mg in total per day administered in two or three divided doses.
Nurse monitoring
See the section on tricyclic antidepressant drugs.

General notes
Capsules and liquid containing Trazidone may be stored at room temperature.

TRIAMCINOLONE (Adcortyl, Kenalog, Ledecort, Lederspan)
Presentation
Tablets—4 mg
Deep intramuscular injection—40 mg in 1 ml. 80 mg in 2 ml
Intra-articular injection—10 mg in 1 ml. 50 mg in 5 ml
Cream, ointment, lotion and dental paste—0.1%
Topical spray—0.006%
Actions and uses
Triamcinolone is a corticosteroid drug and has actions and uses as described in the section on these drugs. It is used by a number of routes for conditions as follows:
1. It is administered topically for the management of inflammatory skin conditions.
2. It may be given orally as a dental paste.
3. It may be taken orally or administered by deep intramuscular injection for hay fever or asthma.
4. Direct intra-articular injection may be given where appropriate for such conditions as arthritis, bursitis and tendonitis.

Dosage
1. Topical applications are applied two to four times daily sparingly.
2. Dental paste is applied two to four times daily.
3. Oral doses depend on the type of disease under treatment and the severity of the symptoms and it is impossible to give relevant instances.
4. For intra-articular injection, 2–20 mg is given according to joint size.

Nurse monitoring
See the section on corticosteroid drugs.
General notes
1. Preparations containing Triamcinolone may be stored at room temperature.

2. Tablets must be protected from moisture.

TRIAMTERENE (Dytac)

Presentation
Capsules—50 mg
Also combined with thiazide diuretics in Dyazide and Dytide.

Actions and uses
Triamterene has a very mild diuretic action. It achieves this by inhibition of sodium excretion in the distal tubules with resultant sodium and water loss in the urine. As a diuretic alone it is of little use. However, it has an action on the renal tubule which reduces potassium excretion and it may therefore be used usefully in combination with thiazide diuretics to prevent the common dangerous side effect of hypokalaemia encountered when thiazide diuretics are given alone. Hypokalaemia is particularly serious in patients who are on Digoxin treatment or in those with serious hepatic dysfunction such as cirrhosis.

Dosage
The usual daily dose is 50 mg once or twice daily. Triamterene produces maximum effect after 8 hours and its actions may continue for 2–3 days after therapy is withdrawn.

Nurse monitoring
1. By far the most important problem which may arise in patients on Triamterene is the development of hyperkalaemia which is especially likely to occur if patients have impaired renal function. Hyperkalaemia is difficult to detect clinically and is extremely dangerous because of the possibility of precipitation of cardiac arrest.
2. Side effects are infrequent but nausea, vomiting, leg cramps and dizziness may occur.
3. In common with other diuretics Triamterene may alter blood glucose levels and therefore treatment requirements in patients with diabetes mellitus may be altered.

General notes
Triamterene capsules may be stored at room temperature.

TRIAZOLAM (Halcion)

Presentation
Tablets—0.125 mg, 0.25 mg

Actions and uses
Triazolam is a benzodiazepine-like compound (q.v.) which has a marked sedative effect and is taken at night as an hypnotic. Of particular interest is the very short action of this drug in the body which tends to reduce the hang-over effect which occasionally extends into the following day with other hypnotics. It may have a particular role therefore in producing sleep in elderly patients who are very sensitive to the prolonged sedative effect of similar hypnotics.

Dosage
0.125–0.25 mg taken on retiring. The lower dose is recommended for elderly patients.

Nurse monitoring
1. See the section on benzodiazepines.
2. A few reports have suggested that this drug may be associated with an unusual range of central excitatory effects such as agitation, and acute psychotic reaction. These effects are only usually seen with high dosage.

General notes
Tablets containing Triazolam may be stored at room temperature.

TRICLOFOS

Presentation
Elixir—500 mg in 5 ml

Actions and uses
Triclofos is a general central nervous system sedative which is used to induce sleep and which is particularly favoured for young and elderly patients. It owes its activity to its conversion in the body to trichloroethanol and in this respect it is similar to Chloral Hydrate.

Triclofos is, however, usually preferred to Chloral Hydrate since it is more palatable and produces a lower incidence of gastrointestinal upset.

Dosage
1. *Adults*: Usually 1 g on retiring though 2 g may occasionally be necessary.
2. *Children*:
   Up to 1 year—25–30 mg/kg body weight
   1–5 years—250–500 mg
   Up to 12 years—500 mg–1 g

Nurse monitoring
1. Triclofos mixture is generally palatable and non-irritant to the gastrointestinal tract. There are therefore few patients who are unable to tolerate this drug.
2. Triclofos and Chloral Hydrate are converted in the body to the same active substance and, for this reason, patients unable to tolerate Chloral Hydrate may receive Triclofos as an alternative. In such cases it should be noted that 1 g Triclofos is equivalent to 600 mg Chloral Hydrate.
3. Where the standard mixture is diluted for ease of administration, e.g. young children, diluted elixir can not be used more than 2 weeks after dilution and any unused quantity should therefore be discarded.

General notes
Triclofos elixir should be stored in room temperature.

TRICYCLIC ANTIDEPRESSANTS

Amitriptyline
Butriptyline
Clomipramine
Desipramine
Dothiepin
Doxepin
Imipramine
Iprindole
Maprotiline
Nortriptyline
Protriptyline
Trimipramine

Actions and uses.
1. These drugs are used for the treatment of depression caused by either pscychotic disturbance (endogenous depression) or as a reaction to a precipitating factor such as the death of a close relative (reactive depression). The precise mechanism of action of tricyclic antidepressants is not clearly understood.
2. Some tricyclic antidepressants have marked sedative properties and are therefore very effective in treating depressed patients who also have features of agitation or anxiety. Conversely other drugs in the group tend to raise mood and are particularly useful when depression is accompanied by marked retardation.
3. This group of drugs has been used in other situations which are as follows:
   a. They have been used successfully in the treatment of enuresis in childhood
   b. Trimipramine has been used in the treatment of peptic ulcer disease.

Dosage
See individual drugs.

Nurse monitoring
1. Perhaps the most important point to make about tricyclic drugs is that they take a number of weeks to exert their antidepressant effect. As the effect is delayed and as depressed patients may be particularly prone to fail to comply with treatment, the nurse may play an important role in ensuring that the patient knows that the drug is not meant to take effect for a number of weeks and in encouraging the patient to continue with treatment during this period.
2. Tricyclic drugs lower the seizure threshold and therefore increase the frequency of fitting in epileptic patients. They should therefore be avoided in epileptic patients if at all possible.
3. The total daily dose may be

taken once in the evening if a sedative effect during the day is not required. This has the added benefit of helping patients get to sleep.
4. Tricyclic drugs have anticholinergic or 'atropine-like' effects, which are particularly likely to occur during the early period of treatment and may be particularly troublesome in elderly patients. These effects include dry mouth, blurred vision, constipation, urinary retention and tachycardia.
   a. Constipation may lead to paralytic ileus
   b. Blurred vision is due to pupillary dilatation and these drugs should be used with caution in patients with glaucoma
   c. Urinary retention may be particularly troublesome in patients with symptoms of prostatism.
5. Other side effects include gastrointestinal upset such as gastric pain, anorexia, nausea and vomiting, fatigue, malaise, dizziness, confusion, cardiac conduction defects and hypotension. The latter two effects indicate that the drug should be used with caution in patients with a history of heart disease.
6. It is recommended that patients receiving tricyclic antidepressants should not concurrently receive a monoamine oxidase inhibitor antidepressant.
7. Large doses of tricyclic antidepressants have caused hyperpyrexia, convulsions, circulatory failure, cardiac arrest, respiratory failure, cyanosis, coma and death.
8. Deaths have also occurred from agranulocytosis and jaundice.

TRIFLUOPERAZINE (Stelazine)

Presentation
Tablets—1 mg, 5 mg
Capsules—2 mg, 10 mg, 15 mg (all slow release)
Syrup—1 mg in 5 ml
Concentrated syrup—10 mg in 1 ml
Injection—1 mg in 1 ml

Actions and uses
Trifluoperazine is a member of the phenothiazine group of drugs and its actions and uses are described in the section on these drugs.

Dosage
1. *Adults*:
   a. Orally: 2–15 mg per day in total is given either in two divided doses or as a single dose of the slow release capsule
   b. 1–6 mg daily has been given by deep intramuscular injection.
2. *Children*:
   Less than 5 years: Up to 1 mg in total per day can be administered.
   5–12 years: Up to 4 mg per day in divided doses is administered. Intramuscularly a dose of 1 mg/20 kg body weight daily should be administered and the dosage thereafter should be adjusted according to individual response.

Nurse monitoring
See the section on phenothiazines.

General notes
1. The drug should be stored at room temperature.
2. Liquid preparations should be protected from direct sunlight.

TRIMEPRAZINE (Vallergan)

Presentation
Tablets—10 mg
Syrup — 7.5 mg in 5 ml
         30 mg in 5 ml

Actions and uses
Trimeprazine is a member of the phenothiazine group of drugs which is particularly valuable in the following situations:
1. It is widely used for its

antiemetic and sedative effect in the treatment of children with vomiting.
2. It is widely used as an antipruritic drug for the treatment of itch associated with dermatological conditions such as urticaria and jaundice.
3. It is also used for the preoperative medication of children.

Dosage
1. When used as a sedative in children:
Less than 1 year old: 0.25 mg/kg is administered three times daily. Between 1 and 7 years of age: 2.5–5 mg is administered three times daily.
2. For the treatment of pruritis: 10–40 mg per day for adults and 7.5–25 mg daily for children in three or four divided doses is given. In severe cases adults may receive up to 100 mg per day.
3. For pre-operative medication of children either 2–5 mg/kg body weight by mouth or 600–900 μ/kg by deep intramuscular injection is administered.

Nurse monitoring
Apart from unwanted drowsiness or sedation Trimeprazine does not cause any of the many problems caused by other phenothiazines (q.v.).

General notes
1. The drug should be stored at room temperature.
2. Liquid preparations should be protected from direct sunlight.

TRIMETHOPRIM (Ipral, Trimopan)

(*See also Co-trimoxazole and Note 3, p. 310*)

Presentation
Tablets—100 mg
Suspension—10 mg in 1 ml

Actions and uses
Trimethoprim is an antibacterial agent which prevents the growth of bacteria by inhibiting the synthesis of the cellular constituent folinic acid within the cell. This substance is essential for growth and division of bacteria. The drug has two main uses:
1. It is used in combination with a sulphonamide under the name Co-trimoxazole (q.v.)
2. It can be used alone for the prevention and treatment of urinary tract infections.

Dosage
1. For the treatment of urinary tract infection:
   a. The adult dose is 200 mg twice daily orally
   b. Children's dosages should be calculated on the basis of 3 mg/kg twice daily.
2. For prophylaxis of urinary tract infections:
   a. The adult dose should be 100 mg at night.
   b. Children's doses should be calculated on the basis of 2.5 mg/kg given in a single dose at night.

Nurse monitoring
1. If taken in short courses, very few problems are encountered with this drug. Occasionally nausea and vomiting occur and more rarely megaloblastic anaemia. This latter effect may be prevented by concurrent administration of folinic acid.
2. Because of its potential to interfere with the metabolism of folic acid in cells, the drug is not recommended for use during pregnancy or for administration to very young children.

General notes
The drug may be stored at room temperature.

TRIMIPRAMINE (Surmontil)

Presentation
Tablets—10 mg, 25 mg
Capsules—50 mg

Actions and uses
Trimipramine is a tricyclic antidepressant drug. Its actions and uses in general are described in the section on these drugs. It should be

noted that Trimipramine has a marked sedative action and is particularly useful where depression is associated with sleep disturbance, anxiety or agitation.

Dosage
For the treatment of depression in adults 50–100 mg is given at night two hours before retiring. Alternatively the dose may be given twice a day i.e. 25 mg at mid-day and 50 mg late in the evening.

Nurse monitoring
1. See the general Nurse monitoring notes in the section on tricyclic antidepressant drugs.
2. As this drug has a marked sedative action it should only be given during the day if it is felt that the sedative action would be advantageous i.e. if patients are particularly anxious or agitated.

General notes
Trimipramine tablets may be stored at room temperature.

TRIPROLIDINE (Actidil, Pro-Actidil)

Presentation
Tablets — 2.5 mg
10 mg (slow release)
Elixir—2 mg in 5 ml

Actions and uses
Triprolidine is an antihistamine. The actions and uses of antihistamines in general are described in the section on these drugs. In clinical practice it is used as a nasal decongestant i.e. in the treatment of allergic rhinitis and hay fever. It is occasionally added to proprietary cough preparations, again because of its decongestant action.

Dosage
1. *Adults*: 2.5–5 mg 4 to 6-hourly or 10 mg slow release tablet once per day.
2. *Children*: 1–3 mg of standard preparation 4–6 hourly.

Nurse monitoring
See the section on antihistamines.

General notes
The drug may be stored at room temperature.

TRI-POTASSIUM DI-CITRATO BISMUTHATE (De-Nol)

Presentation
Tablets—120 mg
Liquid—120 mg in 5 ml

Actions and uses
When this drug is exposed to the acid in the stomach it forms a complex which is thought to coat the surface of the ulcer bed preventing further acid from reaching it and therefore reducing further damage to that area. It is effective in the treatment of both gastric and duodenal ulcers.

Dosage
1. *Adults*: 120 mg (5 ml) is diluted to 15 ml with water and taken four times a day on an empty stomach half an hour before each of the three main meals and 2 hours after the last meal of the day. A higher dosage i.e. 240 mg six times daily taken half an hour before and 2 hours after each of the main meals is sometimes necessary, especially in the treatment of duodenal ulcers. The recommended length of treatment is 28 days.
2. *Adults*: One tablet is chewed and swallowed with water four times a day 30 minutes before meals and two hours after the last meal of the day.
3. *Children*: Adult dosages have been used.

Nurse monitoring
1. It is important to note that the drug causes a dark staining of the tongue and tends to blacken the colour of the stool. Patients may find this distressing especially if they have not been warned of the possibility of these effects occurring prior to starting the drug.
2. Difficulties with compliance are often experienced because the drug has a foul taste and ammoniacal odour.
3. Apart from the inconvenient effects mentioned above, the drug is not associated with any major side effects.

General notes
Tri-potassium di-citrato bismuthate liquid may be stored at room temperature.

TROXIDONE (Tridione)

Presentation
Capsules—300 mg

Actions and uses
This drug has in the past been found to be useful for the treatment of petit mal epilepsy but in clinical practice it is now rarely used.

Dosage
N.B. Individual dosage requirements vary greatly. The following doses are given as a guide only.
1. *adults*: An initial dose of 900 mg per day in divided doses is recommended. This should be increased at weekly or fortnightly intervals by 300 mg per day until the disorder has been controlled or toxic symptoms appear. A maximum dosage of 1800 mg per day is recommended.
2. *Children*: An initial dose of 600 mg per day in divided doses should be given and increased at weekly or fortnightly intervals to a maximum of 1200 mg per day.

Nurse monitoring
1. The Nurse monitoring aspects of anticonvulsants in general are discussed in the section on these drugs.
2. The commonest side effect seen with this drug is drowsiness, which tends to subside with continued treatment and patients should be encouraged to continue with their treatment if this is the only side effect produced.
3. The drug is associated with many other less frequent side effects including gastrointestinal upset, skin rash, bleeding of the gums and nose, haemorrhage into the skin and retina, vaginal bleeding, and blood disorders including thrombocytopenia, leucopenia, aplastic anaemia, neutropenia and agranulocytosis. Fluctuations in blood pressure, hepatitis, renal damage and seizure are less common side effects. As a result of these many and varied side effects it is essential that patients on this drug be strictly medically supervised and have blood and urine tests at monthly intervals. If jaundice or other signs of hepatitis appear or albumin appears in the urine the drug should be immediately withdrawn.
4. The drug should not be used in patients with severe liver or renal impairment or blood dyscrasias.
5. The drug should be used with great caution in patients who have disease of the retina or optic nerve.
6. The drug is not recommended for use in pregnancy.

General notes
The drug should be stored at room temperature.

U

UROKINASE

Presentation
Single ampoules of 5000, 25 000 and 100 000 Ploug units

Actions and uses
This enzyme stimulates the process by which blood clots are dissolved. In clinical practice it is administered locally for the treatment of secondary hyphema, vitreous haemorrhage and clotted arteriovenous shunts. It has a number of other uses which are as yet at the experimental stage.

Dosage
1. Hyphema: 5000 units are dissolved in 2 ml of sterile saline and instilled locally.
2. Vitreous haemorrhage: 5000–25 000 units of Urokinase dissolved in 0.5–1.5 ml of sterile water are introduced into the eye.
3. Clotted arterio-venous shunt: 5000–25 000 units of Urokinase in 2–3 ml of saline are instilled into the effective limb of the shunt which is then clamped off for 2–4 hours.

Nurse monitoring
1. Any evidence of active bleeding or a bleeding disorder is an absolute contraindication to the administration of this drug.
2. High-dosage Urokinase therapy carries the risk of inducing haemorrhage, particularly cerebral haemorrahge in patients with severe hypertension.

General notes
1. Lyophilised Urokinase is extremely stable and may be stored at 4 °C for at least 5 years.
2. Aqueous sulotions at 4 °C retain their activity for 3–4 days.

URSODEOXYCHOLIC ACID (Destolit)

Presentation
Tablets—150 mg

Actions and uses
This drug is chemically related to Chenodeoxycholic Acid and has the actions and uses described in the section on Chenodeoxycholic Acid.

Dosage
Adults: The effective range is 4–10 mg/kg body weight which approximates to 3 or 4 tablets daily in two divided doses (after meals) for most cases. Treatment should not extend beyond 2 years and should continue for 3–4 months after radiological disappearance of the gallstones.

Nurse monitoring
1. The Nurse monitoring aspects of Chenodeoxycholic Acid apply to this drug.
2. It should be noted that a lesser incidence of diarrhoea than with Chenodeoxycholic Acid occurs.

General notes
Tablets should be stored at room temperature when they have a shelf life of 3 years.

V

VANCOMYCIN (Vancocin)

(See Note 3, p. 310)

Presentation
Injection—500 mg
Powder for oral use—10 g quantities

Actions and uses
This antibiotic has a bactericidal action i.e. it kills bacteria present in the body. It is effective against a wide range of Gram-positive bacteria. At present its use is limited to situations where other less toxic antibiotics such as Penicillins or Cephalosporins have been shown to be ineffective or where patients with severe infection are known to be allergic to Penicillin or Cephalosporins.

Dosage
1. Oral: The adult oral dosage is 500 mg four times a day.
2. Intravenous infusion:
   a. *Adults*: 500 mg 6-hourly or 1 g 12-hourly
   b. *Children*: 20 mg/lb body weight daily.

Nurse monitoring
1. As noted above Vancomycin is a highly toxic drug and its use should be restricted to the situations described above.
2. The intravenous administration of Vancomycin leads to frequent toxic effects including nausea, chill, fever, urticaria, other skin rashes and occasionally anaphylaxis with resultant shock.
3. The intravenous injections are very irritant and frequently produce severe pain and thrombophlebitis at injection sites.
4. Intravenous injections should be diluted to a volume of at least 200 ml with normal saline or 5% dextrose and given over 20–30 minutes at appropriate intervals.
5. In high doses the drug is toxic to the auditory nerve (producing deafness) and the kidney. It is therefore contraindicated in patients with renal failure.
6. The oral drug is less well absorbed and produces less severe toxic effects.

General notes
The drug may be stored at room temperature.

VERAPAMIL (Cordilox)

Presentation
Tablets—40 mg, 80 mg, 120 mg
Injection—5 mg in 2 ml

Actions and uses
The actions and uses of Verapamil may be divided into two major groups:
1. It decreases the oxygen requirement of the heart muscle and also reduces peripheral resistance. These two actions make it useful in the treatment of angina pectoris.
2. It has also been found to be useful for the abolition of supraventricular dysrhythmias. It is thought that the drug acts by influencing the movement of calcium ions across cell membranes.

Dosage
1. *Adults*:
   a. Intravenously for cardiac dysrhythmias, 5 mg repeated after intervals of 5–10 minutes until the dysrhythmia

is controlled. It may also be given by infusion in a dose of 5–10 mg per hour up to a total daily dose of 25–100 mg.
  b. The oral maintenance dose for the prophylaxis of angina is 40–120 mg three times a day.
2. *Children*: The intravenous dose for cardiac dysrhythmias is as follows:
   Neonates: 0.75–1 mg
   Infants: 0.75–2 mg
   1–5 years: 2–3 mg
   6–15 years: 2.5–5 mg

Nurse monitoring
1. The most important point to remember with this drug is that it should never be given to patients who are already receiving or have in the immediate past received beta-adrenergic blocking drugs as the combination of these two can lead to complete cessation of heart function.
2. As Verapamil can produce hypotension when given intravenously patients should be placed in the supine position prior to receiving such therapy.
3. The oral preparation of the drug is associated with few side effects of which nausea and vomiting are the commonest.
4. If the drug is given to patients who have heart failure their symptoms are likely to be worsened.

General notes
Verapamil tablets and injection may be stored at room temperature. When given by intravenous infusion the solution may be added to sodium chloride, dextrose or laevulose injections.

VIDARABINE (Vira-A)

Presentation
Injection—200 mg/ml (5 ml vial)
Eye ointment—3%

Actions and uses
1. This anti-viral agent may be given by intravenous injection for the treatment of herpes zoster (shingles) and chickenpox. In normal individuals these diseases are not likely to be life-threatening and therefore the drug should only be given to patients whose body defence systems are compromised by drug treatment or other disease such as patients with immunosuppression disorders, cancer or leukaemia.
2. The eye ointment may be used successfully for the treatment of herpetic keratoconjunctivitis.

Dosage
1. By intravenous injection the drug should be diluted in 500 ml of 5% dextrose or 0.9% sodium chloride or dextrose/saline mixtures. Each 500 ml of infusion fluid should contain, at a maximum, 225 mg. A total daily dose of 10 mg/kg body weight should be administered, slowly over 12–24 hours.
2. Eye ointment should be instilled five times daily initially, reducing subsequently to twice daily.

Nurse monitoring
1. The ophthalmic preparation may lead to lacrimation (excess tear formation), a sense of irritation and a feeling as if there is a foreign body in the eye, a burning sensation, pain and photophobia (pain on exposure to light).
2. Intravenous administration is associated with the following problems:
   a. Anorexia, nausea, vomiting and diarrhoea may commonly occur.
   b. Tremors, dizziness, hallucinations, confusion, psychotic reaction and ataxia may also occur.
   c. The total number of white cells and platelets in the blood may be reduced leading to an increased susceptibility to infection and bleeding disorders.
   d. Less commonly, weight loss, malaise, pruritis, rash and haematemesis may occur
   e. Pain at injection sites is common

f. The drug should be administered with great caution to patients with impaired renal function.

General notes
1. The injection may be stored at room temperature.
2. The ophthalmic preparation should be stored in a refrigerator.

VINBLASTINE (Velbe)

Presentation
Injection—10 mg vials with 10 ml special solvent

Actions and uses
Vinblastine's actions are similar to those described for Vincristine (q.v.). Its uses are as follows:
1. It has been found to be of most value in the management of Hodgkin's disease and other lymphomas.
2. It has also been used in combination with other drugs in the treatment of a variety of solid tumours including neuroblastoma, breast cancer, testicular cancer and resistant choriocarcinoma.

Dosage
The drug is given by intravenous injection at weekly intervals. The dose range is 1–10 mg and varies with the type of condition treated and the state of the patient.

Nurse monitoring
1. Vinblastine more commonly affects the bone marrow than Vincristine and therefore patients receiving this drug are at increased risk of severe infection and haemorrhage.
2. Vinblastine may cause slight neurotoxicity but this effect is not as severe as that seen with Vincristine.
3. Gastrointestinal effects include blistering in the mouth, anorexia, nausea, vomiting, constipation, paralytic ileus, abdominal pain, pharyngitis, bleeding from the healed peptic ulcer sites.
4. Other adverse effects include hair loss, malaise, weakness, dizziness and pain at the tumour site.
5. Leakage from intravenous injection sites produces severe irritation, cellulitis and phlebitis.
6. The drug is contraindicated in pregnancy.
7. The nurse should be constantly aware that most cytotoxic drugs are irritant to the skin and mucous surfaces, and are in general very toxic. Great care should therefore be exercised when handling these drugs, and in particular spillage or contamination of personnel or the environment must be avoided. If cytotoxic drugs are handled regularly it is theoretically possible that repeated skin contact or inhalation may produce systemic toxic effects and in nurses who have developed hypersensitivity, severe local and general hypersensitivity reactions.

General notes
1. Vinblastine ampoules should be stored in a refrigerator.
2. It is given by intravenous injection either directly or via the drip tubing of a running 0.9% sodium chloride infusion.
3. Reconstituted solutions may be stored in a refrigerator for up to 30 days if the special diluent (containing a bacteriocide) is used. Alternatively reconstituted solution should not be used after 48 hours.

VINCRISTINE (Oncovin)

Presentation
Injection—1 mg, 2 mg and 5 mg vials with 10 ml special solvent. Also available as ready mixed solutions.

Actions and uses
Vincristine is a cytotoxic drug, the action of which is incompletely understood. It has, however, been shown to interfere with the synthesis of both DNA and RNA and to affect chromosome multiplication all of which are necessary for cell division. Its uses are as follows:
1. It has been found to be

particularly of value in inducing remission in acute lymphatic leukaemia.
2. It has also been found particularly useful in the management of advanced Hodgkin's disease and other lymphomas.
3. Other malignancies which have been shown to respond to treatment with this drug include neuroblastoma, Wilms' tumour (kidney tumour occurring mainly in children) and rhabdomyosarcoma (a tumour affecting skeletal muscles).

Dosage

Vincristine is given by intravenous injection:
1. For the treatment of acute leukaemias in children:
   a. Initial dosage is 0.05 mg/kg body weight. This is gradually increased to a maximum of 0.15 mg/kg body weight by sequential injection.
   b. Weekly maintenance doses of 0.05–0.075 mg/kg body weight may be given following remission.
2. In the treatment of adult leukaemia: A weekly dose of 0.025–0.075 mg/kg body weight is used.
3. In the treatment of other malignancies: Weekly injections of 0.025 mg/kg are given until an effect is obtained and this effect may be maintained with lower weekly doses of about 0.005–0.01 mg/kg.

N.B. Because the difference between therapeutic and toxic doses is very small it is important to establish carefully dosage requirements for individual patients.

Nurse monitoring

1. Bone marrow suppression is less common with this drug than with many other cytotoxics but if it occurs the patient will be at risk of serious infection and haemorrhage.
2. The most important side effect of Vincristine is neurotoxicity which most frequently presents as peripheral neuropathy either sensory, motor or mixed. Initial symptoms may be slight and patients may complain of tingling or numbness in the fingers and toes. Subsequently tendon reflexes may disappear. If the early signs of neurotoxicity are ignored damage may progress and be irreversible. Thus patients must be closely questioned about the development of these symptoms and if present the drug should be immediately stopped.
3. Gastrointestinal effects may occur and include anorexia, nausea, vomiting, constipation or diarrhoea. Oral ulceration and abdominal cramps are also known to occur. Constipation may be particularly severe in the elderly and may give rise to intestinal obstruction.
4. The most common side effects include diplopia, malaise, depression, headache and psychotic reactions. Alopecia, weight loss and fluid retention, or low serum sodium due to inappropriate secretion of antidiuretic hormone have been known to occur.
5. Leakage into surrounding tissues after intravenous injection causes severe irritation. If administered via the drip tubing of a running 0.9% sodium chloride infusion it is important to check first whether the infusion is working correctly and to look for signs of local leakage before administering the drug.
6. The drug is contraindicated in pregnancy.
7. The nurse should be constantly aware that most cytotoxic drugs are irritant to the skin and mucous surfaces, and are in general very toxic. Great care should therefore be exercised when handling these drugs, and in particular spillage or contamination of personnel or the environment must be avoided. If cytotoxic drugs are handled regularly it is theoretically possible that repeated skin contact or

inhalation may produce systemic toxic effects and in nurses who have developed hypersensitivity, severe local and general hypersensitivity reactions.

General notes
1. Vincristine vials should be stored in a refrigerator.
2. When given intravenously a suitable injection time is about one minute.
3. Reconstituted solution may be stored in a refrigerator for up to 14 days without significant loss of potency, providing the special solvent (containing a bactericide) is used in its preparation. If this is inconvenient, ready mixed solutions may be used.

VINDESINE (Eldesine)

Presentation
Injection—5 mg vials with 5 ml special solvent

Actions and uses
Vindesine's actions are similar to those described for Vincristine. Its uses are as follows:
1. In the treatment of acute lymphoblastic leukaemia in childhood resistant to standard treatments.
2. In blast crisis phases of chronic myeloid leukaemia.
3. In malignant melanoma resistant to standard treatments.

Dosage
Usually 3–5 mg per square metre of body surface area, given by bolus intravenous injection at weekly intervals.

Nurse monitoring
See the section on Vincristine.

General notes
1. Vindesine ampoules should be stored in a refrigerator.
2. It is given by intravenous injection either directly or via the drip tubing of a running 0.9% sodium chloride infusion.
3. Reconstituted solutions may be stored in a refrigerator for up to 30 days if the special diluent (containing a bacteriocide) is used. Alternatively reconstituted solution should not be used after 48 hours.

VITAMIN A (Retinol)

Presentation
Vitamin A is available in a preparation of fish liver oil in doses expressed in terms of international units.

Actions and uses
In the normal body Vitamin A is produced from precursors in the diet and is essential for maintenance of healthy mucus secreting epithelial surfaces and for the maintenance of normal vision via the production of a retinal pigment known as Rhodopsin. In clinical practice, Vitamin A is indicated only for the treatment of deficiency states which are very rare in this country. Symptoms of deficiency states include night blindness, drying and change in the microscopic make-up of skin and other body surfaces, drying and degeneration of the superficial layers of the eye.

Dosage
For the treatment of xerophthalmia: 50–70 000 international units should be given.

Nurse monitoring
Excessive doses of Vitamin A may be toxic:
1. If large doses are taken acutely, nausea, vomiting, abdominal pain, drowsiness and headache may occur.
2. In Chronic overdosage, fatigue, insomnia, bone pain, loss of hair and abnormal pigmentation of the skin may occur.

VITAMIN B COMPLEX

Presentation
Vitamin B complex is available either as preparations of its components (see below) or in multivitamin preparations. Vitamin B complex comprises B_1 (aneurine or thiamine), B_2 (riboflavine) B_6 (pyridoxine), B_5 (pantothenic acid).

Actions and uses
Vitamin B complex is indicated for the treatment of deficiency disorders of components of the complex, Symptoms of deficiency disorders are as follows:
1. Thiamine deficiency may present as:
   a. Beriberi characterised by anorexia, emaciation, cardiac arrhythmias and in the 'wet' form of the disease oedema.
   b. Neurological symptoms due to Thiamine deficiency are known as Wernicke's encephalopathy and these include: agitation, behavioural disturbance, loss of memory and confusion.
2. Riboflavine deficiency: Causes a rough scaly skin on the face, red swollen cracked lips, stomatitis and a swollen red tongue. Congestion of conjunctival blood vessels may also be seen.
3. Nicotinamide deficiency produces diarrhoea, dermatitis and dementia.
4. Pyridoxine: Pyridoxine deficiency may produce roughening of the skin or anaemia.

Dosage
1. For the treatment of beriberi: 5–10 mg of Thiamine daily produces good clinical response.
2. For the treatment of nicotinamide deficiency: between 40 and 200 mg per day produces good clinical response.

Nurse monitoring
No problems have been identified with the administration of these compounds.

VITAMIN C (Ascorbic Acid)

Presentation
Vitamin C is available in many preparations either singly or in combinations of multivitamins.

Actions and uses
Vitamin C is essential for the maintenance of normal body function. Its sole real indication in clinical practice is for the treatment of Vitamin C deficiency known commonly as scurvy. The clinical features of this are weakness, tiredness, lassitude, bleeding and diseased gums, haemorrhage around the hairs of the legs, peripheral oedema and sudden cardiac failure. In addition wounds heal very poorly and bones may be affected by osteoporosis. Anaemia may also occur.

Dosage
For the treatment of scurvy: 500 mg–1 g three times dialy in adults. Children over 12 years should receive three-quarters of the adult dose. Children of 4–12 years should receive half the adult dose. Children under 4 years should receive one-quarter of the adult dose.

Nurse monitoring
There are no problems associated with the administration of this drug.

VITAMIN D

Alfacalcidol (One-Alpha)
Calciferol (Ergocalciferol, Cholecalciferol, Sterogyl)
Calcitriol (Rocaltrol)
Dihydrotachysterol (Tachyrol, AT 10)

Presentation
See individual drugs.

Actions and uses
The drugs listed above are all preparations of various forms of Vitamin D.
1. Vitamin D is essential for the normal growth of bones and teeth. It should only be sued in clinical practice if Vitamin D deficiency has been clearly demonstrated. Vitamin D deficiency causes rickets in children and osteomalacia in adults. The commonest cause in European communities is steatorrhoea. In immigrants inadequate intake in the diet and poor exposure to sun (which stimulates the production of Vitamin D in the body) may be contributory features.
2. Vitamin D may also be used to

treat the rare condition of hypoparathyroidism.
3. In chronic renal disease the body is incapable of producing the active derivatives of Vitamin D necessary to maintain normal healthy bones and it is for the treatment of the resultant condition, renal osteodystrophy, that One-Alpha Hydroxycalciferol is particularly indicated.

Dosage
See individual drugs.

Nurse monitoring
1. An excess of Vitamin D causes high blood calcium. This may cause anorexia, nausea, vomiting, constipation, abdominal pain and increased urine output and subsequently renal stones and renal failure.
2. One-Alpha hydroxycalciferol is the most active of the group of drugs which may be used in Vitamin D deficiency states and, therefore, patients should be carefully monitored by regular estimations of blood calcium.
3. In clinical practice children appear to be at the greatest risk of receiving an excessive dose of Vitamin D.

General notes
All preparations of Vitamin D may be stored at room temperature.

VITAMIN E (Ephynal)

Presentation
Tablets—3 mg, 10 mg, 50 mg, 200 mg
N.B. Vitamin E is also available in a number of proprietary multivitamin preparations.

Actions and uses
The actual function of Vitamin E is yet to be identified. It has been used prophylactically to prevent habitual abortion but its efficacy in this context is in doubt.

Dosage
There are no dosage recommendations for this drug.

Nurse monitoring
There are no problems as yet identified in association with the administration of this drug.

General notes
Nil.

VITAMIN K

Presentation
10 mg Phytomenadione tablets (Konakion)
Ampoules—1 mg Phytomenadione in 0.5 ml.
10 mg Phytomenadione in 1 ml

Actions and uses
1. Vitamin K is indicated for the treatment of Vitamin K deficiency which is usually manifest as an increased bleeding tendency. The commonest cause of Vitamin K deficiency is malabsorption.
2. Vitamin K may also be used to reverse the effect of Warfarin.
3. Premature infants may have a relative deficiency to Vitamin K and are often given therapeutic Vitamin K to avoid the development of bleeding complications.

Dosage
1. To treat Vitamin K deficiency due to malabsorption: 10 mg is given by intramuscular injection until clotting studies have been shown to be normalised.
2. As an antidote to anticoagulant drugs: 10–20 mg is given as a slow intravenous injection. The clotting function of the blood should be estimated three hours later and if still abnormal a second dose of 10–20 mg may be given but not more than 40 mg should be given intravenously in 24 hours.
3. For the prophylactic treatment of newborn infants: 1 mg should be administered by intramuscular injection.

Nurse monitoring
The too rapid intravenous

administration of Vitamin K has caused reactions including facial flushing, sweating, a sense of chest constriction, cyanosis and peripheral vascular collapse.

General notes
1. Konakion ampoule solutions should be protected from light and should not be allowed to freeze.
2. Konakion tablets should be stored in a well closed container, protected from light and in a cool place.

W

WARFARIN (Marevan)

Presentation
Tablets—1 mg, 3 mg, 5 mg, 10 mg

Actions and uses
A number of the substances present in blood which play an important part in preventing bleeding by forming clots are produced by the liver from Vitamin K. Warfarin inhibits the synthesis of these substances (known as clotting factors) and therefore reduces the ability of the blood to clot. Its principal uses are for the prevention and treatment of thromboembolic states such as deep venous thrombosis and pulmonary embolus. They are also used to prevent the formation of clot in cardiovascular disease either on artificial heart valves or in the atria of patients who have atrial dysrhythmias.

Dosage
The general principle is to give a loading dose over 48 hours and subsequently adjust the dosage to the patient's individual requirements as gauged on the results of clotting tests such as the thrombotest or prothrombin time.
1. *Adults*:
   a. Loading dose: 10–20 mg on the first day followed by 10 mg on the second day. The dosage on the third day should depend on the result of the clotting test used.
   b. Maintenance: This depends on results of clotting tests.
2. *Children*:
   a. Loading dose: 2 weeks to 1 year: 0.75 mg/kg
   1–7 years: 7.5–15 mg on the first day. On the second day half of the above dose. On the third day the dose should be adjusted according to the result of the clotting test.
   b. Maintenance dosage: depends on the results of clotting tests.

Nurse monitoring
1. The daily maintenance dose of Warfarin is, as noted above, determined by the results of clotting studies. As the effects of bleeding due to overcoagulation or thrombosis due to undercoagulation can be so rapidly catastrophic strict adherence to the recommended dose is mandatory and the nurse may play an important role in ensuring that patients are aware of this.
2. The effects of Warfarin may be influenced by a number of factors listed below and the nurse may play an important role by identifying their occurrence and alerting both the patient and medical staff. The following circumstances may lead to a requirement for alteration in dosage:
   a. Acute illness such as chest infection or viral infection
   b. Sudden weight loss
   c. The concurrent administration of other drugs: A number of drugs may affect the patient's dosage requirements. Where drugs are known to interfere with anticoagulant control this has been noted in the Nurse monitoring sections of the drugs in this book.
3. The occurrence of haemorrhage in a patient on Warfarin is an

indication for immediate withdrawal of the drug and if the haemorrhage is at all serious or repetitive the patient should be immediately referred to hospital for further assessment and, if necessary, they may be given Vitamin K which accelerates a return to normal clotting function.
4. Warfarin is relatively contraindicated in patients with severe liver or kidney disease, haemorrhagic conditions or uncontrolled hypertension. It should also be used with great caution immediately after surgery or labour.
5. Hair loss, skin rash and diarrhoea may rarely occur.

General notes

The drug may be stored at room temperature.

X

XIPAMIDE (Diurexan)
Presentation
Tablets—20 mg
Actions and uses
Xipamide is a drug which has both a useful diuretic and hypotensive action. It may therefore be used in the treatment of hypertension and also in the management of heart failure (see thiazide diuretics section, actions and uses).
Dosage
The usualy daily adult dose is 20–40 mg taken once daily in the morning.

Nurse monitoring
1. The major points on Nurse monitoring are identical for thiazide diuretics (q.v.).
2. This drug may also produce gastrointestinal upset and dizziness.

General notes
Xipamide tablets may be stored at room temperature.

Z

ZINC SULPHATE (Zincomed, Solvazinc)

Presentation
Eye drops—0.25% (also in combinations with Phenylephrine as 'Zincfrin' and Adrenaline)
Capsules—220 mg
Tablets—200 mg effervescent
Lotion—1%
Mouthwash—2%

Actions and uses
1. Topical: Zinc sulphate possesses a soothing (astringent) action and aids granulation which renders it useful when applied locally in inflammatory conditions e.g. applied to indolent ulcers and to the cornea in conjunctivitis.
2. Oral: Oral tablets or capsules are used to correct zinc deficiency (zinc is an essential trace element in the diet), to aid wound healing and in the treatment of acrodermatitis enteropathica.

Dosage
1. Topical:
    a. Lotion: Apply to inflammatory lesions twice daily.
    b. Eye drops: Apply up to 4 times daily.
2. Oral:
Adults: Once capsule or effervescent tablet is taken three times daily after meals.
Children: Under 10 kg body weight: 100 mg as dissolved table once daily. 10–30 kg: Take half adult dose.

Nurse monitoring
1. The only side effect of note is the production of gastrointestinal upsets. It is for this reason that the drug was formerly used as an emetic, though at somewhat higher doses than described above.
2. Gastrointestinal upsets are reduced if dosages are taken immediately after meals.
3. Melaena and anaemia following haemorrhagic gastric erosion have been reported.
4. It is important to note that zinc sulphate was formerly used as an emetic but this indication is no longer valid.

General notes
Preparations containing Zinc Sulphate may be stored at room temperature.

SPECIAL NOTES

Note 1

NURSING ASPECTS OF INTRAVENOUS INFUSION FLUID THERAPY AND DRUG ADDITIVES TO INTRAVENOUS INFUSION

Nurses are closely involved in the administration of intravenous infusion fluids and should therefore be aware of some general principles related to this form of therapy and in particular the problems with which it may be associated.

Intravenous infusion therapy has several applications:
1. It is a means of rapidly hydrating patients, providing essential electrolytes (sodium, potassium, calcium etc.), adjusting the body's acid base balance and supplying nutrients (see Note 2, p. 306).
2. A number of drugs may be administered at a slow rate in a very dilute form by intravenous infusion. In a number of cases this is the only route by which a particular drug can be administered.

An intravenous infusion fluid is a sterile product supplied either in glass (rigid) containers, plastic (flexible) bags or polythene-like (semi-rigid) 'Polyfusors'. The most common fluids are 0.9% sodium chloride (normal saline), 5% dextrose (glucose) and mixtures of sodium chloride and dextrose (dextrose/saline). These solutions are termed 'isotonic' because they are compatible with body fluids i.e. they mix with blood without damaging red blood cells and do not produce irritation (which is due to the fluid itself) at injection sites. Several other strengths of sodium chloride solutions and dextrose solutions are used less often for more specialised applications; these are however not isotonic.

Other common infusion fluids are solutions of laevulose (fructose), an alternative to dextrose; sodium bicarbonate solutions (1.4%, 1.26%, 4.2% and 8.4%) and sodium lactate solutions including compound sodium lactate or Hartmann's solution (sodium lactate is converted by the body to bicarbonate).

Intravenous infusion fluids are administered through a plastic 'giving set'— a length of tubing running from the container to enter the patient via a cannula inserted into a peripheral vein or after passing along a central venous catheter opening into the great vein (vena cava). The latter is preferred if rapid dilution of the fluid is required, e.g. as in the case of concentrated dextrose solutions which are very irritant if given into peripheral veins. The giving set is fitted with a drip chamber or reservoir to prevent the entry of air bubbles into the system and ultimately therefore the patient and the rate of infusion is controlled by means of a valve which adjusts the drip rate into the reservoir. If infusions in glass bottles are used, a separate airway must be fitted to allow air (filtered through a cotton wool plug) to enter and replace fluid leaving the bottle. Flexible bags or semi-rigid containers require no airway but simply collapse as the internal pressure falls as fluid leaves. It is possible to add drugs to the infusion via an additive port or directly inject them through the wall of a 'Polyfusor'.

Nurse monitoring
1. **Selection of the appropriate fluid:** As previously described, there are a number of different infusion fluids available and there may be several strengths for any one solution. It follows therefore that in a busy hospital ward where limited space results in storage of different infusion fluids in the same area, there is always a possibility that the wrong bottle may be selected, particularly during an emergency situation. It is therefore important that the label attached to the bottle is carefully read and checked against the fluid prescription chart or checked separately by the doctor requesting that infusion fluid.
2. **Contamination by particles:** During the manufacture of intravenous infusion fluids, steps are taken to ensure their quality and sterility. While this minimises contamination by foreign particles, the possibility that occasionally one or more bottles in each batch might be contaminated should not be overlooked. The nurse can provide an important final check by inverting the bottle and examining the solution in bright light. By this method even small particles can be spotted as they fall through the infusion fluid. (Particles which appear to rise through the solution are usually bubbles of air.) Further visual examination of the fluid is important after the rubber closure is punctured, when affixing the administration set and airway. On a few occasions rubber particles from the closure 'bung' may accidentally be forced into the solution.
3. **Contamination by bacteria and fungi:** The contamination of infusion fluids by bacteria and fungi can produce severe and even fatal systemic infections. Contamination may be caused by:
    a. Incorrect sterilisation as mentioned above.
    b. Following the introduction of micro-organisms through a damaged container or closure, i.e. a deep crack in a glass bottle

or a bad seal. If this occurs contaminated solutions may appear cloudy or turbid.

c. Of particular importance to the nurse is the possibility of introducing micro-organisms when puncturing the container while attaching the giving set or during the addition of drugs to the infusion fluid. This risk can be minimised by adequate aseptic techniques.

The nurse should always be alert to the possibility of bacteraemia or fungaemia occurring in patients receiving intravenous infusions and should always consider this as a possibility when patients receiving intravenous infusions develop fever or rigors. Should fever or rigor occur any infusion should be immediately stopped and the remaining solution retained for examination by both the bacteriology and pharmacy departments.

4. **Drug additions to infusion fluids:** Whenever any substance is added to an infusion fluid it is necessary to indicate this by attaching to the bottle an additive label indicating:
   a. The nature of the additive
   b. The quantity added
   c. The date and time of addition.

This information is important since it will prevent the accidental addition of a further dose and is available in the event of any untoward reaction occurring in the patient. Furthermore, it may be necessary to know what is contained in the fluid so that a possible drug interaction can be checked.

Whenever a drug is added to an infusion fluid the possibility that a chemical interaction may occur between the various substances present must be considered. Such an interaction may occur because the added drug and a component of the fluid itself is incompatible, or it may be that two or more additives are incompatible. The following general rules apply:

a. Chemical changes often produce a change in colour and/or loss of clarity in the solution. Often an insoluble precipitate can be clearly seen. Such solutions should not be administered without prior checking.

b. As the number of drugs added to any one solution increases, the possibility of a drug interaction increases considerably. Therefore, avoid adding drugs if at all possible.

c. Drugs should not be added to chemically complex solutions since the possiblity of the chemical change is greatly increased. If possible, drugs should not be added to whole blood, blood products, fat emulsions or amino acid solutions.

d. It is not reasonable to suggest that the nurse should know every possible interaction between either two or more drugs in solutions or the drugs and the solutions themselves. In the list that follows, common problems with drugs and solutions are discussed and there is a section where the more common known interactions between drugs in fluids are listed. Should the nurse be faced with the problem of adding drugs to infusions which are not included in these lists, the information is usually readily available via the Pharmacy Department.

DIRECTIONS FOR THE ADMINISTRATION OF COMMON INJECTIONS

1. Antibiotics

a. Ampicillin — This should preferably be added to sodium chloride injections. It is unstable in solutions of dextrose or sodium lactate containing solutions such as Hartmann's solution. Using dextrose or lactate containing solutions may reduce the efficacy of the antibiotic.

b. Penicillin — As for Ampicillin above

c. Cephalosporins — These may be added to common infusion fluids i.e. sodium chloride 0.9%, dextrose 5%, dextrose/saline etc

d. Cloxacillin — As for Ampicillin above

e. Flucloxacillin — As for Ampicillin above

f. Gentamicin — This drug should never be given by intravenous infusion but should be given, if necessary, by intravenous bolus injection. It should never be mixed in the same syringe with a member of the Penicillin group.

g. Kanamycin — This drug is preferably given by the intramuscular route. If absolutely necessary, intravenous infusions in dextrose 5%, sodium chloride 0.9% or dextrose/saline mixtures may be administered.

h. Erythromycin — This may be added to dextrose 5%, sodium chloride 0.9% or dextrose/saline mixtures. It is important that the injection be initially reconstituted to a 5% stock solution by

302 *A Handbook of Drugs*

		adding 6 ml Water for Injection or dextrose 5% to each 300 mg vial.
i.	Oxytetracycline or Tetracycline	Vials should be reconstituted with Water for Injection and added to dextrose 5%, sodium chloride 0.9% or dextrose/saline. The concentration of infusion must not exceed 0.05% and the rate of administration should not exceed 20 ml/minute and infusions should if possible be administered within 12 hours.
2.	**Aminophylline**	This may be added to dextrose 5%, sodium chloride 0.9%, dextrose/saline or Hartmann's solution.
3.	**Chlorpromazine**	Preferably given by intramuscular injection. If the intravenous route must be used, Chlorpromazine may be administered in sodium chloride 0.9% injection. Do not add other drugs to the infusion fluid.
4.	**Cytotoxic drugs**	These drugs have a highly specialised use and the preferred method of intravenous administration may be critical and should be carefully checked in each case. Cytotoxic drugs are highly reactive chemically and should generally not be mixed together for ease of administration.
5.	**Diazepam**	Direct (slow) intravenous bolus injection is preferred. If necessary, an intravenous infusion containing up to a maximum of 40 mg in 500 ml of dextrose 5%, sodium chloride 0.9% or dextrose/saline solution may be given. Do not mix with any other drugs.
6.	**Digoxin**	Digoxin may be infused in 5% dextrose, 0.9% sodium chloride or dextrose/saline mixtures. A concentration of up to 1 mg in 500 ml may be used where appropriate. The total dosage depends on factors discussed under Digoxin (q.v.).

7. Frusemide	When high dose intravenous therapy is contemplated, the drug may be infused at a rate of 4 mg/minute in either sodium chloride 0.9%, Hartmann's solution or Ringer's solution. Other drugs should not be added to Frusemide infusions.
8. Heparin	This may be given by intravenous infusion in 5% dextrose, 0.9% sodium chloride or dextrose/saline mixtures.
9. Hydrocortisone	100 mg, 500 mg and 1 g vials of Hydrocortisone should be reconstituted with 2, 4 and 8 ml of Water for Injection respectively and these solutions may then be added to dextrose 5%, sodium chloride 0.9% or dextrose/saline mixtures to give a fluid concentration of 0.1% or less.
10. Insulin	It is important to note that only soluble or neutral insulin should be given intravenously. Either of these are compatible with 0.9% sodium chloride. A small proportion of the insulin may be inactivated by absorption on to the glass container.
11. Isoprenaline	Should preferably be added to 5% dextrose. It should be diluted in a large volume of fluid according to manufacturers instructions and must never be administered by bolus injection.
12. Lignocaine	For infusion a 20% solution (200 mg in 1 ml) should be added to 500 ml of 5% dextrose or 0.9% sodium chloride or dextrose/saline mixtures or 5% laevulose. It is also compatible with dextran and Ringer's solutions.
13. Potassium chloride	Potassium chloride should be diluted in such a way that its maximum concentration in the infusion fluid is not greater than 20 mmol/l and a maximum infusion rate of 20 mmol/hr is recommended. The total dose administered

within any 24 hour period should not exceed 3 mmol/kg body weight. Potassium chloride solution may be added to dextrose 5%, sodium chloride 0.9%, dextrose/saline or Hartmann's solution.

14. Vitamins (compound) — The contents of each pair of ampoules should be added to dextrose 5%, sodium chloride 0.9% or dextrose/saline mixtures. It should not be mixed with other drugs in the infusion fluid.

INCOMPATIBILITIES OF COMMON DRUGS ARISING WHEN THEY ARE MIXED IN SYRINGES OR INFUSION FLUIDS

Drug	Known Incompatibility
Aminophylline	Erythromycin Cephalosporins Tetracyclines Penicillins
Calcium Gluconate (Calcium Sandoz)	Magnesium Sulphate
Calcium Salts (general)	Tetracyclines
Cephalosporins	Gentamicin Aminophylline Tetracyclines Erythromycin Heparin Hydrocortisone
Chloramphenicol	Erythromycin Tetracyclines Hydrocortisone
Erythromycin	Aminophylline Penicillins Heparin Chloramphenicol Cephalosporins Sodium salts Tetracyclines

Incompatibilities of common drugs (*continued*)

Drug	Known Incompatibility
Gentamicin	Penicillins Cephalosporins Heparin
Heparin	Erythromycin Gentamicin Hydrocortisone Tetracyclines Penicillin Cephalosporins
Hydrocortisone	Heparin Chloramphenicol Penicillin Cephalosporins
Magnesium Sulphate	Tetracyclines Calcium Gluconate (Calcium Sandoz)
Penicillins	Gentamicin Aminophylline Erythromycin Heparin Hydrocortisone Tetracyclines
Sodium Salts	Erythromycin
Tetracyclines	Aminophylline Calcium Salts Magnesium Salts Heparin Erythromycin Cephalosporins Penicillin Chloramphenicol

Note 2

INTRAVENOUS (PARENTERAL) FEEDING

Introduction
When food, even in its most basic form, cannot be taken by mouth, or if the intestinal absorption of food is seriously impaired, intravenous feeding becomes necessary to preserve life. Common situations in which this occurs include the immediate postoperative period of major surgery especially surgery to the bowel, as part of the intensive care of ventilated or comatose patients and in the treatment of persistent severe vomiting or malabsorption syndromes.

Actions and uses
Parenteral feeding should be designed to provide the patient with an adequate amount of all essential components of a diet. In the following scheme, quantities of the components necessary are quoted and the nurse should bear in mind that these are not the daily requirements of an average fit human being, but they are designed to give seriously ill patients who may, through previous prolonged ill-health or present multiple medical and surgical problems require far more in the way of nutrition in order to prevent further physical deterioration. The essential components of any parenteral feeding regime are as follows:

1. **Amino acids:** Amino acids are a group of chemicals which are essential for production of protein. Almost every structure and functional component of the body requires protein. Amino acids in total comprise more than 20, but a number of these may be produced from other proteins and amino acids by the body itself. There are, however, eight amino acids which the body cannot produce and amino acid solutions are designed to provide both total protein requirements and also sufficient of these eight essential amino acids for the body's use. Many solutions of amino acids are available and these include: Vamin solutions, Aminoplex, Aminofusins, Freamine, Synthamins.
2. **Carbohydrate:** Carbohydrate in the normal diet is derived from

various sugars and starches. The main function of carbohydrate is to provide a high energy source of calories. For intravenous parenteral nutrition, carbohydrates are available alone or in combination with amino acids. For parenteral feeding the simplest sugar, glucose, is available in varying concentrations including Dextrose 5%, Dextrose 10%, Dextrose 30%, Dextrose 50%.
3. **Fat:** Fat is another important source of energy and essential components necessary for body function. It is available as a suspension of fat globules in water and has a creamy, milk-like appearance. Available suspensions include Intralipid 10%, Intralipid 20%.
4. **Vitamins:** All the essential vitamins (see vitamin section) must be included in a parenteral feeding regime. They may be included in any regime either singly or by using compound solutions such as Parentrovite and they may be given either by intravenous bolus injection or intramuscular injection. It should be noted that vitamin D is not included in multiple preparations and should be given separately as required at intervals of approximately one month.
5. **Minerals:** Just as vitamins are necessary for many bodily functions, so are a number of minerals which are present in tiny, yet essential, quantities in the normal diet. These include sodium (Na), potassium (K), magnesium (Mg), zinc (Zn), calcium (Ca), iron (Fe), manganese (Mn), copper (Cu), fluoride (Fl), phosphate (PO_4). There are available preparations which contain all of these essential minerals and these preparations include:
   a. *Addamel*: A compound mineral supplement for injection which is added to Dextrose mixtures
   b. *Pedel*: A solution like Addamel which is appropriate for paediatric use.
6. **Alcohol:** Although alcohol itself is by no means a necessary part of the diet, it has been used frequently in the past as it is an excellent source of energy. There are, however, other suitable preparations available which are not associated with some of the side effects found with alcohol solutions and it is sufficient that the nurse know that alcohol is occasionally included in these regimes, but is not absolutely essential.

Dosage
For seriously ill patients and in order to ensure that catabolism (breakdown of the muscle and tissues of the body) does not occur, it is recommended that patients receive each day:
1. Sufficient amino acid to provide 15–20 g of nitrogen per day
2. 3000 kcal per day

3. Three litres of fluid per day (the nurse should be careful to note that any patient with impaired renal function must have a strictly controlled fluid intake as discussed with the medical staff and the figure quoted is for patients with normal renal function)
4. Vitamin supplementation as required above
5. Mineral supplementation as required above.

Method of administration

Two methods of administration are available:
1. An intravenous infusion line is connected to a 'Y' connector and through each of the lines the feeding regime is administered. An example of a suitable 24 hour regime is as follows:
Line 1: 1 × 8 hour Vamin solution (500 ml); 1 × 8 hour Intralipid (500 m); 1 = 8 hour Vamin solution (500 ml).
Line 2: 1 × 8 hour Dextrose 30% (500 ml); 1 × 8 hour Dextrose 30% (500 ml); 1 × 8 hour Dextrose 30% (500 ml)
This provides all protein, calorie, fat and fluid requirements for 24 hours as described below.
2. **Big bag technique:** This simple technique involves placing the total amount of solutions required for 24 hours in one large bag, mixing them together and infusing them through a single infusion line over 24 hours. The system requires to be prepared in a special sterile laboratory suite, usually within a Pharmacy Department.

Nurse monitoring

1. Many of the solutions used in parenteral feeding cause severe, local irritation and in practice it is usual for an intravenous catheter to be implanted via a peripheral vein into the large central vein such as the superior vena cava.
2. All patients on intravenous parenteral feeding are usually in a poor physical state and the consequences of infection may be diastrous. The nurse plays an important part in ensuring that these regimes are administered in as rigorously an asceptic technique as can be managed. This is of particular importance when the 'big bag technique' is being used with infusions over 24 hours during which time any contaminating bacteria may grow.
3. Because contamination by micro-organisms and subsequent infection is such a high risk, the nurse should always remember the possibility of this complication arising when patients become pyrexial.
4. Prior to setting up an Intralipid infusion the nurse should always examine the consistency of the solution carefully. If the fat glob-

ules in the solution have coalesced and produced a creamy effect on the surface, then the solution should be discarded immediately.
5. It is a useful working rule to remember that all parenteral feeding solutions may contain, if examined under bright light, minute particles but any solution containing particles that are clearly visible should be considered to be contaminated and discarded.

Note 3

ANTIBIOTICS AND SULPHONAMIDES

Antibiotics and sulphonamides are used for the prevention or treatment of infection by bacteria and to a lesser extent other organisms. When antibiotics and sulphonamides are discussed in the text, a number of terms are used, a knowledge of which is important in order to be able to understand the actions and uses of the drugs. These are as follows:

1. **Bacteriostatic:** Possessing an action which prevents the growth of bacterial micro-organisms.
2. **Bacteriocidal:** Possessing an action which kills bacterial micro-organisms.
3. **Classification of bacterial micro-organisms:** A bacteriologist by the name of Gram invented a staining technique whereby most common bacterial micro-organisms fell into one of two groups, designated Gram-positive and Gram-negative on the results of the staining test. This has proved to be an immensely useful test in clinical practice, as many antibiotics seem to have spectrums of activity related to either one or the other group. These are listed below:
   a. Gram-positive:
      i. Cocci: *Staphylococcus aureus*
         other staphylococci
         Streptococcus viridans
         Streptococcus pyogenes
         Streptococcus faecalis
         Streptococcus bovis
         Streptococcus pneumoniae
      ii. Gram-positve bacilli: *Bacillus anthracis*
         Corynebacterium diphtheriae
         Listeria monocytogenes
         Clostridium tetani
         Clostridium welchii

b. Gram-negative:
   i. Cocci: *Neisserria gonorrhoeae*
      Neisserria meningitidis
   ii. Gram-negative bacilli: *Haemophilus influenzae*
       Klebsiella pneumoniae
       E. coli
       Enterobacter species
       Proteus species
       Pseudomonas aeruginosa
       Pseudomonas pyocynaea
4. **Pathogen:** This is a common term for a bacterial micro-organism which produces infection.
5. **Strain:** By using various staining and other techniques, major groups of pathogens such as staphylococci may be divided into sub-groups known as strains. This is useful in that differing strains of organisms can produce different patterns of disease and also have differing antibiotic sensitivity.
6. **Resistance:** When antibiotics or sulphonamides are found to be ineffective against a particular micro-organism, the micro-organism is said to be resistant to the drug. Organisms have different means of acquiring resistance but such a discussion is beyond the scope of this text.

INFECTIONS CAUSED BY BACTERIA

Infection	Infecting micro-organism (pathogen)
Bacteraemia or septicaemia	Coliforms Enterobacter species *Staphylococcus aureus* Streptococcus species
Bacterial meningitis	*Streptococcus pneumoniae* *Neisseria meningitidis*

N.B. Many micro-organisms may cause meningitis in neonates

Endocarditis (acute)	*Staphylococcus aureus* *Streptococcus pyogenes* Gram-negative bacilli
(sub-acute)	Streptoccus species *Staphylococcus epidermidis* Gram-negative bacilli

Infections caused by bacteria (continued)

Infection	Infecting micro-organism (pathogen)
Enteric fever	Salmonellae
Cholecystitis	Coliforms *Streptococcus faecalis* Salmonellae
Enterocolitis	*Staphylococcus aureus*
Food poisoning	Salmonellae *Clostridium welchii*
Gastroenteritis	Salmonellae (as for food poisoning) *E. coli*
Peritonitis	Mixed organisms commonly found in bowel including: Coliforms Proteus species *Streptococcus faecalis* Clostridia
Impetigo	*Streptococcus pyogenes* *Staphylococcus aureus*
Post-operative wound infections	*Staphylococcus aureus* Coliforms *Pseudomonas aeruginosa*

Urinary tract:
  i. Cystitis   Coliforms
                      Proteus
                      Streptococcus faecalis

    N.B. *Staphylococcus epidermidis* is often the cause of cystitis resulting from bladder catheterisation.

  ii. Acute and chronic pyelonephritis   Gram-negative bacilli

Venereal disease
  i. Gonorrhoea   *Neisseria gonorrhoea*
  ii. Non-specific urethritis   Chlamydia
  iii. Vaginitis   Normally fungal infection

Infections caused by bacteria (continued)

Infection	Infecting micro-organism (pathogen)
Tuberculosis	*Mycobacterium tuberculosis*
Respiratory tract:	
i. Exacerbation of chronic bronchitis	*Haemophilus influenzae* *Streptococcus pneumoniae*
ii. Pneumonia (previously healthy chest)	*Streptococcus pneumoniae* *Staphylococcus aureus*
iii. Pneumonia (previously unhealthy chest)	*Streptococcus pneumoniae* *Staphylococcus aureus* *Haemophilus influenzae*

  N.B. *Staphylococcus aureus* infections commonly occur after respiratory viral infections e.g. influenza.

E.N.T.—

i. Tonsilitis	*Streptococcus pyogenes*

    N.B. Often caused by virus infection.

ii. Otitis media	*Streptococcus pyogenes* *Streptococcus pneumoniae* *Haemophilus influenzae* (infants)
iii. Sinusitis	*Streptococcus pyogenes* *Streptococcus pneumoniae* *Haemophilus influenzae* (infants)

Note 4

DRUGS IN BREAST MILK

When a nursing mother ingests a drug a proportion of that drug may appear in her breast milk. The actual amount of drug appearing depends on the type of drug, the amount ingested and its metabolism in the body. Although only small amounts of these drugs or their metabolites are excreted in breast milk they may still be relevant. Firstly, because the infants receiving these drugs are very small, so even small dosages can affect them. Secondly, young infants have immature liver and renal function and this can delay drug metabolism and therefore increase the drug's effect. It is obvious, therefore, that when drugs are given to a nursing mother a number of basic important principles must be adhered to by the doctor, and the nurse should be aware of them. They include:
1. Never prescribe a drug unless it is absolutely necessary
2. Whenever possible use the safest alternative
3. Use the lowest possible dose for the shortest possible time
4. Ensure that the mother understands the dose regime and is aware of any recognisable effects on the baby.

The information available on the effect on babies of drugs given to mothers who are breast feeding is limited. A number of important groups, however, may be identified. These are:
1. Drugs which can safely be given to nursing mothers:
    Aminoglycoside antibiotics
    Aminophylline slow (Phyllocontin)
    Antacids
    Carbamazepine (Tegretol)
    Cephalosporin antibiotics
    Chloral hydrate (noctec)
    Chloroquine (Avloclor, Nivaquine)
    Codeine phosphate
    Colchicine

Corticotrophin
Dextropropoxyphene (in Distalgesic)
Dichloralphenazine (Welldorm)
Oigoxin
Erythromycin
Ethambutol (Myambutol)
Ethosuximide (Zarontin)
Fenoterol (Berotec)
Flufenamic acid (Meralen)
Folic acid
Guanethidine (Ismelin)
Haloperidol (Serenace)
Heparin
Ibuprofen (Brufen)
Insulin
Iron
Ketoprofen
Liothyronine (Tertroxin)
Loperamide (Imodium)
Mefenamic acid (Ponstan)
Methyldopa (Aldomet)
Metoclopramide (Maxolon)
Metronidazole (Flagyl)
Paracetamol
Penicillins
Pentazocine
Pethidine
Phenothiazines
Progestogens
Propantheline (Pro Banthine)
Propranolol
Rifampicin
Rimiterol (Pulmadil)
Salbutamol
Sodium Valproate (Epilim)
Spironolactone (Aldactone)
Terbutaline (Bricanyl)
Theophylline slow (Theocontin, Nuelin SA)
Thyroxine
Triclofos
Tricyclic antidepressants
Vitamins B complex and C
Warfarin (Marevan)

2. Drugs which definitely should not be administered to nursing mothers:
   Atropine (in some gastrointestinal sedatives/antispasmodics)
   Belladonna (as for Atropine)
   Carbimazole (Neo Mercazole)
   Danthron (Dorbanex)
   Gold injection (Myocrisin)
   Hyoscine (as for Atropine)
   Hyoscyamine (as for Atropine)
   Iodides
   Meprobamate
   Phenindione (Dindevan)
   Reserpine (Serpasil, Decaserpyl)
   Senna (Senokot)
   Tetracyclines
   Thiazide diuretics

It is worth also looking at this problem from another viewpoint and taking selected drug groups in turn:

1. **Anti-inflammatory and analgesic drugs:**
   a. Only Phenylbutazone and Oxphenbutazone of the non-steroidal anti-inflammatory drugs are absolutely contra-indicated.
   b. Breast milk concentration of opiates such as Morphine and Diamorphine are very low and unless the mother takes high doses there is negligible effect on the breast-fed baby. However, the infants appear to be particularly affected by the constipating action of these drugs.
   c. In high dosage salicylates given to the mother may cause skin rash and a bleeding tendency in the child.
   d. Gold injections given to the mother may produce skin rash in the infant.

2. **Anticoagulants:**
   a. Phenindione has produced fatal haematoma in one infant.
   b. Warfarin may safely be taken by nursing mothers.
   c. Heparin, although excreted in breast milk, is inactivated in the infant's gastrointestinal tract and is therefore safe.

3. **Anti-infective agents:**
   a. Sulphonamides if given to the mother may lead to jaundice in the infant. They are relatively contraindicated.
   b. Penicillin and cephalosporin antibiotics may be given. Very few problems are likely to arise although diarrhoea and hyper-sensitivity reactions may occur.

c. Erythromycin, Ethambutol, Rifampicin and Metronidazole have safely been given to breast-feeding mothers.
   d. Isoniazid enters breast milk in high concentration and produces restlessness and neuropathies. The drug should not be given unless prophylactic vitamin B_6 supplements are given to the child.
   e. Chloramphenicol even in low doses can produce serious toxic effects in the infant and an alternative drug should be used, or if this is not possible breast feeding should be stopped.
   f. Tetracyclines are not thought to be safe for administration to breast-feeding mothers as they may, via this route, affect the growth of long bones and stain teeth in infants.
   g. Nitrofurantoin will accumulate in infants of breast-feeding mothers who receive this drug and, therefore, it should not be given.
   h. Aminoglycoside antibiotics (Gentamicin, Kanamycin, Amikacin) are destroyed in the gastrointestinal tract of breast-fed infants and, therefore, are safe.
4. **Drugs acting on the central nervous system:**
   a. Major tranquillisers of the phenothiazine group (q.v.) Haloperidol (q.v.) and tricyclic antidepressant drugs (q.v.) may be safely used during the nursing period.
   b. Of the benzodiazepines, Diazepam has been most widely studied and it is quite clear that the drug accumulates in breast-fed infants and may produce lethargy and weight loss. It also prolongs neonatal jaundice. It is, therefore, relatively contraindicated.
   c. Meprobamate produces high levels in breast milk and is contraindicated.
   d. Barbiturates are excreted in breast milk and cause drowsiness in the infant. They are therefore relatively contraindicated.
   e. Phenytoin has caused methaemoglobinaemia in one infant.
   f. Carbamazepine and sodium valproate appear safe but information is limited.
5. **Drugs acting on the cardiovascular system:**
   a. Diuretics suppress lactation by producing dehydration. There is also a risk of thrombocytopenia in the infant. Spironolactone, however, may be taken safely.
   b. There is no evidence that beta-blockers are harmful to the infant.
   c. Reserpine, a drug now rarely used, is relatively contraindicated because it produces nasal stuffiness and increased bronchial secretions in the infant.

d. Methyldopa appears to be safe for administration to nursing mothers.
e. Guanethidine does not appear to enter breast milk and is, therefore, safe for administration to nursing mothers.
f. Digoxin enters breast milk in such low concentrations that it would appear safe for administration to breast feeding mothers.
g. Ergot and its derivatives used for the treatment of migraine are contraindicated as side effects may be produced in the infant.

6. **Corticosteroids and other hormonal agents:**
   a. If drugs of this group are taken in physiological doses i.e. replacement therapy, there is little risk to breast-fed infants. However, there is a potential risk of growth retardation if doses are higher than those of physiological replacement doses.
   b. The very low doses of oestrogens contained in most oral contraceptives present little risk to the breast-fed infant. However, oestrogens will tend to suppress lactation.
   c. Thyroxine and liothyronine are used to replace a physiological deficit and do not cause problems in the suckling infant. However, iodides and Carbimazole may produce goitre. Propylthiouracil appears to be useful in low dose, provided the circulating thyroid hormones in the baby are regularly checked.
   d. Of the oral hypoglycaemic drugs studied, only small amounts of Tolbutamide and Phenformin have been detected and these do not appear to affect the infant's blood glucose.

7. **Gastrointestinal drugs:**
   a. Anthraquinine laxatives such as Senna and Danthron (q.v.) can produce diarrhoea in breast-fed infants. Thus, non-absorbable bulk laxatives such as bran or Methylcellulose are preferable.
   b. Cimetidine, widely used for the treatment of peptic ulcer disease, is present in breast milk in high concentrations. Thus it is relatively contraindicated as long term effects of such exposure are not as yet known.
   c. Anticholinergic drugs do not appear to cause problems.
   d. Antacids do not appear to cause problems.
   e. Metoclopramide may be safely taken and may in fact increase milk flow.
   f. The anti-diarrhoeal preparation 'Lomotil' contains diphenoxylate and atropine, both of which could have profound effects on the breast-fed infant and it is therefore contraindicated.

Respiratory drugs:
   1. Xanthine drugs i.e. Aminophylline, Theophylline etc., when

given to mothers may produce irritability, insomnia and fretfulness in the infant. In general oral slow-release xanthine preparations are less likely to produce this effect and, therefore, are relatively safer.

   b. Drugs taken by inhalation in asthma, chronic bronchitis such as beta agonists (Salbutamol, Terbutaline) and steroids (Becotide and Bextasol) produce minimal blood levels and, therefore, appear safe.

9. **Vitamins and mineral supplements:**
   a. Fat soluble vitamins A and D, if taken in excess, may accumulate in the breast-fed infant and produce symptoms of hypervitaminosis.
   b. There are no such problems with water soluble vitamins (B complex and vitamin C).
   c. Iron preparations appear safe.
   d. Folate preparations appear safe.
   e. It is interesting to note that mothers who are thiamine-deficient (i.e. have beri-beri) produce milk which is toxic to infants.

10. **Social factors:**

    Nicotine and regular high alcohol consumption reduce milk flow. A high alcohol intake may also produce CNS depression and reduce clotting factor synthesis in the infant.

Note 5

OPHTHALMIC PREPARATIONS

Introduction
The following definitions are frequently encountered when dealing with ophthalmic preparations:
1. **Accommodation:** The means by which the eye adapts for near or distant vision.
2. **Cycloplegia:** Paralysis of accommodation.
3. **Myosis:** Constriction of the pupil, (usually performed in clinical practice to facilitate drainage of ocular fluid in the treatment of glaucoma).
4. **Mydriasis:** Dilatation of the pupil (usually performed to facilitate the examination of the interior of the eye).

Actions and uses
There are five major groups of ophthalmic preparations:
1. Those used to treat ophthalmic infection:
   a. Antibacterial drugs: Tetracycline, Chloramphenicol, Aminoglycosides, Sulphacetamide.
   b. Antiviral drugs: Idoxuridine, Vidarabine Acyclovir

   These drugs are primarily to treat superficial infection of the eye and the surrounding structures.
2. To reduce inflammation and allergic inflammatory response. There are four groups of drugs useful for the treatment of inflammation and allergy:
   a. Corticosteroids, including Betamethasone, Dexamethasone, Hydrocortisone, Prednisolone
   b. Non-steroidal anti-inflammatory drugs, including Oxyphenbutazone, and Zinc Sulphate
   c. Antihistamines including Xylometazoline and Antazoline
   d. Sodium Cromoglycate.

The first two groups of drugs are used primarily for the treatment of inflammatory disorders, whereas the latter two are used for the treatment of allergic conditions.
3. Drugs used in the management of glaucoma (raised intra-ocular pressure): Glaucoma may be treated by oral administration of drugs (see Acetazolamide and Dichlorphenamide) or by topical applications which include: Adrenaline acid tartrate 0.5%, 1% and 2% (Simplene); Adrenaline (neutral) 1% (Eppy); Carbachol 3% (Isopto Carbachol); Demacarium 0.25% and 0.5% (Tosmelin); Ecthiopate 0.03%, 0.06%, 0.125% and 0.25% (Phospholine); Guanethidine 5.0% (Ismelin); Neostigmine 3% (Prostigmin); Physostigmine 1% (Eserine); Pilocarpine 1%, 2%, 3% and 4%; Timolol 0.25% and 0.5% (Timoptol).
4. Drugs used to aid examination of the eye and operative techniques:
   a. *Mydriatics and cycloplegics*: These drugs are used in the pre-operative preparation of the eye, for refraction ophthalmoscopy and photography of the fundus. They include: Atropine sulphate 1% and 2%; Cyclopentolate 0.1%, 0.5% and 1%; Homatropine hydrobromide 1% and 2%; Hyoscine hydrobromide 0.2%; Phenylephrine 10%; Tropicamide 0.5% and 1%
   b. *Local anaesthetics*: These drugs are applied to the eye before minor ophthalmic surgery, prior to removal of foreign bodies and during other investigative procedures. They include: Amethocaine 0.5% and 1%; Cocaine (various strengths); Benoxinate 0.4%; Lignocaine 4%
   c. *Stains*: Staining the surface of the eye assists in the identification of corneal lesions and the presence of foreign bodies. Common stains are: Fluorescein sodium 2%; Rose Bengal 1%.
5. In the treatment of anterior uveitis:
   Mydriatics: e.g. Atropine sulphate 1% and 2%; Cyclopentilate 0.1%, 0.5% and 1%; Homatropine hydrobromide 1% and 2%; Hyoscine hydrobromide 0.2%.

Nurse monitoring
1. Most drugs available for direct application to the eye will come in the form of single dose units (minims) without an added bacteriocide, or as a multidose bottle, in which case they will have a bacteriocide and fungicide added. Multidose containers should be discarded after:
   a. 24 hours if used in an operating theatre
   b. One week from the date of opening if used in a hospital ward

c. Four weeks from the date of opening when used in domiciliary practice.
2. It is always worth noting that to prevent cross-contamination from an infected eye to the other eye, in hospital use one bottle should be made available for the treatment of each eye, and should be labelled so that each bottle is applied to the appropriate eye.

Note 6

ANTI-CANCER DRUGS—THEIR SAFE HANDLING

Introduction

In recent years great concern has been expressed by nurses and other Health Service professionals about the possible danger they face when handling drugs used in the treatment of malignant and some auto-immune diseases. These drugs, collectively termed cytotoxic agents, are by definition potentially harmful to all cells of the body, be they cancer cells in the patient or 'healthy' cells in those providing the treatment. Such has been the concern expressed by different groups, including the Royal College of Nursing, that in December, 1983, the Health and Safety Executive (an official government body) published a Guidance Note which set out precautions to be observed when handling cytotoxic drugs (Guidance Note MS 21, H.M.S.O. Price 50 pence). Thus all staff preparing and administering cancer chemotherapy should now do so within the terms of a strict policy aimed at minimising the risk of contaminating themselves or their environment. This Note summarises basic concepts for the safe handling of anti-cancer drugs. The nurse's attention is also drawn to local policies which are likely to exist in individual Health Service Areas or Regions.

Possible dangers to staff

It is important to appreciate the significant increase in the number of anti-cancer drugs available, their wider application in the treatment of malignant and other diseases, and the increasing numbers of patients treated outwith specialist oncology units and indeed often in the home. Thus concern is not only for the specialist oncology nurse but also with the general nurse in hospital and community practice.

The basic action of any cytotoxic drug is to suppress the growth of cancer cells, producing regression and ultimately death of the cells. Inevitably, other healthy cells can be similarly affected. This is evident from the wide range of side effects attributed to cycotoxic therapy. The decision to use cancer chemotherapy is based on the fact that the beneficial effects of the drug (cancer cell kill) outweighs the risks to the patient (drug adverse effects).

The risks to nursing, medical, pharmaceutical and other personnel after exposure to drugs of this type depend on the site of contact and the duration of exposure. On contact with the skin, eyes and mucous surfaces many cytotoxic drugs are vesicants or powerful irritants capable of blistering or producing severe lesions.

In individuals reconstituting injectable cytotoxic drugs who have not had direct contact with the drugs, symptoms reported include dizziness or lightheadedness, headaches, facial flushing, nausea, development of nasal mucosal sores and hair loss.

Chronic low level exposure in situations where these drugs are regularly prepared and administered may theoretically result in a degree of progressive drug absorption after accidental ingestion or inhalation or penetration via the transcutaneous route. Most fears expressed by nurses and others relate to the possible development, through this exposure, of infertility, fetal malformation (in the case of the pregnant subject), bone marrow suppression and the development of cancers. It is important to stress that adverse effects due to this type of exposure have never been demonstrated in practice.

Prevention of risks
There are many ways by which accidental contamination of self or environment can be prevented by simple protective measures and application of good common sense. These include the following.
1. **Personnel**
   The handling, reconstitution and administration of cytotoxic drugs, should be delegated to nominated, trained nursing personnel who fully understand the risks involved.
2. **Location**
   a. Cytotoxic drugs should be prepared in designated areas only, be they in an area set aside in the ward or out-patient unit, or confined to a sophisticated centralised pharmacy-based service. The latter is clearly desirable in a situation where this form of therapy is regularly administered.
   b. The work surface should be clear, easily cleaned and should not have other drugs, equipment, food, drink, etc. stored in the immediate vicinity.
   c. There should be no through traffic of personnel in the area and draughts should be excluded as far as possible.
   d. In the event of accidental contamination of the skin or eyes the initial measure is to wash off the drug with a copious amount of water. Thus a running water supply should be available in the

vicinity and also purpose-made eye wash bottles can be supplied.

3. **Techniques and precautions**
   a. Equipment used in all processes should be disposable if possible.
   b. It may be necessary for the individual preparing a product which is likely to contaminate the work area to ensure protection by wearing protective clothing e.g. covering gown, face mask, goggles and gloves.
   c. It should be noted that the use of transfer needles, luer-lock syringes and special venting filters (which prevent spray or droplet contamination) is possible and can minimise considerably many of the risks. Nurses supervising cytotoxic chemotherapy should confirm the availability of these and other devices through their pharmacy/surgical stores department.
   d. The nurse must *never* break tablets or open capsules in order to facilitate the administration of solid oral dosage forms to patients.

4. **Disposal**
   a. It is absolutely essential to clean adequately all work surfaces after any cytotoxic drug has been prepared.
   b. Disposable equipment, syringes, needles, ampoules and vials should be disposed of into a plastic or polypropylene sharps box which is suitably labelled 'Cytotoxic waste' and disposed of by incineration. Other items, disposable gloves, face masks, gowns, etc., should also be incinerated after placing in a polythene bag suitably labelled 'Cytotoxic waste'.
   c. It is also important to ensure extra care when disposing of patient waste i.e. urine and faeces, which might also contain traces of cytotoxic drug or drug metabolites.

Summary

It is understandable that given the theoretical risks facing workers handling anti-cancer drugs that most nurses have become extremely concerned. Given the benefits of extensive education and training in the handling of these drugs, many fears can be allayed. Locally established codes of practice must always be followed and, if necessary, advice sought from apppropriate expert bodies.

APPENDICES

Appendix 1

THE SECURITY AND ADMINISTRATION OF MEDICINES IN HOSPITAL

The nurse should be familiar with a few important general points related to the security of medicines in the ward.
1. *All* medicines should be locked up to prevent access by unauthorised persons. This is particularly important where there is freedom of movement for patients in the ward area.
2. Special considerations apply to controlled drugs which are covered by the Misuse of Drugs Act, 1971—they are designated M.D.A. or C.D. These drugs usually have a powerful addictive potential and are particularly liable to misuse or abuse. The following points are important with regard to the storage and administration of controlled drugs.
    a. They should be stored on the ward in a locked cupboard within a locked cupboard and the keys held by the ward sister or nurse-in-charge.
    b. They may *only* be supplied against an order bearing the signature of the ward sister or the nurse-in-charge. For this purpose a special controlled drugs order book is available. When administering to the patient, two nurses, one of whom must be state-registered, check the drug, then an appropriate entry is made in the controlled drugs record book. This entry indicates date and time of administration; the patient's name; the amount given; the amount discarded (if any) and the balance remaining in stock. The entry is made at the time of administration and is witnessed by the second nurse.
    c. The controlled drugs record book indicates the balance remaining in stock of individual preparations and these amounts should be checked regularly against the actual stock in the controlled drugs cupboard.
    d. When checking the amounts of controlled drugs remaining in stock, the nurse should pay particular attention to expiry dates whenever they appear on the label.

e. A hospital pharmacist or ward pharmacist should carry out regular independent checks of controlled drugs against the controlled drugs record book. In addition he/she will take charge of the removal or destruction of out-of-date medicines and supervise the record book entry.
3. Prescription Only Medicines (designated P.O.M.) is a term which indicates that the medicine can only be supplied by the pharmacy on the written order of the ward sister or nurse-in-charge. These drugs must be kept in a locked cupboard although the very strict regulations for controlled drugs (see above) do not apply. The term 'Prescription Only' indicates the need for a doctor's prescription before such medicines are supplied to patients in the community.
4. Oral medicines, injections, ointment, creams and lotions and eye preparations should each be stored in separate areas to avoid confusion when selecting drugs. *Note* that disinfectants must be stored in a separate area away from all medicines.

The Pharmacist should advise on any matter relating to the security and administration of medicines in the ward.

Appendix 2

METRIC WEIGHTS AND OTHER MEASURES

In recent years the introduction of metrication into medical practice has altered the ways in which drug dosages and concentrations, patient data (including height, weight and body surface area), drug levels in the body and other measurements are expressed. The following are those units of measurement which the nurse will commonly encounter in every day practice.

1. **Weight.** The unit of weight is the kilogram (kg). This is made up of 1000 grams (g) and each gram is composed of 1000 milligrams (mg). Each milligram in turn is composed of 1000 micrograms (μg or mcg)—hence, 1 kg = 1000 g; 1 g = 1000 mg; 1 mg = 1000 μg or mcg. When converting from or to the imperial system 1 kg = 2.2 lb. N.B. Whenever drugs are prescribed in microgram dosages it is good practice to write the units in full i.e. Digoxin 250 micrograms as the use of the contracted terms μg or mcg may in practice be mistaken for mg and as this dose is one thousand times greater disastrous consequences may follow.

   Drug dosages are often described in terms of unit dose per kg of body weight i.e. mg/kg, μg/kg etc. This method of dosage is frequently used in paediatric medicine and allows doses to be tailored to the individual patient's size.

2. **Volume.** The unit of volume is the litre which is denoted by the symbol 'l'. One litre comprises 1000 millilitres (ml). Occasionally the term decilitre (dl) is used. 1 l = 10 dl; 1 dl = 100 ml and 1 l = 1000 ml. When converting from or to the imperial system 1 l = 35.2 fluid ounces (fl oz) or 1 ml = 0.0352 fl oz. The symbols 'l' or 'ml' account for almost all measurements expressed in unit volume for the prescription and administration of drugs.

3. **Concentration.** When expressing concentration or dosages of a medicine in liquid form, several methods are available:
   a. **Unit weight per unit volume:** This describes the unit of weight of a drug contained in unit volume e.g. 1 mg in 1 ml; 2 mg in 1 l; 40 mg in 2 ml etc. Examples of drugs in common use expressed in these terms: Diazepam injection 10 mg in

1 ml; Chloral Hydrate Mixture 1 g in 10 ml; Penicillin suspension 250 mg in 5 ml.
b. **Percentage (weight in volume):** This describes the weight of a drug expressed in grams (g) which is contained in 100 ml or 1 dl of solution. Common examples are: Lignocaine hydrochloride injection 2%; this contains 2 g in each 100 ml of solution or 0.2 g (200 mg) in each 10 ml of solution or 0.02 g (20 mg) in each 1 ml of solution, etc. Calcium gluconate injection 10%: this contains 10 g in each 100 ml of solution or 1 g in each 10 ml or 0.1 g (100 mg) in each 1 ml, etc.
c. **Percentage (weight in weight):** This describes the weight of a drug expressed in grams (g) which is contained in 100 g of a solid or semi-solid medicament e.g. ointments and creams. Examples are: Fucidin ointment 2% which contains 2 g of fusidic acid in each 100 g of ointment. Betnovate cream 25% in Aqueous cream which contains 25 g of Betnovate cream mixed with 75 g of Aqueous cream (overall weight 100 g).
d. **Volume containing '1 part':** A few liquids and to a lesser extent gases, particularly those containing drugs in very low concentrations, are often described as containing 1 part per 'x' units of volume. For liquids 'parts' are equivalent to grams and volume to millitres, e.g. Adrenaline injection 1 in 1000 which contains 1 g in 1000 ml or expressed as a percentage (w/v): 0.1%.
e. **Molar concentration:** Only very occasionally are drugs in liquid form expressed in molar concentration. The mole is the molecular weight of a drug expressed in grams and a one molar (1 M) solution contains this weight dissolved in each litre. More often the term millimole (mmol) is used to describe a medicinal product. 1000 mmol = 1 mole. e.g. Potassium chloride solution 15 mmol in 10 ml indicates a solution containing the molecular weight of potassium chloride in milligrams × 15 dissolved in 10 ml of solution. Molar concentrations are most commonly seen in the results of biochemical investigations.

4. **Body height and surface area:** Occasionally drug doses are expressed in terms of microgram, milligram or gram per unit of body surface area. This is frequently the case where precise dosages tailored to individual patient's needs are required. Typical examples may be seen in cytotoxic chemotherapy or in drugs used in paediatric problems. Body surface area is expressed as square metres of m^2 and drug dosages as units/m^2 or units per square metre. Examples are: Cytarabine injection 100 mg/m^2 (q.v.); Dacarbazine injection 250 mg/m^2 (q.v.). The surface area is calculated from the patient's body weight (in kilograms, kg) and height (in centimetres, cm), as follows:

BODY SURFACE AREA OF CHILDREN
NOMOGRAM FOR DETERMINATION OF BODY SURFACE AREA FROM HEIGHT AND WEIGHT

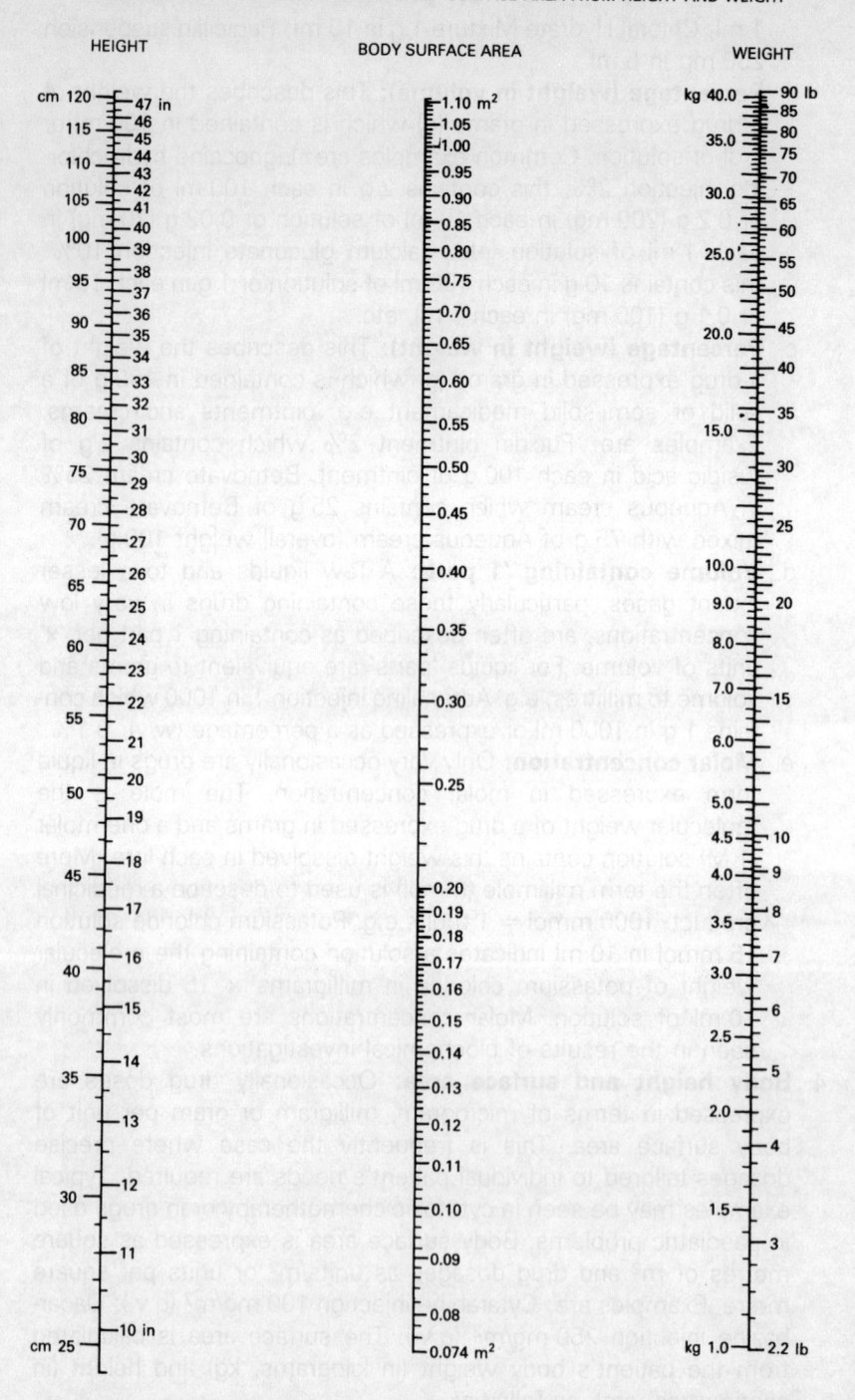

BODY SURFACE AREA OF ADULTS
NOMOGRAM FOR DETERMINATION OF BODY SURFACE AREA FROM HEIGHT AND WEIGHT

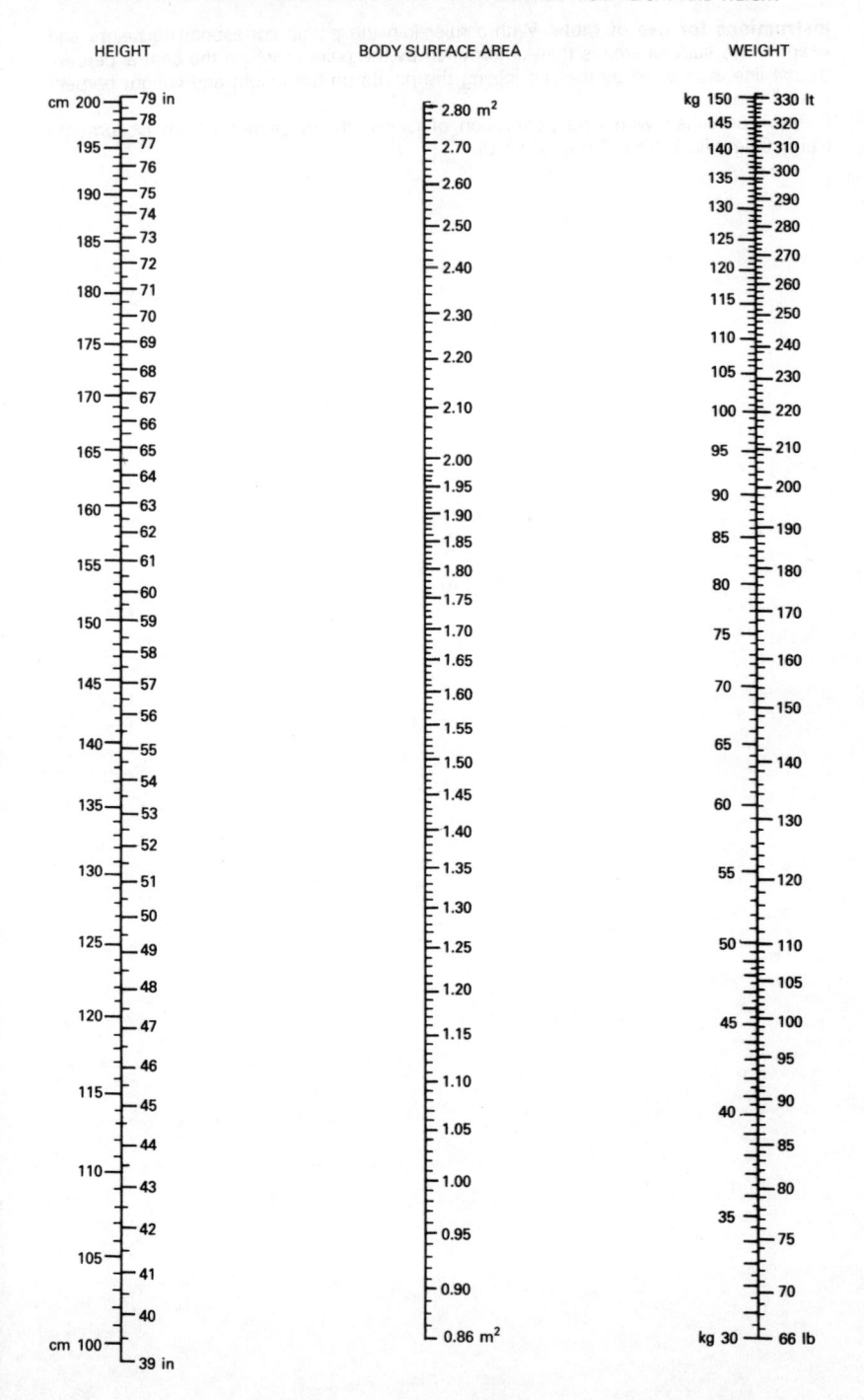

334 A Handbook of Drugs

Instructions for use of table: With a ruler join the points corresponding height and weight. The surface area is then determined by the point at which the central perpendicular line is crossed by the line joining the points on the height and weight perpendicular lines.
(Table reproduced with kind permission of Geigy Pharmaceuticals from Documenta Geigy Scientific Tables, 7th edn. 1970).

INDEX OF DRUGS BY PROPRIETARY AND OTHER COMMON NAMES

Index of drugs by proprietary and other common names

Achromycin (Antibiotic) see Tetracycline
Actidil (Antihistamine) see Tripolidine
Actrapid MC (Insulin) see Insulin
Acupan (Analgesic) see Nefopam
Adalat (Anti-anginal) see Nifedipine
Adcortyl (Corticosteroid) see Triamcinolone
Adriamycin (Cytotoxic agent) see Doxorubicin
Airbron (Mucolytic agent) see Acetylcysteine
Albucid (Sulphonamide) see Sulphacetamide
Alcobon (Anti-fungal) see Flucytosine
Alcopar (Anthelmintic) see Bephenium
Aldactone (Diuretic) see Spironolactone
Aldomet (Antihypertensive) see Methydopa
Alexan (Cytotoxic agent) see Cytarabine
Alkeran (Cytotoxic agent) see Melphalan
Allegron (Antidepressant) see Nortriptyline
Alrheumat (Anti-inflammatory agent) see Ketoprofen
Alu-cap (Antacid) see Aluminium Hydroxide
Aludrox (Antacid) see Aluminium Hydroxide
Alupent (Bronchodilator) see Orciprenaline
Amikin (Antibiotic) see Amikacin
Amoxil (Antibiotic) see Amoxycillin
Amytal (Barbiturate) see Amylobarbitone
Anafranil (Antidepressant) see Clomipramine
Ananase Forte (Enzyme) see Bromelains
Anapolon (Anabolic steroid) see Oxymetholone
Androcur (Anti-androgen) see Cyproterone
Anovlar 21 (Contraceptive) see Contraceptives, oral

Anquil (Tranquilliser) see Benperidol
Antepar (Anthelmintic) see Piperazine
Antepsin (Ulcer healing agent) see Sucralfate
Anthipen (Anthelmintic) see Dichlorophen
Anthisan (Antihistamine) see Mepyramine
Antisin-Privine (Antihistamine) see Antazoline
Anturan (Antiplatelet and Anti-inflammatory agent) see Sulphinpyrazone
Anxon (Tranquilliser) see Ketazolam
Apisate (Appetite suppressant) see Diethylpropion
Apresoline (Antihypertensive) see Hydralazine
Ara-C (Cytotoxic agent) see Cytarabine
Artane (Anticholinergic) see Benzhexol
AT 10 (Vitamin) see Dihydrotachysterol
Atarax (Sedative) see Hydroxyzine
Ativan (Tranquilliser) see Lorazepam
Atromid-S (Lipid lowering agent) see Clofibrate
Atrovent (Bronchodilator) see Ipratropium Bromide
Augmentin (Antibiotic with Clavulanic Acid) see Augmentin
Aureomycin (Antibiotic) see Chlortetracycline
Aventyl (Antidepressant) see Nortriptyline
Avloclor (Antimalarial and Anti-inflammatory agent) see Chloroquine
Avomine (Anti-emetic) see Promethazine

Bactrim (Anti-bacterial) see Co-Trimoxazole
Banistyl (Antihistamine) see Dimethothiczine
Banocide (Anthelmintic) see Diethylcarbamazine

Baxan (Antibiotic) see Cefadroxil
Baycaron (Diuretic) see Mefruside
Baypen (Antibiotic) see Mezlocillin
BC 500 with Iron (Iron and Vitamins) see Ferrous Fumarate
Beconase (Corticosteroid) see Beclomethasone
Becotide (Corticosteroid) see Beclomethasone
Benadryl (Antihistamine) see Diphenhydramine
Benemid (Urate lowering drug and penicillin potentiator) see Probenecid
Benoral (Analgesic) see Benorylate
Berotec (Bronchodilator) see Fenoterol
Beta-Cardone (Beta-blocker) see Sotalol
Betaloc (Beta-blocker) see Metoprolol
Betnelan (Corticosteroid) see Betamethasone
Betnesol (Corticosterioid) see Betamethasone
Betnovate (Corticosteroid) see Betamethasone
Bextasol (Corticosteroid) see Betamethasone
Biogastrone (Ulcer healing agent) see Carbenoxolone
Bisolvon (Mucolytic agent) see Bromhexine
Blocadren (Beta-blocker) see Timolol
Bolvidon (Antidepressant) see Mianserin
Bradilan (Peripheral vasodilator) see Nicofuranose
Bretylate (Antidysrhythmic) see Bretylium
Brevinor (Contraceptive) see Contraceptives, Oral
Bricanyl (Bronchodilator) see Terbutaline
Brietal (Barbiturate) see Methohexitone
Bronchodil (Bronchodilator) see Reproterol
Broxil (Antibiotic) see Phenethicillin
Brufen (Anti-inflammatory agent) see ibuprofen
Burinex (Diuretic) see Bumetanide
Buscopan (Antispasmodic) see Hyoscine-N-Butylbromide

Cafergot (Vasoconstrictor) see Ergotamine
Calciparine (Anticoagulant) see Heparin
Calpol (Analgesic) see Paracetamol
Camcolit (Antidepressant) see Lithium Carbonate
Canesten (Antifungal) see Clotrimazole

Capastat (Antitubercule) see Capreomycin
Capoten (Antihypertensive) see Captopril
Carbocaine (Local anaesthetic) see Mepivacaine
Catapres (Antihypertensive) see Clonidine
Caved-S (Ulcer healing agent) see Deglycyrrhizinsed Liquorice
CCNU (Cytotoxic agent) see Lomustine
Cedocard (Anti-anginal) see Isosorbide Dinitrate
Ceftizoxime (Antibiotic) see Cefizoxime
Celbenin (Antibiotic) see Methicillin
Celevac (Laxative) see Methylcellulose
Centrax (Tranquilliser) see Prazepam
Ceporex (Antibiotic) see cephalexin
Ceporin (Antibiotic) see Cephaloridine
Cerubidin (Cytotoxic agent) see Daunorubicin
Cesamet (Anti-emetic) see Nabilone
Chendol (Gallstone dissolving agent) see Chenodeoxycholic Acid
Chloromycetin (Antibiotic) see Chloramphenicol
Choledyl (Bronchodilator) see Choline Theophyllinate
Chymar (Enzyme) see Chymotrypsin
Cidomycin (Antibiotic) see Gentamicin
Citanest (Local anaesthetic) see Prilocaine
Claforan (Antibiotic) see Cefotaxime
Clinoral (Anti-inflammatory agent) see Sulindac
Clomid (Anti-oestrogen) see Clomiphene
Clopixol (Tranquilliser) see Clopenthixol
Cobalin-H (Vitamin) see Vitamin B_{12}
Co-Ferol (Iron salt) see Ferrous Fumarate
Cogentin (Anticholinergic) see Benztropine
Colofac (Antispasmodic) see Mebeverine
Cologel (Laxative) see Methylcellulose
Combizym (Pancreatic enzyme) see Pancreatin
Combizym Compositum (Pancreatic enzyme) see Pancreatin
Concordin (Antidepressant) see Protriptyline
Conova 30 (Contraceptive) see Contraceptives, Oral
Cordarone X (Antidysrthythmic) see Amiodarone
Cordilox (Anti-anginal and Antidysrhythmic agent) see Verapamil

Corgard (Beta-blocker) see Nadolol
Cortelan (Corticosteroid) see Cortisone
Cortistab (Corticosteroid) see Cortisone
Cortisyl (Corticosteroid) see Cortisone
Cosmogen Lyovac (Cytotoxic agent) see Actinomycin D
Cotazyme (Pancreatic enzyme) see Pancreatin
Cotazyme B (Pancreatic enzyme) see Pancreatin
Cream of Magnesia (Antacid) see Magnesium Hydroxide
Crystapen G (Antibiotic) see Benzylpenicillin
Cycloberal (Cerebral vasodilator) see Cyclandelate
Cyclogest (Progestational hormone) see Progesterone
Cyclokapron (Antifibrinolytic agent) see Tranexamic acid
Cyclospasmol (Cerebral vasodilator) see Cyclandelate
Cytacon (Vitamin) see Vitamin B_{12}
Cytamen (Vitamin) see Vitamin B_{12}
Cytosar (Cytotoxic agent) see Cytarabine
Cytosine Arabinoside (Cytotoxic agent) see Cytarabine

Dactinomycin (Cytotoxic agent) see Actinomycin D
Daktarin (Anti-fungal) see Miconazole
Dalacin-C (Antibiotic) see Clindamycin
Dalmane (Hypnotic) see Flurazepam
Danol (Steroid blocker) see Danazol
Daonil (Hypoglycaemic agent) see Glibenclamide
Daranide (Carbonic anhydrase inhibitor) see Dichlorophenamide
Daraprim (Antimalarial) see Pyrimethamine
Dartalan (Phenothiazine) see Thiopropazate
Deca-Durabolin (Anabolic steroid) see Nandrolone
Decadron (Corticosteroid) see Dexamethasone
Declinax (Antihypertensive) see Debrisoquine
Decoderm (Corticosteroid) see Fluprednylidene
Decortisyl (Corticosteroid) see Prednisone
Defencin (Peripheral vasodilator) see Isoxsuprine
Deltacortone (corticosteroid) see Prednisone

Deltacortril (Corticosteroid) see Prednisolone
Dendrid (Antiviral agent) see Idoxuridine
De-Nol (Ulcer healing agent) see Tri-Potassium Di-Citrato Bismuthate
Depixol (Tranquilliser) see Flupenthixol
Depocillin (Antibiotic) see Procaine Penicillin G
Depot-Medrone (Corticosteroid) see Methylprednisolone
Depot-Provera (Progestational hormone) see Medroxyprogesterone Acetate
Dermovate (Corticosteroid) see Clobetasol
Deseril (Antiserotonin agent) see Methysergide
Destolit (Gallstone dissolving agent) see Ursodeoxycholic Acid
DF 118 (Analgesic) see Dihydrocodeine
Diabenese (Hypoglycaemic agent) see Chlorpropamide
Diamicron (Hypoglycaemic agent) see Gliclazide
Diamox (Carbonic anhydrase inhibitor) see Acetazolamide
Diazemuls (Tranquilliser) see Diazepam
Dibenyline (Vasodilator) see Phenoxybenzamine
Dibromomannitol (Cytotoxic agent) see Mitobronitol
Diconal (Narcotic analgesic) see Dipipanone
Digitaline Nativelle (Cardiac stimulant) see Digitoxin
Dimelor (Hypoglycaemic agent) see Acetohexamide
Dimotane (Antihistamine) see Brompheniramine
Dindevan (Anticoagulant) see Phenindione
Dinoprost (Prostaglandin) see Prostaglandin F_2 Alpha
Dinoprostone (Prostaglandin) see Prostaglandin E_2
Dioctyl Medo (Laxative) see Dioctyl Sodium Sulphosuccinate
Dipidolor (Narcotic analgesic) see Piritramide
Disalcid (Anti-inflammatory) see Salsalate
Disipal (Anticholinergic) see Orphenadrine
Distaclor (Antibiotic) see Cefaclor
Distalgesic (Analgesic) see Dextropropoxyphene
Distamine (Antirheumatic and heavy

metal poison antidote) see Penicillamine
Diurexan (Diuretic) see Xipamide
Dixarit (Migraine prophylactic) see Clonidine
Dobutrex (Cardiac stimulant) see Dobutamine
Dolobid (Analgesic) see Diflunisal
Doloxene (Analgesic) see Dextropropoxyphene
Dopram (Respiratory stimulant) see Doxapram
Dorbanex (Laxative) see Danthron
Dormonoct (Hypnotic) see Loprazolam
Dramamine (Antihistamine) see Dimenhydrinate
Dromoran (Narcotic analgesic) see Levorphanol Tartrate
DTIC (Cytotoxic agent) see Dacarbazine
Dulcolax (Laxative) see Bisacodyl
Duogastrone (Ulcer healing agent) see Carbenoxolone
Duphalac (Laxative) see Lactulose
Duphaston (Progestational hormone) see Dydrogesterone
Durabolin (Anabolic steroid) see Nandrolone
Duromine (Appetite suppressant) see Phentermine
Duvadilan (Peripheral vasodilator) see Isoxsuprine
Dyazide (Diuretic) see Triamterene
Dytac (Diuretic) see Triamterene
Dytide (Diuretic) see Triamterene

Ecostatin (Anti-fungal) see Econazole
Edecrin (Diuretic) see Ethacrynic Acid
Efcortelan (Corticosteroid) see Hydrocortisone
Efcortesol (Corticosteroid) see Hydrocortisone
Elantan (Anti-anginal agent) see Isosorbide Mononitrate
Eldepryl (Anti-Parkinson agent) see Selegiline
Eldesine (Cytotoxic agent) see Vindesime
Eltroxin (Thyroid hormone) see Thyroxine
Emeside (Anticonvulsant) see Ethosuximide
Endoxana (Cytotoxic agent) see Cyclophosphamide
Enduron (Diuretic) see Methyclothiazide
Enzypan (Pancreatic enzyme) see Pancreatin

Epanutin (Anticonvulsant and Antidysrhythmic agent) see Phenytoin
Ephynal (Vitamin) see Vitamin E
Epilim (Anticonvulsant) see Sodium Valproate
Epsikapron (Antifibrinolytic) see Aminocaproic Acid
Equanil (Tranquilliser) see Meprobamate
Erythrocin (Antibiotic) see Erythromycin
Esbatal (Antihypertensive) see Bethanidine
Estracyt (Cytotoxic agent) see Estramustine
Estrovis (Oestrogen) see Quinestrol
Eudamine (Antihypertensive) see Diazoxide
Euglucon (Hypoglycaemic) see Glibenclamide
Eugynon (Contraceptive) see Contraceptives, Oral
Euhypnos (Hypnotic) see Temazepam
Eumovate (Corticosteroid) see Clobetasone
Evadyne (Antidepressant) see Butriptyline
Exirel (Bronchodilator) see Pirbuterol

Fabahistin (Antihistamine) see Mebhydrolin
Feac (Iron and vitamins) see Ferrous Sulphate
Fe-Cap (Iron salt) see Ferrous Sulphate
Fe-Cap C (Iron and vitamin) see Ferrous Sulphate
FE-Cap Folic (Iron and vitamin) see Ferrous Sulphate
Fefol (Iron salt) see Ferrous Sulphate
Fefol Vit (Iron and vitamins) see Ferrous Sulphate
Feldene (Anti-inflammatory agent) see Piroxicam
Femulen (Contraceptive) see Contraceptives, Oral
Fenopren (Anti-inflammatory agent) see Fenoprofen
Fenostil Retard (Antihistamine) see Dimethindene
Fentazin (Phenothiazine) see Perphenazine
Feospan (Iron salt) see Ferrous Sulphate
Ferfolic (Iron and vitamin) see Ferrous Gluconate
Fergluvite (Iron and vitamins) see Ferrous Gluconate
Fergon (Iron salt) see Ferrous Gluconate

Ferraplex B (Iron and vitamin) see Ferrous Sulphate
Ferrlecit 100 (Iron salt) see Ferrous Sulphate
Ferrocap (Iron salt) see Ferrous Fumarate
Ferrocap-F 350 (Iron and vitamin) see Ferrous Fumarate
Ferrocontin (Iron salt) see Ferrous Sulphate
Ferrocontin Folic (Iron and vitamin) see Ferrous Sulphate
Ferrograd C (Iron and vitamin) see Ferrous Sulphate
Ferrograd Folic (Iron and vitamin) see Ferrous Sulphate
Ferro-Gradumet (Iron salt) see Ferrous Sulphate
Ferromyn (Iron salt) see Ferrous Succinate
Ferromyn B (Iron and vitamin) see Ferrous Succinate
Ferromyn S (Iron salt) see Ferrous Succinate
Ferromyn S Folic (Iron and vitamin) see Ferrous Succinate
Fersaday (Iron and vitamin) see Ferrous Fumarate
Fersamal (Iron salt) see Ferrous Fumarate
Fesovit (Iron and vitamins) see Ferrous Sulphate
Flagyl (Antibiotic) see Metronidazole
Florinef (Corticosteroid) see Fludrocortisone
Floxapen (Antibiotic) see Flucloxacillin
Fluanxol (Tranquilliser) see Flupenthixol
Folex 350 (Iron and vitamin) see Ferrous Fumarate
Folicin (Iron and vitamin) see Ferrous Sulphate
Folvron (Iron salt) see Ferrous Sulphate
Fortral (Analgesic) see Pentazocine
Fortum (Antibiotic) see Ceftazidime
Fortunan (Tranquilliser) see Haloperidol
Frisium (Tranquilliser) see Clobazam
Froben (Anti-inflammatory agent) see Flurbiprofen
Fucidin (Antibiotic) see Fusidic Acid/Sodium Fusidate
Fulcin (Anti-fungal) see Griseofulvin
Fungilin (Anti-fungal) see Amphotericin B
Fungizone (Anti-fungal) see Amphotericin B
Furadantin (Antibacterial) see Nitrofurantoin
Fybogel (Laxative) see Ispaghula

Galfer (Iron salt) see Ferrous Fumarate
Gantrisin (Sulphonamide) see Sulphafurazole
Gastrocote (Antacid) see Alginic Acid
Gastrovite (Iron and vitamins) see Ferrous Sulphate
Gaviscon (Antacid) see Alginic Acid
Genticin (Antibiotic) see Gentamicin
Gerifit (Iron and salt) see Ferrous Fumarate
Gestanin (Progestational hormone) see Allyloestrenol
Givitol (Iron salt) see Ferrous Fumarate
Glibenese (Hypoglycaemic agent) see Glipizide
Globin Insulin (Insulin) see Insulin
Glucophage (Hypoglycaemic agent) see Metformin
Glurenorm (Hypoglycaemic agent) see Gliquidone
Glutril (Hypoglycaemic agent) see Glibornuride
Gondafon (Hypoglycaemic agent) see Glymidine
Grisovin (Anti-fungal) see Griseofulvin
Gynovlar 21 (Contraceptive) see Contraceptives, Oral

Haelan (Corticosteroid) see Flurandrenolone
Halciderm (Corticosteroid) see Halcinonide
Halcion (Hypnotic) see Triazolam
Halcort (Corticosteroid) see Halcinonide
Haldol (Tranquilliser) see Haloperidol
Harmogen (Oestrogen) see Piperazine Oestrone Sulphate
Heminevrine (sedative) see Chlormethiazole
Hepacon (Vitamin) see Vitamin B^{12}
Heroin (Narcotic analgesic) see Diamorphine
Herpid (Antiviral agent) see Idoxuridine
Hexopal (Peripheral vasodilator) see Inositol Nicotinate
Hismanal (Antihistamine) see Astemizole
Histryl (Antihistamine) see Diphenylpyraline
Hyalase (Enzyme) see Hyaluronidase
Hydrenox (Diuretic) see Hydroflumethiazide
Hydrocortone (Corticosteroid) see Hydrocortisone
Hydrosaluric (Diuretic) see Hydrochlorothiazide

Hygroton (Diuretic) see Chlorthalidone
Hypovase (Antihypertensive) see Prazosin
Hypurin Isophane (Insulin) see Insulin
Hypurin Lente (Insulin) see Insulin
Hypurin Neutral (Insulin) see Insulin
Hypurin Protamine Zinc (Insulin) see Insulin

Iberet 500 (Iron salt) see Ferrous Sulphate
Ilosone (Antibiotic) see Erythromycin
Ilotycin (Antibiotic) see Erythromycin
Imferon (Iron salt) see Iron (Parenteral)
Imodium (Anti-diarrhoeal) see Loperamide
Impericin (Antibiotic) see Oxytetracycline
Imuran (Immunosuppressant) see Azathioprine
Inapasade (Antitubercule) see sodium Aminosalicylate
Inderal (Beta-blocker) see Propranolol
Indocid (Anti-inflammatory agent) see Indomethacin
Initard (Insulin) see Insulin
Insulatard MC (Insulin) see Insulin
Intal (Anti-allergic agent) see Sodium Cromoglycate
Intraval (Barbiturate) see Thiopentone
Intropin (Cardiac stimulant) see Dopamine
Ionamin (Appetite suppressant) see Phentermine
Ipral (Antibacterial) see Trimethoprim
Irofol C (Iron and vitamins) see Ferrous Sulphate
Ismelin (Antihypertensive) see Guanethidine
Ismo (Anti-anginal agent) see Isosorbide Mononitrate
Isogel (Laxative) see Ispaghula
Isophane NPH (Insulin) see Insulin
Isordil (Anti-anginal) see Isosorbide Dinitrate

Jectofer (Iron salt) see Iron (Parenteral)

Kabikinase (Fibrinolytic agent) see Streptokinase
Kantrex (Antibiotic) see Kanamycin
Kefadol (Antibiotic) see Cefamandole
Keflex (Antibiotic) see Cephalexin
Keflin (Antibiotic) see Cephalothin
Kefzol (Antibiotic) see Cephazolin
Kelferon (Iron salt) see Ferrous Sulphate
Kelfezine W (Sulphonamide) see Sulphametopyrazine
Kelfolate (Iron and vitamin) see Ferrous Sulphate
Kemadrin (Anticholinergic) see Procyclidine
Kenalog (Corticosteroid) see Triamcinolone
Kinidin (Antidysrhythmic agent) see Quinidine
Konakion (Vitamin) see Vitamin K

Lanitop (Cardiac stimulant) see Medigoxin
Lanoxin (Cardiac stimulant) see Digoxin
Lanvis (Cytotoxic agent) see Thioguanine
Largactil (Phenothiazine) see Chlorpromazine
Larodopa (Anti-Parkinso agent) see Levodopa
Lasix (Diuretic) see Frusemide
Laxoberal (Laxative) see Sodium Picosulphate
Ledecort (Corticosteroid) see Triamcinolone
Lederfen (Anti-Parkinson agent) see Fenbufen
Lederkyne (Sulphonamide) see Sulphamethoxypyridazine
Ledermycin (Antibitotic) see Demethylchlortetracycline
Lederspan (Corticosteroid) see Triamcinolone
Lentard MC (Insulin) see Insulin
Lente Insulin (Insulin) see Insulin
Leukeran (Cytotoxic agent) see Chlorambucil
Librium (Tranquilliser) see Chlordiazepoxide
Lidothesin (Local anaesthetic) see Lignocaine
Lignostab (Local anaesthetic) see Lignocaine
Lincocin (Antibiotic) see Lincomycin
Loestrin (Contraceptive) see Contraceptives, Oral
Lomotil (Anti-diarrhoeal) see Diphenoxylate
Loramet (Hypnotic) see Lormetazepam
Ludiomil (Antidepressant) see Maprotiline

M & B 693 (Sulphonamide) see Sulphapyridine
Macrodantin (Antibacterial) see Nitrofurantoin
Madopar (Anti-Parkinson agent) see Madopar
Madribon (Sulphonamide) see Sulphadimethoxine
Marcaine (Local anaesthetic) see Bupivacaine
Marevan (Anticoagulant) see Warfarin
Marplan (Antidepressant) see Isocarboxazid
Marsilid (Antidepressant) see Iproniazid
Masteril (Androgen) see Drostanolone
Maxolon (Gastric emptier and anti-emetic) see Metoclopramide
Medomin (Barbiturate) see Heptabarbitone
Medrone (Corticosteroid) see Methylprednisolone
Mefoxin (Antibiotic) see Cefoxitin
Megace (Progestogen) see Megestrol Acetate
Melatase (Hypoglycaemic) see Chlorpropamide
Melleril (Phenothiazine) see Thioridazine
Menophase (Oestrogen) see Mestranol
Merbentyl (Antispasmodic) see Dicyclomine
Merital (Antidepressant) see Nomifensine
Mestinon (Anticholinesterase) see Pyridostigmine
Metenix (Diuretic) see Metolazone
Metosyn (Corticosteroid) see Fluocinonide
Mexitil (Antidysrhythmic agent) see Mexiletine
Microgynon 30 (Contraceptive) see Contraceptives, Oral
Micronor (Contraceptive) see Contraceptives, Oral
Microval (Contraceptive) see Contraceptives, Oral
Midamor (Diuretic) see Amiloride
Migril (Vasoconstrictor) see Ergotamine
Milk of Magnesia (Antacid) see Magnesium Hydroxide
Milonorm (Tranquilliser) see Meprobamate
Minihep (Anticoagulant) see Heparin
Minilyn (Contraceptive) see Contraceptives, Oral
Minocin (Antibiotic) see Minocycline
Minodiab (Hypoglycaemic) see Glipizide
Minoviar (Contraceptive) see Contraceptives, Oral
Minovlar ED (Contraceptive) see Contraceptives, Oral
Mintezol (Anthelminitic) see Thiabendazole
Mixtard Insulin (Insulin) see Insulin
Modecate (Phenothiazine) see Fluphenazine
Moditen (Phenothiazine) see Fluphenazine
Mogadon (Hypnotic) see Nitrazepam
Molipaxin (Antidepressant) see Trazidone
Monaspor (Antibiotic) see Cefsulodin
Monit (Anti-anginal agent) see Isosorbide Mononitrate
Mono-cedocard (Anti-anginal agent) see Isosorbide Mononitrate
Monotard MC (Insulin) see Insulin
Moxalactam (Antibiotic) see Latamoxef
MST Continus (Analgesic) see Morphine
Motilium (Anti-emetic) see Domperidone
Mucaine (Antacid with local anaesthetic) see Oxethazine
Myambutol (Antitubercule) see Ethambutol
Mycardol (Anti-anginal) see Pentaerythritol Tetranitrate
Myelobromol (Cytotoxic agent) see Mitobronitol
Myleran (Cytotoxic agent) see Busulphan
Myocrisin (Gold salt) see Sodium Aurothiomalate
Myotonine (Sympathomimetic) see Bethanecol
Mysoline (Anticonvulsant) see Primidone

Nacton (Anticholinergic) see Poldine Sulphate
Nalcrom (Anti-allergic agent) see Sodium Cromoglycate
Naprosyn (Anti-inflammatory agent) see Naproxen
Nardil (Antidepressant) see Phenelzine
Narphen (Narcotic analgesic) see Phenazocine
Natrilix (Antihypertensive) see Indapamide
Natulan (Cytotoxic agent) see Procarbazine

Navidrex (Diuretic) see Cyclopenthiazide
Nebcin (Antibiotic) see Tobramycin
Negram (Antibacterial) see Nalidixic Acid
Nembutal (Barbiturate) see Pentobarbitone
Neo-Cytamen (Vitamin) see Vitamin B_{12}
Neogest (Contraceptive) see Contraceptives, Oral
Neo-Mercazole (Antithyroid) see Carbimazole
Neo-Naclex (Diuretic) see Bendrofluazide
Neoplatin (Cytotoxic agent) see Cisplatin
Nephril (Diuretic) see Polythiazide
Nerisone (Corticosteroid) see Diflucortolone
Netillin (Antibiotic) see Netilmicin
Neulactil (Tranquilliser) see Pericyazine
Neulente (Insulin) see Insulin
Neuphane (Insulin) see Insulin
Neusilin (Insulin) see Insulin
Nipride (Antihypertensive) see Sodium Nitroprusside
Nitrocine (Anti-anginal agent) see Glyceryl Trinitrate
Nitrocontin (Anti-anginal agent) see Glyceryl Trinitrate
Nitrolingual (Anti-anginal agent) see Glyceryl Trinitrate
Nivaquine (Antimalarial and anti-inflammatory agent) see Hydroxychloroquine
Nizoral (Antifungal) see Ketoconazole
Nobrium (Tranquilliser) see Medazepam
Noctamid (Hypnotic) see Lormetazepam
Noctec (Hypnotic) see Chloral Hydrate
Nolvadex (Anti-oestrogen) see Tamoxifen
Norgeston (Contraceptive) see Contraceptives, Oral
Noriday (Contraceptive) see Contraceptives, Oral
Norimin (Contraceptive) see Contraceptives, Oral
Norinyl 1 (Contraceptive) see Contraceptives, Oral
Norinyl 1/28 (Contraceptive) see Contraceptives, Oral
Norlestrin (Contraceptives) see Contraceptives, Oral
Normison (Hypnotic) see Temazepam
Norval (Antidepressant) see Mianserin
Nuelin (Bronchodilator) see Theophylline
Nuso Neutral (Insulin) see Insulin

Nutrizym (Pancreatic enzyme) see Pancreatic
Nydrane (Anticonvulsant) see Beclamide
Nystan (Anti-fungal) see Nystatin

Omnopon (Narcotic analgesic) see Papveretum
Oncovin (Cytotoxic agent) see Vincristine
One-Alpha (Vitamin) see Alfacalcidol
One-Alpha Hydroxy Cholecalciferol (Vitamin) see Alfacalcidol
Opilon (Vasodilator) see Thymoxamine
Opticrom (Anti-allergic agent) see Sodium Cromoglycate
Optimine (Antihistamine) see Azatadine
Oradexon (Corticosteroid) see Dexamethasone
Orap (Tranquilliser) see Pimozide
Orbenin (Antibiotic) see Cloxacillin
Orisulf (Sulphonamide) see Sulphaphenazole
Orlest 21 (Contraceptive) see Contraceptives, Oral
Ortho-Novin 1/50 (Contraceptive) see Contraceptives, Oral
Orudis (Anti-inflammatery agent) see Ketoprofen
Ospolot (Anticonvulsant) see Sulthiame
Otrivine-Antistin (Antihistamine) see Antazoline
Ovestin (Oestrogen) see Oestriol
Ovran (Contraceptive) see Contraceptives, Oral
Ovran 30 (Contraceptive) see Contraceptives, Oral
Ovranette (Contraceptive) see Contraceptives, Oral
Ovulen 50 (Contraceptive) see Contraceptives, Oral
Ovysmen (Contraceptive) see Contraceptives, Oral

Palaprin Forte (Analgesic) see Aloxiprin
Palfium (Narcotic analgesic) see Dextromoramide
Panadol (Analgesic) see Paracetamol
Pancrex V (Pancreatic enzyme) see Pancreatin
Pancrex V Forte (Pancreatic enzyme) see Pancreatin
Paramisan (Antitubercule) see Sodium Aminosalicylate
Parentrovite (Vitamin) see Multivitamins

Parlodel (Dopamine-like drug) see Bromocriptine
Parnate (Antidepressant) see Tranylcypromine
Parvolex (Paracetamol antidote) see Acetylcysteine
P.A.S. (Antitubercule) see Sodium Aminosalicylate
Peganone (Anticonvulsant) see Ethotoin
Penbritin (Antibiotic) see Ampicillin
Penidural (Antibitotic) see Benzathine Penicillin
Pentovis (Oestrogen) see Quinestradol
Percutol (Anti-anginal agent) see Glyceryl Trinitrate
Periactin (Antiserotonin) see Cyproheptadine
Peritrate (Anti-anginal) see Pentaerythritol Tetranitrate
Peroidin (Antithyroid agent) see Potassium Perchlorate
Persantin (Antiplatelet and Anti-anginal) see Dipyridamole
Pertofran (Antidepressant) see Desipramine
Pevaryl (Anti-fungal) see Econazole
Pexid (Anti-anginal) see Perhexiline
Phandorm (Barbiturate) see Cyclobarbitone
Phasal (Antidepressant) see Lithium Carbonate
Phenergan (Antihistamine) see Promethazine
Phyllocontin (Bronchodilator) see Aminophylline
Physeptone (Narcotic analgesic) see Methadone
Piriton (Antihistamine) see Chlorpheniramine
Plaquenil (Antimalarial and Anti-inflammatory agent) see Hydroxychloroquine
Plesmet (Iron salt) see Ferrous Sulphate
Ponderax (Appetite suppressant) see Fenfluramine
Ponstan (Anti-inflammatory agent) see Mefenamic Acid
Pramidex (Hypoglycaemic agent) see Tolbutamide
Praxilene (Peripheral vasodilator) see Naftidrofuryl
Precortisyl (Corticosteroid) see Prednisolone
Prednesol (Corticosteroid) see Prednisolone

Predsol (Corticosteroid) see Prednisolone
Pregaday (Iron and vitamin) see Ferrous Fumarate
Pregfol (Iron and vitamin) see Ferrous Sulphate
Pregnavite Forte (Iron and vitamins) see Ferrous Sulphate
Pregnavite Forte F (Iron and vitamins) see Ferrous Sulphate
Premarin (Oestrogen) see Oestrogens, Conjugated (Equine)
Pressimune (Immunosuppressant) see Antilymphyocyte Immunoglobulins
Priadel (Antidepressant) see Lithium Carbonate
Primalan (Antihistamine) see Mequitazine
Primoteston (Androgen) see Testosterone
Pripsen (Anthelmintic) see Piperazine
Pro-Actidil (Antihistamine) see Tripolidine
Pro-Banthine (Anticholinergic) see Propantheline
Progynova (Oestrogen) see Oestradiol Valerate
Proluton Depot (Progestational hormone) see Hydroxyprogesterone Hexanoate
Prominal (Anticonvulsant) see Methylphenobarbitone
Prondol (Antidepressant) see Iprindole
Pronestyl (Antidysrhythmic agent) see Procainamide
Prostigmin (Anticholinesterase) see Neostigmine
Prostin E$_2$ (Prostaglandin) see Prostaglandin E$_2$
Prothiaden (Antidepressant) see Dothiepin
Pro-vent (Bronchodilator) see Theophylline
Provera (Progestational hormone) see Medroxyprogesterone Acetate
Pro-Viron (Androgen) see Mesterolone
Pularin (Anticoagulant) see Heparin
Pulmadil (Bronchodilator) see Rimiterol
Pri-Nethol (Immunosuppressant) see Mercaptopurine
Pyopen (Antibiotic) see Carbenicillin
Pyrogastrone (Ulcer healing agent) see Carbenoxolone
P.Z.I. (Insulin) see Insulin

Questran (Ion exchange resin) see Cholestyramine

Yomesan (Anthelmintic) see Niclosamide
Yutopar (Uterine relaxant) see Ritodrine

Zantac (Ulcer healing agent) see Ranitidine
Zarontin (Anticonvulsant) see Ethosuximide
Zinacef (Antibiotic) see Cefuroxime
Zinamide (Antitubercule) see Pyrizinamide
Zincomed (Mineral) see Zinc Sulphate
Zonulysin (Enzyme) see Chymotrysin
Zovirax (Antiviral agent) see Acyclovir
Zyloric (Urate lowering agent) see Allopurinol